DERMATOLOGY

CONTEMPORARY ISSUES IN SMALL ANIMAL PRACTICE VOLUME 8

Volumes Already Published

Vol. 1 Medical Emergencies
Robert G. Sherding, D.V.M., Guest Editor
Vol. 2 Surgical Emergencies
Ronald M. Bright, D.V.M., Guest Editor
Vol. 3 Infectious Diseases
Frederic W. Scott, D.V.M., Ph.D., Guest Editor
Vol. 4 Nephrology and Urology
Edward B. Breitschwerdt, D.V.M., Guest Editor
Vol. 5 Neurologic Disorders
Joe M. Kornegay, D.V.M., Ph.D., Guest Editor
Vol. 6 Oncology
Neil T. Gorman, B.V.Sc., Ph.D., Guest Editor
Vol. 7 Cardiology
John D. Bonagura, D.V.M., Guest Editor

Forthcoming Volumes in the Series

Vol. 9 Disorders of Exotic Animals
Elliot R. Jacobson, D.V.M., Ph.D., and
George V. Kollias, Jr., D.V.M., Ph.D.,
Guest Editors

DERMATOLOGY

Edited by

Gene H. Nesbitt, D.V.M., M.S.

Diplomate, American College of
Veterinary Dermatology
Veterinary Referral Associates, P.C.
West Caldwell, New Jersey

Churchill Livingstone
New York, Edinburgh, London, Melbourne 1987

ISBN 0-443-08447-5

Distributed in the United Kingdom by Churchill Livingstone, Robert Stevenson House, 1-3 Baxter's Place, Leith Walk, Edinburgh EH1 3AF, and by associated companies, branches, and representatives throughout the world.

Accurate indications, adverse reactions, and dosage schedules for drugs are provided in this book, but it is possible that they may change. The reader is urged to review the package information data of the manufacturers of the medications mentioned.

Copy Editor: *Julia Muiño*
Production Designer: *Angela Cirnigliaro*
Production Supervisor: *Jocelyn Eckstein*

Printed in the United States of America

First published in 1987

Contributors

Donna Walton Angarano, D.V.M. Diplomate, American College of Veterinary Dermatology. Associate Professor, Department of Small Animal Surgery and Medicine, College of Veterinary Medicine, Auburn University, Auburn, Alabama

Diane E. Bevier, D.V.M. Diplomate, American College of Veterinary Dermatology. Associate Professor, Department of Medical Science, College of Veterinary Medicine, University of Florida, Gainesville, Florida; Consultant in Dermatology, Animal Skin Disease Clinic, Rockville, Maryland

David K. Chester, D.V.M., M.S. Diplomate, American College of Veterinary Dermatology. Professor, Department of Veterinary Medicine and Surgery, Texas A&M University College of Veterinary Medicine, College Station, Texas

Bobby R. Collins, D.V.M., M.S. Diplomate, American College of Laboratory Animal Medicine. Assistant Professor, Department of Special Clinical Sciences, University of Florida College of Veterinary Medicine, Gainesville, Florida; Associate Director, Health Center Animal Resources Department, J. Hillis Miller Health Center, University of Florida College of Medicine, Gainesville, Florida

Carol S. Foil, D.V.M., M.S. Diplomate, American College of Veterinary Dermatology. Associate Professor, Department of Veterinary Clinical Sciences, School of Veterinary Medicine, Louisiana State University, Baton Rouge, Louisiana; Veterinary Dermatologist, Veterinary Teaching Hospital and Clinics, Louisiana State University, Baton Rouge, Louisiana

Craig E. Griffin, D.V.M. Diplomate, American College of Veterinary Dermatology. Clinical Instructor, Department of Dermatology, School of Medicine, University of California, Irvine, Irvine, California; Director, Animal Dermatology Clinic, Garden Grove, California

Peter J. Ihrke, V.M.D. Diplomate, American College of Veterinary Dermatology. Associate Professor of Dermatology, School of Veterinary Medicine, University of California, Davis, Davis, California; Staff Member, Dermatology

Service, Small and Large Animal Clinic Veterinary Medical Teaching Hospital, School of Veterinary Medicine, University of California, Davis, Davis, California

Kenneth W. Kwochka, D.V.M. Diplomate, American College of Veterinary Dermatology. Assistant Professor, Department of Veterinary Clinical Sciences, College of Veterinary Medicine, The Ohio State University, Columbus, Ohio; Consultant in Dermatology, Berwyn Veterinary Associates, Berwyn, Illinois

Sharron L. Martin, D.V.M., M.S. Professor, Department of Veterinary Clinical Sciences, The Ohio State University College of Veterinary Medicine, Columbus, Ohio

Gene H. Nesbitt, D.V.M., M.S. Diplomate, American College of Veterinary Dermatology. Veterinary Referral Associates, P.C., West Caldwell, New Jersey

Candace A. Sousa, D.V.M. Diplomate, American College of Veterinary Dermatology. Diplomate, American Board of Veterinary Practitioners. Elvas Avenue Animal Hospital, Sacramento, California

Stephen D. White, D.V.M. Diplomate, American College of Veterinary Dermatology. Assistant Professor, Department of Medicine, Tufts University School of Veterinary Medicine, North Grafton, Massachusetts

Ton A. Willemse, D.V.M., Ph.D. Associate Professor of Veterinary Dermatology, State University of Utrecht, Small Animal Clinic, Dermatology Section, Utrecht, The Netherlands

Preface

The veterinary clinician is called upon to diagnose and treat a myriad of dermatoses on a daily basis. In the majority of practices the diagnosis and treatment of these dermatologic diseases represents a major time commitment and economic return.

Almost daily advances are made in the identification of specific causes, enhancement of diagnostic procedures, and improvement of therapeutic protocols. This expansion of knowledge is built upon a solid understanding of the basic principles of diagnosis and treatment of dermatologic disorders.

The purpose of this volume is to present state-of-the-art clinical veterinary dermatologic information in a useful format for the busy clinician. To achieve this, contributions from skilled clinicians, clinical researchers, and educators in private and institutional practices have been solicited.

Chapter 1 is a comprehensive review of the basic principles of diagnosis. Chapters 2 through 8 focus on specific diseases based on etiology. In several areas, especially flea allergies and atopic dermatitis, there have been major achievements in the understanding of the pathogenesis of the diseases, thus enabling the clinician to utilize better diagnostic and therapeutic protocols. Although great strides have been made in feline dermatology, the clinician is still often frustrated. Where applicable, specific feline dermatoses have been discussed under disease chapter headings. In Chapter 9 the feline dermatoses are reviewed with emphasis on a diagnostic approach.

Until recently, dermatologic disorders of exotic and avian species have not received adequate attention. Chapters 10 and 11 present a first in the veterinary medical literature. The current knowledge is presented in a useful format for the practicing veterinarian.

The editor acknowledges the efforts expended by all of the contributing authors to present state-of-the-art information about their selected topics. Appreciation is expressed to all.

Gene H. Nesbitt, D.V.M.

Contents

1 Diagnostic Approach to Dermatologic Disease

Craig E. Griffin

Dermatologic problems are frequently encountered in clinical practice and are often viewed as frustrating and difficult cases. Many clinicians prefer not to get involved with a major workup of skin diseases, but rather seek short-term alternatives. Actually, skin problems are a challenging group of diseases that should stimulate a diagnostic interest.

When dealing with skin diseases the clinician has a tremendous advantage as compared to working with other organ systems. The advantage is that both the client and the clinician can see all the gross pathology without a necropsy. More importantly the pathology can frequently be visualized in all its various stages of development. However, to consistently achieve an accurate diagnosis the clinician must develop and follow a systematic approach to dermatologic diseases.

The systematic approach starts by obtaining a thorough history, which is followed by a routine physical examination and complete dermatologic examination. Following the history and physical and dermatologic examinations the clinician should be able to list the differential diagnoses and make a tentative diagnosis. Based upon the list of differentials, diagnostic tests and/or specific trial therapies should be performed. Prior to advanced testing, simple diagnostics such as skin scrapings, smears, and fungal cultures should be completed. If a diagnosis is not evident from these test results further tests and/or trial therapies should be pursued. This process is continued to eliminate differential diagnoses until a definitive diagnosis is made. This systematic approach may be better visualized by examining Figure 1-1 for a systematic approach to dermatologic disease.

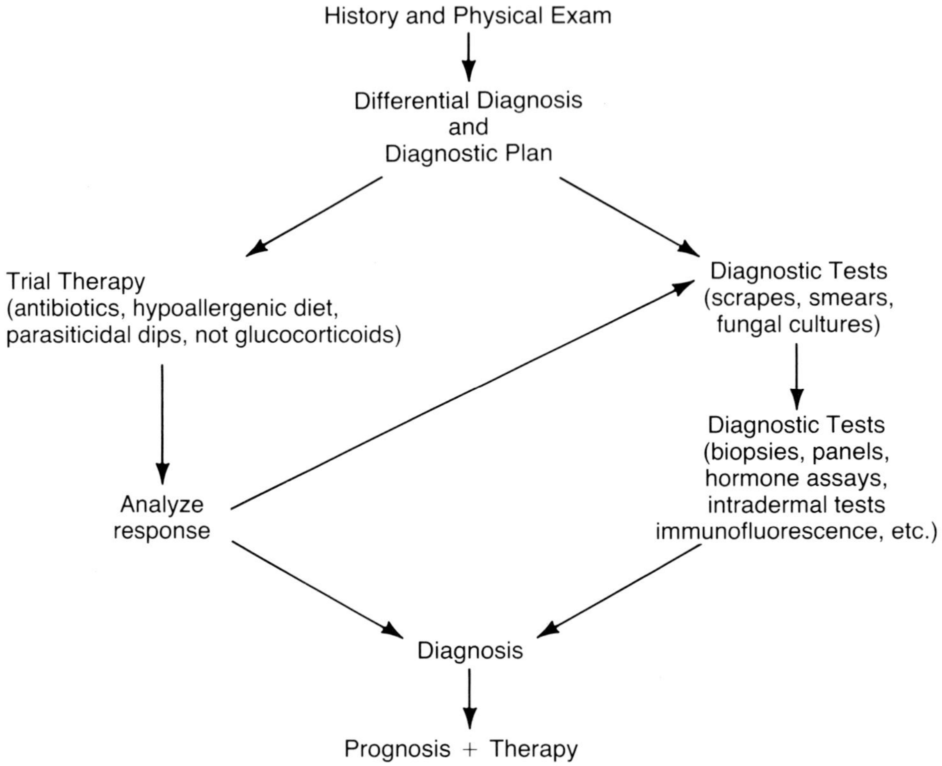

Fig. 1-1. Algorithm for systematic approach to dermatologic disease.

HISTORY

The complete medical and dermatologic history of the patient is absolutely vital in establishing a diagnosis. Much of the information used in making a dermatologic diagnosis is derived from the history. In some cases the history may be so classic that a diagnosis can be made from it alone. Obviously, it is important that the history is accurate and thorough. In most instances the dermatologic history is so involved that it takes longer to complete a good history than to do a physical and dermatologic examination.

The majority of dermatologic problems are chronic resulting in multiple visits to one or more veterinarians. If accurate, detailed notes have been recorded in the animal's chart, most of the information pertaining to the dermatologic history can be obtained by reviewing the multiple entries in the patient history. Often, good records have not been kept. In addition the client may have a different perspective of the condition than that suggested by the chronological notations in records. It is advantageous to have the client fill out a dermatologic history form prior to the office visit (Fig. 1-2). The client's thoughts are recorded on the questionnaire prior to being influenced by the

DERMATOLOGY HISTORY FORM

Date ____________

Client ____________ Animal's name ____________

Animal's Age ______ Sex ______ Breed ____________

1. *What is the skin problem?*
   Itching ______ Loss of Hair ______ Rash ______
   Oily Skin ______ Dry Skin ______ Dandruff ______
   Redness ______ Odor ______ Other ______
2. *At what age did you first notice problem?* ______
3. *Are the symptoms worse any time of year?*
   Spring ____ Summer ____ Fall ____ Winter ____
4. *What did problem look like when it first started?*
   Itching ______ Hair Loss ______ Rash ______
   Pimples ______ Redness ______ Other ______
5. *Where did it start?* Nose ____ Eyes ____ Ears ____ Neck ____
   Back ____ Tail ____ Rump ____ Legs ____ Paws ____ Chest ____
   Stomach ____ Groin ____
6. *Has it spread?* Yes ____ No ____ *If so, where?* Explain ______
7. *Does your pet scratch, rub, chew, lick or bite?*
   Yes ____ No ____ Where? Nose ____ Muzzle ____ Eyes ____ Ears ____
   Neck ____ Back ____ Rump ____ Tail ____ Axilla ("Arm Pit") ____
   Front legs ____ Back legs ____ Paws ____ Chest ____ Abdomen ____
   Groin ____
8. *Was itching first thing noticed?* Yes ____ No ____
9. *Do you have other pets in house?* List ______
10. *Do you have any skin problem?* Explain ______
11. *Do any people in your household have a skin problem?*
    Explain ______
12. *Percent of time your pet is confined:* Indoors ____ Outdoors ____
13. *Are symptoms worse:* Indoors ____ Outdoors ____ Night ____ Morning ____
14. *Has your pet been neutered?* If so, what age? ____
15. *If female, has she had normal heat cycles?* Yes ____ No ____
    When last appeared ____ Any Problems ____
16. *If male, does he have normal interest in females?* Yes ____ No ____
17. *Does your pet have fleas?* Yes ____ No ____ Did have ____
18. *Do you or did you use any of the following?*
    Flea Spray ____ Flea Dips ____ Flea Powder ____ Flea Collar ____
    Powders ____ Baths ____ Name products ______
19. *Any other parasite problems?* Ticks ____ Mites ____ Flies ____
20. *Do you use insecticides in your home?* ____ Yard ____
21. *Has your pet been out of his/her normal area (vacation-visit-boarded, etc.)?*
    No ____ Yes ____ Where ______ When ______
22. *What medications has your pet been using since problem started?*
    Oral ______ Topical ______ Injection ______
23. *Did these medications help or cure the problem?*
    Yes ____ No ____ Some ____ For Awhile ____
24. *Does your pet use food supplements or vitamins?*
    Yes ____ What ______ No ____
25. *What type and brand of food do you feed your pet?*
    Canned ______ Dry ______
    Table Scraps ______ Other ______
26. *Does your pet do or have any of the following?*
    Cough ____ Sneeze ____ Runny nose ____ Runny eyes ____
    Vomit ____ Diarrhea ____ Poor Appetite ____ Worms ____
    Excessive Appetite ____ Regular exercise ____
    Shake head ____
27. *Has your pet had any other illnesses?* Explain

Fig. 1-2. Sample questionnaire for obtaining a patient's dermatological history. Reprinted with permission. Allerderm, Inc. Hurst, TX.

veterinarian's comments. After reviewing the answers, the clinician should review and verify the important or leading responses. It is often helpful to ask a question in several ways and at different times. Repetitive questioning gives the clinician a feel for the client's accuracy, reliability, and ability of observation, all of which are important in weighing the historical information.

When reviewing the client history form and/or the patient history the importance of key questions and previous observations should be emphasized to the client. The clinician should clarify these questions and verify previous clinical signs and responses to therapies. This is especially important in chronic or recurrent disorders and evaluating trial therapies.

Information that should be ascertained in a dermatologic history includes signalment, initial problem, course, drug history, general health and diet.

Signalment

The signalment of the animal may be very helpful to prioritize the various differential diagnoses.

Age

The patient's age at the time of disease onset can be used to eliminate some differentials and increase the index of suspicion about others (Table 1-1). The age of onset is especially important when considering pruritus. The most frequent causes of pruritus are flea allergy, atopy, pyoderma, scabies, and food allergy. In dogs demonstrating abnormal pruritus prior to 4 months of age, atopy, flea allergy, and food allergy are rarely seen while scabies must always be considered. From 4 to 9 months, atopy is still uncommon, but flea and food allergies may have developed. At the other end of the spectrum it is very unlikely to see allergies develop in dogs over 8 years of age. However, a recent change in environment could transform a mildly allergic skin disease with minimal clinical signs into a clinically significant problem.

Breed

The animal's breed may also be helpful in establishing a differential diagnosis. It is important to realize that even though a breed may have certain disease predilections other diseases can and do occur. More than one cocker spaniel has been misdiagnosed as having seborrhea just because of its breed and presentation with crusts. A complete list of breed predispositions for dermatologic diseases can be found in a standard reference text.[1]

Table 1-1. Diseases Related to Age of Onset

Age	Diseases Considered	Unlikely Diseases
<4 months	Congenital disorders (e.g., ectodermal defects, cutaneous asthenia, hypotrichosis Dermatomyositis Juvenile pyoderma/cellulitis Localized demodex Pituitary dwarf	Allergy Cushing's syndrome Hypothyroidism Neoplasia Immune mediated
<1 year	Localized & generalized demodex Food allergy Flea allergy Zinc responsive dermatoses Viral papillomatosis Pruritus from parasite migration Color mutant alopecia Follicular dysplasia Canine acne	Cushing's syndrome Neoplasia Atopy[a]
1–3 years	Atopy Food allergy Flea allergy Adult onset hyposomatotropism	Congenital defect Neoplasia except histiocytoma Cushing's syndrome Sex hormone
3–8 years	Allergy Hypothyroidism Immune mediated	Congenital
Over 8 years	Endocrine Neoplasia Immune deficiency	Congenital Atopy

[a] Atopy usually starts after 1 year of age. However in regions with heavy allergenic loads (e.g., southern California) atopy may occur with some frequency by 8–9 months of age.

Sex

The animal's sex is primarily helpful in the diagnosis of sex hormone imbalances. If the animal has been altered, the age at which surgery occurred should be recorded. Any abnormalities in the estrus cycle or correlation with disease symptoms should be noted.

Initial Problem/Primary Lesions

Determination of the initial problem and/or lesion is extremely important, but sometimes difficult. In many cases by the time a client seeks veterinary care, secondary changes and complicating factors (e.g., pyoderma) have developed. In cases of pruritus it is helpful to know if there were any lesions or gross inflammation prior to the pruritus. The same is true with alopecia, as postinflammatory alopecia can sometimes be misinterpreted as an endocrine problem, which begins with noninflammatory alopecia. This type of information is usually determined by asking the client several different questions. What did the problem look like initially or was there just itching? What drew your attention to the problem? Ask the client to describe the first lesion or lesions noticed such as redness, bumps, pimples, crusts, hives, and hair loss. Was itching noticed first? Where did it start? It is helpful to give a list of options that the client can check or circle such as nose, eyes, ears, neck, back, rump, and tail.

To determine if a dog is pruritic it is important that different manifestations of pruritus be questioned. Is there any scratching, chewing, biting, licking, or rubbing? Does the pet rub its face, body, or back along objects such as walls, floors, or furniture? The clinician should note the areas that are most pruritic and the areas that are mildly pruritic with no obvious disease.

Course

Disease progression and changes must be determined. The more chronic the problem, the more important this aspect becomes, as this part of the history will give the first clues that more than one skin disease or problem exists. Was the onset rapid or slow. Did the disease spread over the body from one initial focus or did multiple distant sites develop? As the disease spread or became more severe what changes occurred? Did new types of lesions occur? Where did it spread to and how fast has it been spreading? Did pruritus finally develop or become more severe? Has this been a continuous or intermittent problem? If intermittent, is there anything the client can correlate with remissions or flare up such as seasonality, routine chemical spraying, fertilizing, or previous therapies?

If the client reports a continuous problem in a chronic case it is often worthwhile to review history of previous skin problems, ear infections, or pruritus. A client may remark on a pet's previous summertime itch, which was nothing like what it is now. It is common for those early signs to represent the earliest manifestations of atopy or flea allergy dermatitis (FAD) that became severe or secondarily infected. Some clients do not perceive mild disease as abnormal and do not consider it in this type of questioning. This should also be taken into consideration when determining the age of onset.

Drug History

Drug eruptions are a common problem in humans. In the last few years drug eruptions have been recognized as problems in animals and can mimic or cause most skin diseases described in veterinary dermatology.[2] If a drug eruption is suspected, drugs being taken for any reason prior to the onset of a skin disease should be discontinued unless the medication is necessary for sustaining the life of the animal. Many clients perceive drugs as prescribed products only

Table 1-2. Response to Glucocorticoids

Response	Diseases and Doses	
	0.25–0.5 mg/lb prednisone	>1.0 mg/lb prednisone
Complete	Atopy Some food, contact and flea allergy	Allergies Parasitic Some immune mediated
Partial	Most food and flea allergy Parasitic Some bacterial Seborrheic dermatitis Sterile granuloma	Most pyoderma[a] and some fungal Most immune mediated Seborrheic dermatitis
Poor, none, or temporary	Some food[b] and flea allergy Pyoderma Immune mediated Fungal Demodex	Some fungal Some pyoderma Some immune mediated Endocrine Demodex

[a] Usually temporary and later refractory.
[b] Especially in the feline.

and emphasis should be made about other types of medications such as aspirin, vitamins, and heartworm preventatives.

The response to therapies for the disease should also be pursued. This can be especially helpful in ranking suspect differentials. Responses to antibiotics, environmental insecticide use, and topical therapy can be very informative. Most commonly, glucocorticoids have been administered and the clinician should determine how helpful they were. This requires knowledge of the type of glucocorticoid as well as the dose and route of administration. The client needs to be questioned about how helpful the treatments really were. Did the itching stop or decrease? What happened to the lesions, hair growth, and pattern of disease, and how quick was the response? Many clients have reported pruritus stopping but crusted papules and pustules remaining, though they were not as red as prior to treatment. This commonly occurs when pruritic pyodermas are treated with glucocorticoids. Diseases and their response to glucocorticoids are compared in Table 1-2.

Environment

The complete history should also include questions about the environment of the pet. Environmental questioning can be very time-consuming and frequently in-depth questioning may be put off until needed. This type of questioning is most important when one has tentatively diagnosed allergic, traumatic, or contact dermatitis. Diseases with a history of seasonal activity also require indepth environmental questioning.

Contagion

The clinician should ask questions about involvement of other pets and exposed humans. When a positive response is obtained further questioning about that problem should be pursued. Although the involvement of other pets or human disease makes one consider a contagious ectoparasitic or environmental problem, it may be misleading. Skin diseases among animals and humans are common enough that the owner's problems may not be related to that of the animal.

General Health and Diet

A history about the basic health and diet of the pet should be obtained. In cases where systemic diseases are suspected, in-depth questioning about specific organ systems may be required.

PHYSICAL EXAMINATION

A routine physical examination should be performed on all patients. This is particularly important to determine if the skin disease reflects another internal disorder. In addition, other medical problems may be uncovered which might affect the client's decisions about the pursuit and therapy of their pet's skin disease.

DERMATOLOGIC EXAMINATION

A complete dermatologic examination is required in all cases. The clinician that only looks at the client's chief complaint is frequently missing other lesions which may add important diagnostic information. To decrease the likelihood of missing this information, the clinician should develop a systematic approach to all cases, and must always do the examination with suitable lighting. Natural light is ideal, but fluorescent lighting is acceptable if it is bright and even. It may be necessary in some cases to shave or magnify areas to adequately visualize lesions.

The patient should first be viewed from a distance and from all sides, front and back. Attention should be paid to the general health, conformation, and mental attitude of the patient. Any signs of pruritus and the overall coat quality should be noted.

The patient should be examined closely, starting with the hair coat. The hair coat should be examined by petting and brushing the patient's body. Attention should be given to coat thickness, texture, hair quality, and oiliness. How much oil, sebum, and dirt is left on your hands? Can the hair in any region be abnormally epilated, and is abnormal epilation associated with specific lesions or is it diffuse? Abnormal epilation associated with specific lesions is seen with folliculitis and perifollicular inflammatory diseases. More diffuse epilation is seen with hair growth disorders and is most commonly seen with endocrine disorders and telogen effluvium. Any abnormalities should be mentioned to the owner; then determine if the owner noticed the same changes, and for how long.

Following the examination of the coat, the clinician should start at the head and examine all skin, mucocutaneous junctions, mucosa, conjunctiva, nails, pads, and lymph nodes. Special attention should be paid to hard-to-see areas such as lip folds, face folds, interdigital webs, nail beds, genitalia, and heavily haired regions such as the caudal thighs.

The skin examination may be facilitated by rolling the skin between the thumb and index finger and looking from the side. This separates the hair and allows better visualization without the need for shaving. The skin should be checked for texture, thickness, color, elasticity, oiliness, scaliness, and cutaneous markings. The skin and coat should be examined for the presence of any

Table 1-3. Primary Lesions

Lesions	Description	Significance
Macule	Circumscribed flat area of color changes < 1 cm diameter	Pigment changes, hemorrhage, vascular engorgement
Patch	a macule > 1 cm diameter	
Wheal	Sharply marginated, raised flat topped	Dermal edema Urticaria Allergy
Papule	Solid elevated lesion < 1 cm diameter	Localized cellular infiltrates or hyperplasia Folliculitis
Plaque	Flat elevated skin > 1 cm diameter	Coalition of papules, often in chronic cases
Nodule	Palpable, solid, elevated lesion > 1 cm diameter	Cellular infiltrates, usually neoplastic or granulomatous extending into deeper dermis or subcutis
Tumor	Neoplastic mass	Biopsy if not definitely benign
Pustule	Circumscribed elevation of skin containing purulent exudate	Folliculitis Pyoderma Pemphigus foliaceus Subcorneal pustular dermatosis
Vesicle	Circumscribed elevated skin, fluid filled, < 1 cm	Autoimmune Irritants Viral
Bulla	Vesicle > 1 cm	

Table 1-4. Secondary Lesions

Lesion	Description	Significance
Scale	Accumulation of corneocytes[a] and keratin debris	Abnormal keratinization or corneocyte adhesion, post inflammation
Crust	Dried exudate of serum, pus, blood	Frequently with pustular diseases, pyoderma, folliculitis
Excoriation	Superficial excavations of epidermis	Usually linear from scratching or external trauma
Ulcer	Loss of entire epidermis	Implies severe or deep process—results in scarring
Scar	Fibrous tissue defect	Follows after areas of ulceration, post chronic dermal inflammation
Lichenification	Firm, thickened area of skin with exaggerated markings	Chronic lesion—usually area of chronic pruritus and inflammation
Hyper/hypopigmentation	Increase or loss of melanin	Usually post-inflammatory with hyperpigmentation common; may be endocrine
Fissure	Linear cleavages in the skin	Excessive drying and loss of tone

[a] Corneocytes are the anuclear keratinocytes that form the dead cellular layer of the stratum corneum.

ectoparasites, eggs, and excreta. All types of lesions and their location should be noted.

The clinician should become familiar with the different morphologic types of dermatologic lesions (Tables 1-3 and 1-4). Primary lesions are the direct result of the disease process. Secondary lesions result from self-trauma or the degeneration and aging of primary lesions, such as a pustule that dries to a small crust. Primary lesions have more diagnostic significance than secondary lesions. In most cases several different types of lesions at various stages can be found.

The shape or configuration of the lesions should also be recorded. They may be single, grouped, linear, annular, arciform, polycyclic, or serpiginous. The lesions should be closely examined and palpated to determine color changes, consistency, depth, and relationship to hair follicles.

The pattern and distribution of skin lesions is extremely valuable and important in establishing a tentative and definitive diagnosis. The distribution is so important that many differential diagnostic lists are based on a characteristic disease distribution. Some examples are nasal diseases, facial diseases, pododermatitis, otitis, diseases of the perineum, and mucocutaneous diseases. An algorithm used to facilitate the diagnosis of nasal dermatoses is found in Figure 1-3.

The lesions should be characterized as circumscribed, regional or generalized and as symmetrical or asymmetrical. Symmetrical diseases are usually

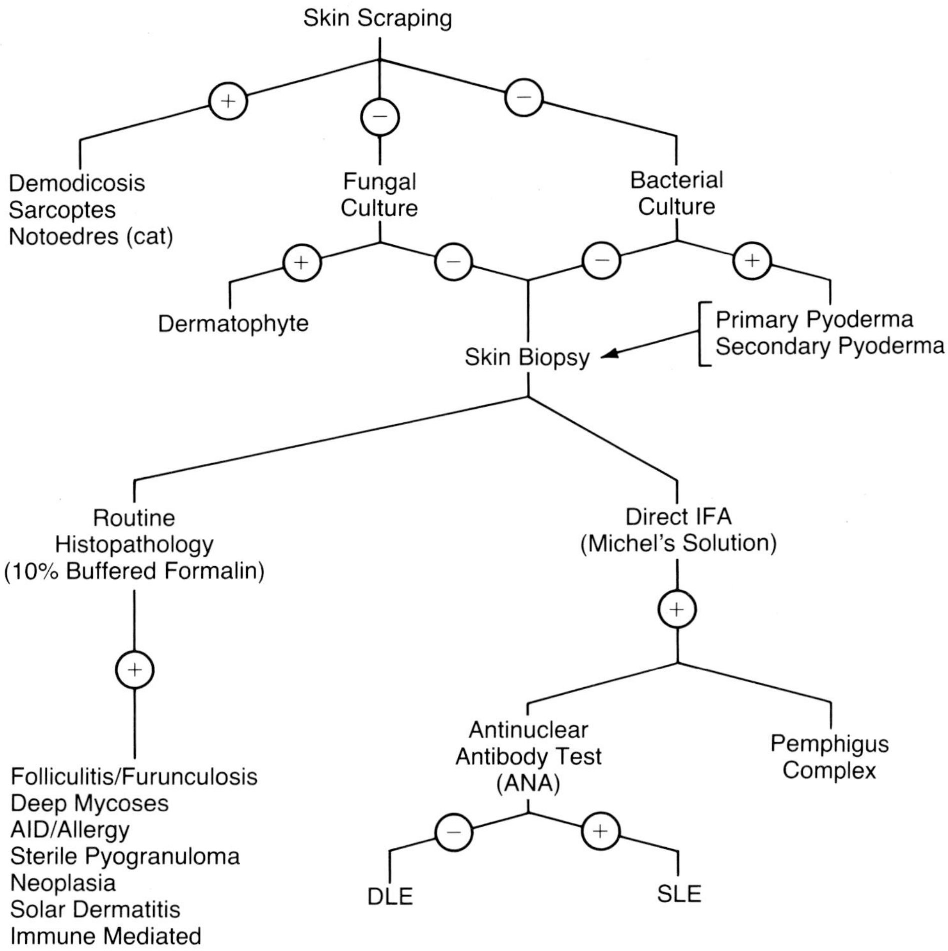

Fig. 1-3. Diagnostic algorithm for nasal dermatoses. (Griffin CE: Nasal Dermatitis, Dermatology Reports, No. 2, 1983.)

associated with diseases of a systemic or "internal" nature. We think of endocrine disorders as symmetrical, but many allergic, immune-mediated, and ecotoparasitic diseases present with strikingly symmetrical disease. Patterns of involvement should be noted such as dorsal or ventral, mucocutaneous junctions, contact areas, pressure points, and intertriginous areas.

Most skin diseases have a characteristic or classic pattern of involvement. Obviously there are many variations based on the chronicity, stage of development, and secondary problems that may occur. The clinician must become familiar with the diseases and their patterns. To list all the diseases and patterns is beyond the scope of this chapter and the reader is referred to discussion of individual diseases that follow in other chapters. In addition, lists and diagrams can be found in standard references.[1,3]

DIFFERENTIAL DIAGNOSIS AND DIAGNOSTIC PLAN

After the history and physical and dermatologic examinations are completed the clinician should have recognized the patient's problems. By identifying the problems and correlating all the available information, a differential diagnosis can be determined. The necessary steps to rule in a tentative diagnosis and/or rule out the differentials can now be planned and explained to the client. It can be helpful for the clinician and the client to visualize a diagnostic plan by using an algorithm. Figure 1-4 is an example of an algorithm for the diagnostic approach to alopecia. As can be seen in this algorithm the initial steps in narrowing down the plan and determining which tests to run are determined from information gathered by the dermatologic examination and history.

When dealing with chronic or recurrent skin diseases it is imperative that the clinician obtains the support and aid of the client. Handouts that include a list of diagnostic tests and their purpose help the client understand the problem, and also promote their cooperation and support for the proposed diagnostic plan.[1,3]

The diagnostic plan will usually involve the use of specific trial therapies, minor or screening office tests, and possibly more advanced laboratory tests or ancillary procedures. The list of differentials should be systematically eliminated until a diagnosis is reached. How this is actually accomplished will vary from case to case depending on the client's motivation, level of frustration, and financial considerations. In some situations a complete battery of tests that address all the differentials may be run at one time. Though not necessarily cost effective this is the quickest route to a diagnosis. More commonly the client will want to limit testing to the most likely differentials, especially in the general practice setting.

Other clients will want to try a therapeutic approach and avoid testing. In chronic cases the therapeutic approach should be limited to specific trial therapies that will provide diagnostic information. The primary concern is that the clinician and client do not lose site of a systematic approach to a diagnosis, prognosis, and the safest effective therapy.

TRIAL THERAPY

Therapeutic trials can be valuable in establishing a diagnosis. In some cases, especially scabies and food allergy, a therapeutic trial may be the only way to achieve a diagnosis. To ensure proper interpretation a trial therapy should be aimed at a specific diagnosis. The therapy should have a narrow spectrum. Glucocorticoids are not very useful for trial therapy as so many different inflammatory or pruritic diseases will respond (Table 1-2). Even dermatophytes and pyodermas can be clinically and temporarily improved by the antiinflammatory effects of glucocorticoids. The most informative trial therapies are antihistamines, hypoallergenic diets, antibiotics, and insecticides. An explanation about the therapy and its purpose must be given to the client.

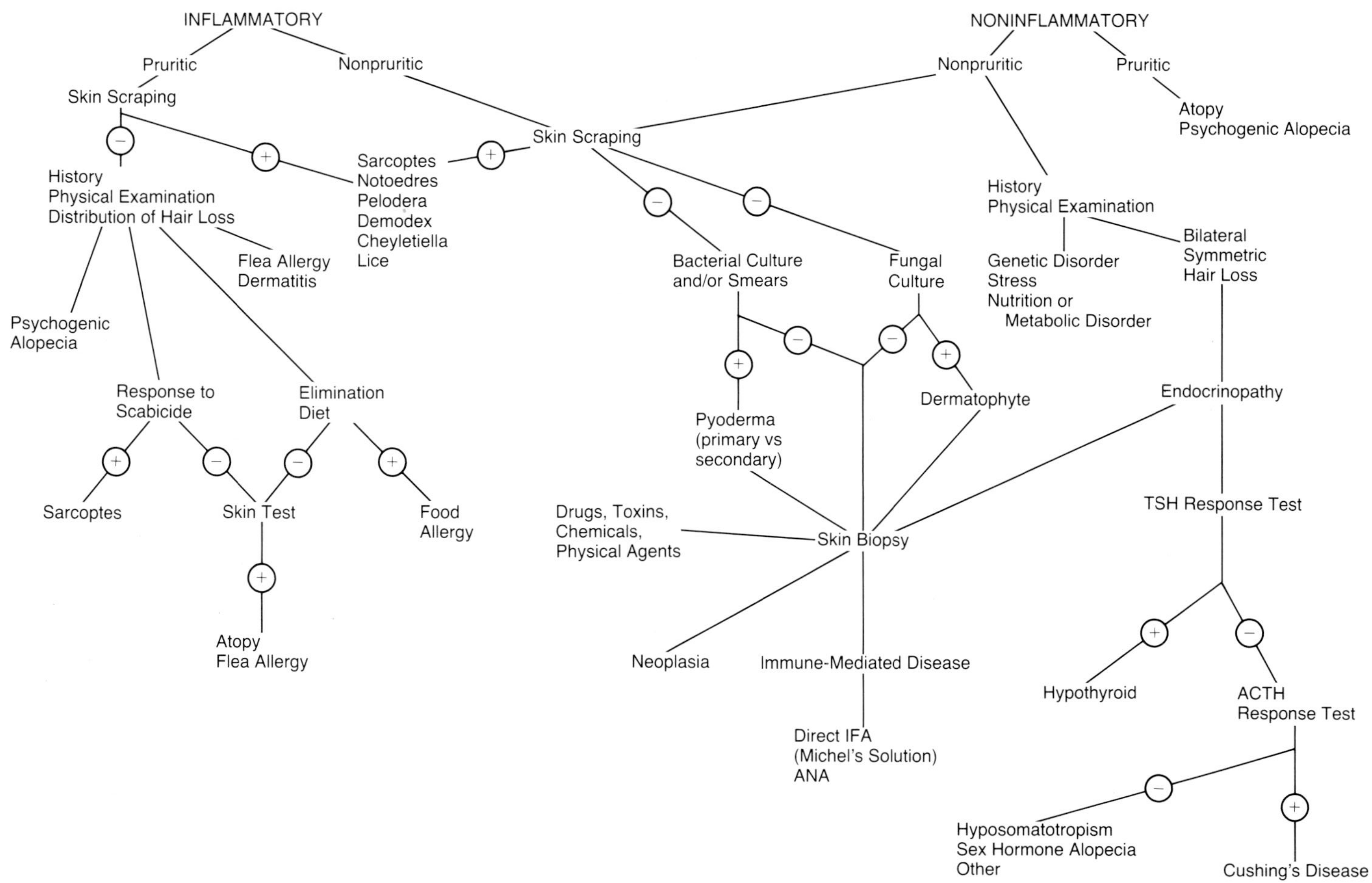

Fig. 1-4. Diagnostic algorithm for alopecia. (Rosenkrantz W, Griffin CE: Dermatology Reports, No. 3, 1984.)

To gain the most information from a trial therapy the client must be involved. The clinician must know what aspects of the disease respond. Does the rash go away, but the itch persist? Are there any changes in the pattern or location of pruritus? Does itching stop or decrease? Are there changes in the type, color, or location of lesions? The client can determine the answers to these questions only if he or she is adequately prepared beforehand. It is the clinician's responsibility to teach the client what to observe. Whenever possible the patient should be examined at the end of a trial therapy so the clinician can support or confirm the client's observations.

In recurrent cases or following the discontinuation of a trial therapy the client again plays a critical role. The client must carefully observe the patient to accurately determine how the disease begins and progresses. This is particularly important when trying to differentiate between pruritic pyodermas and allergic diseases with concurrent pyodermas. The client's daily examination of the dog can help determine what comes first, rash or itch.

Antihistamines may be used as a trial therapy for atopic or IgE mediated diseases. In the author's experience antihistamines are not very helpful for FAD, food allergy, ectoparasitic diseases, or pruritic pyodermas.

Both environmental and topical trial insecticidal therapies are utilized to determine how much fleas and FAD contribute to a patient's problem. Lime sulfur and amitraz dips and ivermectin, which are not effective against fleas, can be used to treat, and at the same time aid in the diagnosis of sarcoptic mange. Trial therapy for sarcoptic mange is particularly useful since a definitive diagnosis by skin scrape is, at best, achieved in 50 percent of the cases.

Antibiotics are used to help diagnose pyodermas, and are especially helpful in determining if pruritus is related to bacterial infections or nonbacterial etiologies.

A trial on a hypoallergenic diet followed by provocative exposure is currently the only way to accurately diagnose food allergy. It is obvious that trial therapies can be very helpful when carefully planned, executed, and observed. However, trial therapy alone can not be relied upon to diagnose every dermatologic problem.

It is important to remember that many drugs have more than one effect. Some antibiotics, such as erythromycin and tetracycline, have antiinflammatory properties. Griseofulvin has some antibacterial effects as well as antifungal. Avlosulfon (Dapsone), once believed to be a specific treatment for subcorneal pustular dermatosis and dermatitis herpetiformis has been found useful in numerous cutaneous diseases. Hormonal therapies are frequently abused. A patient responding to thyroid or sex hormones is not necessarily deficient in those hormones, just as most patients responding to glucocorticoids are not glucocorticoid deficient. Large doses of vitamins and minerals may result in alteration of body functions in addition to correction of a deficiency state. All the known and as yet unknown effects of a drug used as a trial therapy must be considered when interpreting the patient's response.

DIAGNOSTIC TESTS

In the diagnostic approach to dermatologic diseases numerous ancillary tests are available. A brief introduction to common tests will be discussed. More specific tests, such as intradermal skin testing, endocrine function tests, and immunofluorescence testing are covered in their appropriate chapters.

Some simple screening tests (scrapes, cytology, fungal cultures) should be done in the majority of cases and especially prior to more expensive and advanced testing. These simple tests must be done frequently because they rule in or out some very common problems that can present with many different clinical lesions and patterns.

Scrapes

Skin scrapes may be used to diagnose demodicosis, sarcoptic mange, cheyletiella, notoedric mange, trombiculiasis, and pelodera dermatitis. Properly performed negative scrapes rule out demodicosis, notoedric mange, and pelodera dermatitis. *Sarcoptes scabiei* can be very difficult to find in 50 to 70 percent of the cases and even multiple, well-performed negative scrapes do not preclude the diagnosis.

Site selection for scraping is very important. The sites should be unexcoriated, unmedicated areas where the suspect parasite is known to invade. Typical lesions for the parasite should be scraped. As an example, scabies mites primarily live on the pinnal margin yet the most severe lesions may be in other areas. *Cheyletiella* mites are usually recovered from scaly areas of the dorsal trunk.

The type and depth of scrape will vary depending on the parasite suspected. Scrapings for *Demodex* and *Pelodera* must be deep enough to induce superficial diffuse capillary hemorrhage. Scrapes for sarcoptiform mites should cover large areas and need not induce hemorrhage. Superficial scrapes for *Cheyletiella* are satisfactory, though acetate tape impressions and collections of large amounts of scales are the preferred techniques.

Woods Light, Potassium Hydroxide, and Fungal Cultures

Woods light, used to induce fluorescence of arthrospores from some dermatophytes, is valuable only when positive. False-positive fluorescence should not be interpreted as a diagnosis of dermatophytosis. A true positive result is indicated by a bright yellow-green flourescence extending down into the follicular ostia, associated with hair shafts.

Potassium Hydroxide preparations done by an experienced person can be a valuable aid in the rapid diagnosis of dermatophytosis. However, in most general practices this procedure is relatively time consuming and often inaccurate, unless the clinician has spent time learning to rapidly recognize fungal spores.

Fungal cultures are usually the preferred and most cost-effective method of diagnosis. Fungal cultures are more accurate and allow a definitive diagnosis of the dermatophyte species involved. Knowing the species can be valuable in identifying the source of exposure. Appropriate samples and frequent culture observations must be made to achieve the most accurate results.

Samples of hair and scales should be taken from unmedicated lesions. Scales can be scraped from the periphery of lesions. Broken or fragmented hairs should also be plucked and embedded on the surface of the culture medium. Embedding excessive amounts of crust, scales, and hairs should be avoided. For routine purposes the samples should be inocculated on dermatophyte test medium (DTM) and Sabouraud's dextrose agar. The Sab-Duet plates (BactiLab, Mountain View, CA) contain both agars on one plate.

The plate should be stored at room temperature in a dark place. It is important to record the date of sampling and examine the plate at least every 2 days for 10 days. On the DTM the colony growth and red color change should occur at the same time. If the plate is only examined weekly and a color change is seen with substantial fungal growth already present, a positive diagnosis cannot be made. Saprophytic fungi will turn the DTM red once they have exhausted the carbohydrates present in the media. The Sabouraud's agar is utilized to make preparations for microscopic examination. Macroconidia are more likely to be found from colonies growing on Sabouraud's agar. It is often possible to identify macroconidia on colonies grown on DTM.

Cytology

Cytology is an extremly helpful procedure in dermatologic practice and it should be applied to more than neoplastic diseases. Cytology from pustules, vesicles, exudates, and underneath crusts is a very valuable and informative, but underutilized, procedure. Examining cell types can help to rapidly determine if the disease is parasitic, granulomatous, or suppurative. Pemphigus complex, especially foliaceus, may be tentatively diagnosed by the presence of numerous acantholytic cells. Cytology may also lead to a diagnosis by the identification of a specific etiologic agent, especially in fungal and bacterial diseases.

Exudates, impression smears, and the contents of intact pustules or vesicles should be air dried on a microscope slide. The slide can then be stained with a rapid Wright's stain such as Diff Quick (Harleco, Gibbstown, NJ) or a Gram's stain. The slide can then be blotted dry and examined under the microscope within minutes of sampling.

The major benefit of cytology is the determination of bacterial involvement. Over 95 percent of pyodermas are caused by coagulase-positive *Staphylococcus* spp. If the clinician is aware of the typical antimicrobial sensitivity patterns in his geographic area, cytology eliminates the need for the more costly "routine" aerobic culture and sensitivity. Cytology will also help to determine the depth of infection as deeper infections are associated with more mononuclear cells, macrophages, and occasionally plasma cells. Superficial pyodermas are primarily neutrophilic.

Neither cytology nor bacterial culture and sensitivity will determine if a pyoderma is primary or secondary. However, if intracellular cocci are seen, the bacteria are considered significant. When rods are identified, a culture and sensitivity is indicated as different pathogens may be present. In general practice, cytology from an intact pustule is a rapid, accurate, and inexpensive way to diagnose a pyoderma.

Bacterial Culture and Sensitivity

Bacterial culture and sensitivity is indicated when a pyoderma is nonresponsive to appropriate empirical antibiotic therapy. In addition, granulomatous diseases and many deep pyodermas should have cultures and sensitivities performed. In these diseases the author prefers to have tissue samples ground and cultured. Prior to sampling, the site is cleaned with a light surgical scrub. When culturing the skin surface or pustules, care must be taken to avoid contamination of samples by commensal organisms. Anaerobic cultures are indicated in deep lesions or in cases in which cultures have failed to grow any organisms but smears demonstrated bacteria. Whenever mycobacterium or other unusual bacteria are suspected the reference laboratories should be informed.

In general practice the clinician should become familiar with the microbiology reference laboratory since the experience of their technicians and the quality of their microbiology services may vary.

Routine Blood Screens

For most dermatologic diseases routine blood screens are neither diagnostic nor very informative. However, in cases related to systemic diseases or endocrine dermatoses, routine blood screens may be of value. Unless a diagnosis of a systemic disorder is being pursued, routine blood screens are not indicated until other tests such as scrapes, fungal cultures, smears, and biopsies have been completed. Though blood screens can be valuable, their expense and lack of specificity often precludes their use as a routine dermatologic screen.

Dermatopathology

Just as skin lesions are readily available for gross examination they are also easily biopsied for dermatopathologic examination. All skin diseases not readily diagnosed should be biopsied.

Indications for dermatopathology include suspect tumors, nonhealing ulcers, nondiagnosed dermatoses, diagnosed conditions not responding to appropriate therapies, diseases that entail dangerous or expensive therapies, and diseases that require dermatopathology for a definitive diagnosis. Skin biopsies should be performed as soon as indicated. Clinicians often put off a biopsy of an animal while spending valuable time and money performing other less informative tests. For example, the author has seen many cases of suspect autoimmune skin diseases with no biopsies. Instead they have had routine blood panels and immune profiles including Coomb's test, rheumatoid factor, and antinuclear antibody (ANA). In most autoimmune skin diseases these tests (except ANA) will not contribute to a diagnosis. The client's money would have been better spent on biopsies.

Dermatopathologic examination will not always give the clinician a definitive diagnosis. Instead, the microscopic findings will help categorize the disease into a specific type or group of problems. It will also eliminate some or many potential differentials. More importantly it gives the clinician information about the cellular, epidermal, and dermal changes present. This information allows the clinician to determine pathophysiologic changes and recommend more appropriate therapies.

Sample selection is very important if one wishes to get the best results from a biopsy. General guidelines to follow include (1) taking multiple biopsies, unless a solitary lesion or tumor is being biopsied; (2) selecting lesions that are typical of the patient's disease; (3) always including early and primary lesions if various stages are present; (4) removing pustules, vesicles, and bulla intact; and (5) trying to avoid medicated, excoriated, or ulcerative lesions. The most important guideline is to take multiple samples. Many times only one of three or four samples will contain diagnostic information.

Various biopsy techniques are available. In most cases 6 mm punch biopsies will be sufficient. The subcutaneous tissue below the biopsy site should be infiltrated with 2 percent lidocaine. Preparation of the site, other than spraying with alcohol, is contraindicated. Scrubbing and antiseptics may destroy, remove, or otherwise alter important surface pathology. The punch sample should *not* include normal skin as the pathologist may only section the normal part. The sample should always include some subcutaneous tissue.

Once the incision has been made the sample should be removed without crushing it. Thumb forceps, mosquito hemostats, or a needle should be passed down through the incision and into the subcutaneous section of the sample. The sample is then elevated and any attached subcutaneous tissue can be cut. For routine dermatopathology the tissue is placed in 10 percent neutral phosphate buffered formalin. If special procedures or stains are required, special fixatives or transport media should be available at the time of sampling. The biopsy site is then sutured. Even without prepping, postbiopsy infections are extremely rare.

Excisional biopsies are required occasionally for large lesions, lesions involving subcutaneous tissues and some cases with vesicles, bulla, or large pustules. Excisional biopsies are also preferred when sampling through disease margins or junctions. In these cases elliptical samples are required and the junction desired should be near the center of the ellipse. The ellipse can start in normal skin with this type of sample. Whenever possible the direction of hair growth should parallel the long axis of the ellipse. Whenever elliptical or large (>7 mm) punch biopsies are taken, the samples should be placed, subcutaneous side down, on wooden tongue depressors or cardboard. If this is not done, rolling and folding artifacts will occur.

The sample should be sent to a veterinary dermatopathologist, who may be a veterinary pathologist with an expertise in dermatopathology or a clinical veterinary dermatologist with an expertise in dermatopathology. The sample should be accompanied by a description of the lesions biopsied, the anatomic locations that were biopsied, a brief patient dermatologic history, and a differential or tentative diagnosis.

SUMMARY

The patient's prognosis and appropriate therapy can only be determined after a specific diagnosis is reached. Clinicians routinely following a systematic approach will enhance their ability to diagnose even the most complicated dermatologic cases.

To consistently achieve definitive diagnoses, the clinician must routinely follow a systematic approach, the foundations of which are the patient's history and the dermatologic examination. The clinician and client must then interact to determine what approach to follow in each individual case.

REFERENCES

1. Muller GH, Kirk RW, Scott DW: Small Animal Dermatology. 3rd Ed. WB Saunders, Philadelphia, 1983
2. Nesbitt GH: Cutaneous drug reactions in small animals. In Fellner, MJ, Zeide, DA, (Eds). Clinics in Dermatology. JB Lippincott, Philadelphia, 4(Jan-March):190, 1986
3. Nesbitt GH: Canine and Feline Dermatology: A Systematic Approach. Lea & Febiger, Philadelphia, 1983

2 Flea Dermatitis

Kenneth W. Kwochka
Diane E. Bevier

Now here's the happy bounding flea.
You cannot tell the he from she.
The sexes look alike, you see,
But she can tell, and so can he.[1]
R. Young

It seems unusual for us as veterinarians to regard these cursed insects as "happy bounding fleas." However, in spite of continual research and development of new generations of insecticides and better application techniques, in endemic areas the flea population remains just that—happy and bounding. Flea bite dermatitis is unquestionably the most common veterinary dermatologic entity in the world[2,3] and may be the most common overall disease problem of domestic animals.[3] In the southeastern part of the United States where environmental conditions enhance flea survival and reproduction and increased resistance to insecticides has accentuated the problem,[4] flea related diseases may account for over 50 percent of dermatologic cases presented to veterinarians[2] and in excess of 35 percent of the total small animal veterinary effort (R.E.W. Halliwell, Personal communication, 1985).

There are, of course, benefits to be gained from a problem of this magnitude. Research efforts exploring the pathogenesis of flea-allergy dermatitis (FAD) in the dog have provided important information on the immunologic mechanisms of arthropod hypersensitivity in general. Both the domestic animal species and man will benefit from this work. In humans, flea allergy is known to be a major cause of a common and frustrating condition known as papular urticaria.[5,6]

ETIOLOGY

Fleas are ectoparasitic bloodsucking insects of mammals and birds belonging to the order Siphonoptera.[1–4,7] As indicated by their phylogenetic classification, they have an exoskeleton of chitin, three pairs of jointed legs, anatomic division into head, thorax, and abdomen, laterally compressed wingless bodies, suctorial mouthparts, antennae, eyes, and combs.[8,9] The prothoracic and genal combs are useful taxonomically and are found both on *Ctenocephalides canis* and *C. felis*.[8] Many wild rodent fleas have only pronotal combs.[8] Other common fleas including *Echidnophaga gallinacea* (sticktight flea) and *Pulex irritans* (human flea) lack combs.

The adult fleas of domestic animals are generally dark brown, although other species may range from yellow to black. Adults from the many hundreds of classified species may range in size from less than 1 mm to 16 mm.[1] Males are generally smaller than females.

Fossil flea remains from the Paleocene era suggest a long evolutionary history with hundreds of species found on all continents.[10] However, there is much debate over the evolution of the flea. Some have presumed fleas to be related to flies, Diptera, while others have favored a close connection to the Mecoptera, the scorpion flies and hanging flies.[1] The wingless condition is believed to have been a secondary adaptation of ectoparasitic life.[1] The three pairs of strong jointed legs greatly enhance leaping ability, which also contributes to survival in an ectoparasitic existence.[7,9]

There are only a few flea species of importance that regularly bite domestic animals and humans (Table 2-1). *C. felis* is generally regarded as the most common species to parasitize dogs and cats.[1,3,4,7,11–13] Fleas are not considered strongly host specific and, thus, if the preferred hosts are not available they may parasitize a variety of hosts including humans.[1–4,7,11] It appears, however, that human blood is not nutritionally adequate for successful reproduction of *C. felis* which will die out in 6 to 8 weeks without exposure to the dog or cat.[1] *C. canis* is occasionally encountered on dogs and cats but not found as often as *C. felis*. Both *C. felis* and *C. canis* may serve as the intermediate host of the dog tapeworm, *Dipylidium caninum*.[1,9,11] *C. felis* is known to harbor the plague bacillus (*Yersinia pestis*) and the murine typhus and tularemia organisms.[1,9,10,14,15] *C. canis* has been infected with *Salmonella* sp. experimentally but it is unknown whether it can actually transmit the organism.[1]

E. gallinacea, the sticktight flea of poultry, is common in the southeastern United States and parasitizes a great variety of hosts including dogs, cats, rats, wild mammals, and birds.[1–3,9,16] The causative organisms of plague and typhus have been isolated from this species.[1]

P. irritans and *P. simulans* are cosmopolitan pests of humans, occasionally causing a severe allergic hypersensitivity dermatitis known as papular urticaria.[1,5,6,9,17] These species also infest many domestic and wild animals and may serve as a vector for the plague bacillus.[9] *Xenopsylla cheopis* is found throughout the world but primarily parasitizes rats and other rodents. It is of concern as the primary vector of bubonic plague and has been widely dissem-

Table 2-1. Important Flea Species of Domestic Animals and Man

Genus and Species	Common Hosts	Disease Transmission	Seasonal Abundance
Ctenocephalides felis	Cat, dog, opossum, other native mammals, man	Plague bacillis, murine typhus, tularemia, intermediate host of *Dipylidium caninum*	Maximum adult population in late summer and early fall
Ctenocephalides canis	Dog, red fox, gray fox, cat, man	Intermediate host of *Dipylidium caninum,* can be experimentally infected with *Salmonella*	Maximum adult population in late summer and early fall
Echidnophaga gallinacea	Dog, cat, rat, native wild mammals, birds	Plague bacillis, murine typhus	Maximum adult population in March, April, October, and November
Pulex irritans *Pulex simulans*	Man, many domestic and wild mammals	Plague bacillis	Maximum adult population in summer
Xenopsylla cheopis	Rat, other rodents	Murine typhus, primary vector of plague bacillis, alternate host for tapeworm *Hymenolepis diminuta*	Maximum adult population in spring

(Prepared from Benton, AH: An Atlas of the Fleas of the Eastern United States. Marginal Media, Fredonia, NY, 1980.)

inated throughout the world on Norwegian and black rats.[1,8,10,15] This species also serves as a vector for murine typhus and is an alternate host for the tapeworm *Hymenolepis diminuta*.[1,8,10,14]

Flea population surveys have been conducted in various areas of the United States, and it appears that in some areas such as the southeastern United States, *P. irritans* may be the most frequently encountered species of flea on dogs. In a study of 35 dogs from Georgia and Mississippi 5,831 fleas were collected and speciated. *P. irritans* comprised 81.2 percent of the population, *C. felis* 9.9 percent, *C. canis* 8.7 percent, and *E. gallinacea* 0.1 percent.[17] A recent survey from Gainesville, Florida noted *C. felis* and *P. irritans* accounting for most of the population with *E. gallinacea* in small numbers (R.E.W. Halliwell, Personal communication, 1985). Domestic flea species prevalent in human habitations in the San Francisco Bay area were primarily *P. irritans* and *C. felis*.[18]

Most flea species including *Ctenocephalides* spp. differ from many other ectoparasites by their lack of host specificity and by the fact that most of the life cycle is spent off the host in the environment. Although there is not true host specificity to particular species, many fleas may show an association with a particular mammalian or avian taxon.[1] However, these associations vary among different areas of the world.[1] It appears that fleas may inhabit a variety of hosts within a suitable set of environmental conditions and thus be more habitat specific than host specific.[1] Factors such as altitude, temperature, humidity, and location and composition of nests or burrows are important.[1]

The life span of the flea is heavily influenced by environmental factors but usually ranges from 6 to 12 months.[2,4] Temperature and humidity are the two most important factors influencing survival, development, and reproduction of *Ctenocephalides* spp. A moist warm environment with a relative humidity of 75 to 85 percent and temperature of 65 to 80°F is most favorable for rapid completion of the life cycle.[2,7,9,11,12,16] The cycle may be as short as 16 to 21 days under optimal conditions or as long as a year when unfavorable conditions prevail.[2–4,7,9,10,12,16] Fleas may survive but will not thrive in extreme temperatures, in dry conditions, or at high altitudes. Humidity is even more important than nutrition with desiccation occurring within a few days in dry environments. If humidity is high, fleas are reported to live anywhere from 4 to 12 months without nutrition.[7,16]

In order for an adult flea to reach sexual maturity it must ingest a blood meal from the host.[1,11] Several studies have been conducted to investigate mechanisms by which fleas locate a suitable host for feeding. Host odor, body temperature, and low concentrations of exhaled carbon dioxide appear to be important attractants for *C. felis*.[1,19] Air currents set up by wingbeats of birds over the nest have also been postulated as attractions.[1] One very interesting observation is that fleas would jump toward a bird which had landed on a branch above their location, stimulated by the casting of a shadow.[1]

In most cases only adult fleas will be found parasitizing the host.[4,7] After ingestion of the blood meal, mating and oviposition occur. The white oval eggs (0.5 to 2.0 mm) are randomly laid in small groups in the environment, surviving even in cracks and crevices of floors.[1] Those that are laid in the hair coat soon fall off into the bedding and surrounding environment. With frequent blood meals by the female, oviposition may last for several weeks with from 3 to 18 eggs laid at one time with the potential for several hundred over a 1-year period.[7,9,12] After incubation of 2 to 12 days (2 to 4 under optimal conditions) the eggs hatch to small (1 to 2 mm), white, maggot-like larvae, which feed on organic matter including fecal material and dried blood. Locomotion of these legless larvae is assisted by caudal processes called anal struts.[7]

Although in most species the larvae reside in the environment, Molyneux reported that larvae of the rat flea, *Nosopsyllus fasciatus*, attach to the pygidial region of adult fleas.[20] The larvae stimulate defecation and then suck the liquid blood excreted by the adult for nutrition. He also suggested that larvae might be predatory on mites and injured fleas. Flea larvae cannibalizing adults and utilizing blood for nutrition has also been reported but not in association with those species parasitzing domestic animals or humans.

Under optimal environmental conditions the larvae undergo 3 molts over 7 to 14 days. The third-instar larva spins a thin whitish cocoon followed by pupal formation within a few days. The adult flea emerges from the cocoon after several days to several months depending on conditions of temperature and humidity. Environmental disturbances such as vibrations also appear to have a direct stimulatory effect on hatching of adult fleas from the cocoon.[1,19]

The life cycle of the sticktight flea, *E. gallinacea*, is similar to that of *C. felis*. One difference is that during copulation the female burrows and firmly attaches herself to the host's skin. The eggs are laid in an ulcerated nodule but after hatching on the host the larvae fall off into the environment. The life cycle is then completed as previously described.[9]

PATHOPHYSIOLOGY

It is generally felt that a flea bite is capable of inducing significant clinical disease without a true hypersensitivity reaction being involved.[2,3,12,16] Flea saliva contains histamine-like compounds and enzymes which are proteolytic, anticoagulant, and cytolytic and have hyaluronidase-like activity.[2,3] These substances have irritant and pruritogenic properties which may result in digestion and liquefaction of the host tissue with local inflammatory reactions.[12] Recently, the importance of simple flea-bite irritancy without a hypersensitivity reaction has been questioned. Halliwell has indicated that although a flea bite in a normal, unsensitized animal may be somewhat irritating, clinically significant reactions will always involve allergy (Personal communication, 1985). He feels this will become more apparent as the hypersensitivity reactions are better characterized and new techniques are developed for diagnosis.[3]

In the late 1950s flea bites were causing severe problems in the human population in the San Francisco Bay area of California. Extensive studies were undertaken to explore the pathogenesis of the skin reactions. The ultimate goals were to characterize the types of hypersensitivity involved, purify flea antigen,

Table 2-2. The Sequence of Skin Reactivity of Guinea Pigs to Flea Bites Following Repeated Exposure

Reactivity Stage	Type of Hypersensitivity	Time After Initial Exposure (days)
I	Induction with no observable skin reactions	1–4
II	Delayed, cell—mediated immune reactions	5–9
III	Delayed, cell—mediated immune reactions and immediate, IgE mediated immune reactions	10–60
IV	Immediate, IgE mediated immune reactions	61–90
V	Anergy, no skin reactivity	After 90

(Prepared from Feingold BF, Benjamini E, Michaeli D: The allergic responses to insect bites. Ann Rev Entomology 13:137, 1968; and Benjamini E, Feingold BF, Kartman L: Skin reactivity in guinea pigs sensitized to flea bites: The sequence of reactions. Proc Soc Exp Biol Med 108:700, 1961.)

and use it for development of a hyposensitization program for allergic individuals. A large scale, successful hyposensitization program was not achieved but many important things were learned about flea bite hypersensitivity.

A number of investigators working with a guinea pig model determined that flea sensitivity was primarily of the delayed type with any immediate reactions being part of the delayed hypersensitivity response.[21–23] It also appeared that delayed reactions were the most important in human subjects with flea bite hypersensitivity.[18] Benjamini, Feingold, and Kartman further revealed that in the guinea pig there was a definite sequence in the development of reactivity in response to repeated exposure to flea bites or whole flea extract (Table 2-2).[24] Of particular interest was that all animals reached a state of nonreactivity within 140 days as long as at least twice weekly exposure was maintained.[24]

It was also discovered that guinea pigs sensitized to one species of flea reacted to all three species used in the studies (*P. irritans, P. simulans, C. felis*).[18,22] This indicated the presence of a common antigenic factor. The active principle responsible for flea bite reactions was found to be contained in both whole flea extract and oral secretion.[23] At least one of the substances responsible for inducing hypersensitivity is an incomplete antigen or hapten of relatively low molecular weight and stable to heat and acid hydrolysis.[25] This haptenic substance combines with both salt- and acid-soluble fractions of dermal collagen to form a complete antigen which is at least partly responsible for hypersensitivity reactions.[26,27]

It has been assumed for many years that the clinical and experimental findings regarding flea bite hypersensitivity in the guinea pig could be applied to other species including the dog and cat. Halliwell, however, was puzzled by the fact that dogs, unlike guinea pigs, appear to maintain their state of hypersensitivity and never reach anergy (Personal communication, 1985). Based on this observation, he has conducted numerous experiments which have helped to better characterize flea-bite-hypersensitivity in the dog.

The induction of flea allergy was attempted experimentally in flea-naive dogs by exposure to flea bites either continually or intermittently. Skin testing with flea antigen was performed at weekly intervals to document and characterize the development of the hypersensitive state. Animals continually exposed either failed to develop hypersensitivity or developed it later and to a lesser degree. IgG and IgE were absent in the sera or present only at low levels.[28] These animals, however, could still develop allergy if changed from continual to intermittent flea exposure (R.E.W. Halliwell, Personal communication, 1985). This information on the development of tolerance with continual exposure may have important implications for future development of therapeutic programs.

All of the dogs exposed to flea bites intermittently developed positive skin test reactions to fleas within 12 weeks (Halliwell R.E.W.: Personal communication, 1985) and had IgG and IgE antibody levels against flea antigen detectable in their sera.[28] Nine of 20 dogs developed delayed reactions prior to immediate ones. Six animals developed immediate reactions first and five dogs showed immediate and delayed reactions simultaneously. Twelve of 20 dogs showed immediate and delayed reactions concomitantly on most weeks of the 44-week study. Five dogs had predominantly immediate reactions most weeks while three demonstrated delayed reactions most often. Dogs that became allergic maintained their hypersensitivities during the entire 44 weeks of the study (R.E.W. Halliwell, Personal communication, 1985). Thus, it was shown that unlike the guinea pig, flea sensitivity in the dog is not primarily a delayed-type hypersensitivity response. Also, a random sequence of delayed, immediate and mixed reactions occurs in the dog and not the orderly sequence observed in the guinea pig. Furthermore, dogs appear to retain their hypersensitive state over a long period of time without reaching anergy.

Histopathologic examination of skin biopsies from sequential lesions on dogs with experimental flea-bite hypersensitivity revealed that the allergic reaction might be more involved than classical immediate and delayed hypersensitivities. A number of dogs had dermal edema and an eosinophilic perivascular infiltrate for as long as 48 hours after exposure indicating a possible overlap of immunologic mechanisms and a late-onset IgE-mediated response as part of the pathogenesis.[29]

Halliwell also examined glutaraldehyde-fixed skin biopsies from these lesions cut into ultrathin sections and stained with acid Giemsa.[30] He found basophils present in each of 10 animals which had strong delayed reactions. The highest proportion recorded was 22.1 percent with biopsies from 7 of 10 dogs showing greater than 10 percent basophils at some point in the study. Cutaneous basophil hypersensitivity may, therefore, be involved in the immunopathogenesis of flea-bite hypersensitivity in the dog. This cutaneous reaction is involved in the pathogenesis of tick bite hypersensitivity in other species and is in part responsible for parasite immunity.

CLINICAL SIGNS

Clinical syndromes associated with flea infestation in dogs and cats include (1) asymptomatic carriers, (2) flea-bite dermatitis, (3) FAD, (4) *Dipylidium caninum* (tapeworm) infestation, (5) blood loss anemia (especially in puppies, kittens, and debilitated adults), and (6) personality changes (especially in cats: irritability, growling, sudden running and jumping.)[9,12,16] The dermatologic and other clinical signs related to fleas depend on the degree of immunologic sensitivity and the level of flea exposure.[3]

When sensitization to the bite of the flea occurs, the resulting condition is termed flea-allergy dermatitis (FAD). Flea-allergy dermatitis involves lesions that are more severe and pruritus that is more intense than is seen in animals with dermatitis due to infestation only. Although dogs and cats may develop FAD at any age, it is rare to see an affected animal less than 6 months old. The most common age of onset is 3 to 6 years but hypersensitivity may occur even in very old animals.[12] No sex or breed predilection has been reported in FAD.[12,31,32] A recent study showed increased incidence in long-haired dogs,[33] but this point has been controversial in past flea related literature.[12,31,34]

Flea-bite dermatitis and flea-allergy dermatitis are usually distinctly seasonal disorders in areas with cold winters, with the most severe infestation and clinical signs seen in summer and fall. In warm climates, or where household infestation persists, flea infestation and FAD may be nonseasonal problems.[9]

Clinical Signs in the Cat

Flea-infested cats without hypersensitivity may be asymptomatic. If flea-bite dermatitis exists, pruritus is usually of mild to moderate intensity. Lesions, if present, are caused by flea bite irritancy with resultant scratching. Small crusts are located primarily on the head, neck, and dorsum of the body, but papules on the abdomen may be noted. Scaling, crusts, and thinning of the hair may also be present.[35] Focal or patchy alopecia caused by excessive licking with little or no dermatitis may be the presenting complaint.[36] Cats of all ages are affected. In kittens, heavy flea infestation may result in severe anemia and death.

In cats with flea sensitization, a diagnosis of FAD is made. The primary lesion in cats with FAD is an erythematous papule covered by a small reddish-brown crust. Lesions, as with flea-bite irritation, are usually most severe on the head, neck, and dorsal lumbosacral regions but have a tendency to generalize. The degree of alopecia is highly variable, with some cats having a surprisingly full hair coat associated with severe underlying dermatitis. Other cats have localized or generalized patchy or confluent alopecia with associated mild to severe dermatitis. Because of their fastidious grooming habits, it may be difficult to locate fleas or flea debris on a flea-allergic cat with extensive alopecia. Cats generally manifest moderate to severe pruritus by licking, scratching, chewing, shaking of the head, ripping hairs out, rippling of the skin upon stimulation, or turning and violently attacking areas of the skin without visible provocation. Any of these signs may accompany FAD in the cat.[4,16]

Additional clinical signs seen in the cat with flea bite dermatitis or FAD may include the finding of segments of *Dipylidium caninum* in the stool, the presence of gastric trichobezores, peripheral eosinophilia, anemia, and loss of weight or general condition due to the pruritus and scratching combined with the anemia and intestinal parasitism.

Clinical Signs in the Dog

Dogs may be asymptomatic carriers of small or large numbers of fleas. In nonsensitized individuals, response to the bites is minimal and results in mild pruritus, seborrheic changes, and excoriations.[3,37] Some individuals may have staphylococcal folliculitis secondary to flea dermatitis. Even in a nonallergic individual the bite of the flea will cause a transient papular eruption (G.A. Kunkle, Personal communication, 1985).

In the dog with flea-bite hypersensitivity, the severity of the dermatitis is determined by the animal's immunologic status, flea burden, extent of self-trauma, other secondary lesions, duration of the disorder, and prior therapy. Classically, when the flea bites a hypersensitive dog, a small wheal develops at the site of the bite that either resolves, or if the animal has a delayed hypersensitivity response, develops into a papule which later crusts over.[3] This highly pruritic papulocrustous dermatitis is typically confined to the dorsal lumbosacral area, caudomedial thighs, ventral abdomen, flank, and neck.[9,38] In severely hypersensitive animals, generalized cutaneous signs may develop.[39] Erythema, excoriation, and alopecia with stubbled hairs, due to chewing and licking by the dog, are present. Secondary seborrhea may be mild to severe and owners often complain of the dog's offensive odor.[4] Some animals experience recurrent episodes of acute moist dermatitis (''hot spots''.) Long-standing pruritus and self-trauma may lead to marked secondary changes of acanthosis, hyperkeratosis, lichenification, and hyperpigmentation. Severely affected animals may develop redundant folds of skin over the caudal back and caudomedial thighs. The chronic changes function as a protective mechanism in some cases with diminution of the pruritus during this stage of the dermatitis.

Some dogs develop a staphylococcal folliculitis whenever infested with fleas, although the frequency of this accompanying sign is debatable. One study reports a 10 percent incidence of superficial folliculitis lesions occurring in 330 cases of FAD.[12] Others, who practice in areas with heavy flea burdens, feel the incidence of flea-associated staphylococcal infection may be higher (G.A. Kunkle, Personal communication, 1985.)

As noted for the cat, additional clinical signs in the dog with flea dermatitis or FAD may include the finding of segments of *Dipylidium caninum* in the stool, peripheral eosinophilia, anemia and loss of weight or general condition due to the pruritus and scratching.

DIAGNOSIS

The aforementioned history and clinical findings are highly suggestive of flea-bite dermatitis or FAD. Nonallergic dogs may be infested with fleas but will have no signs of FAD.[4] Observation of fleas and/or flea dirt is beneficial, but the diagnosis should not be abandoned if fleas are not present on the patient at the time of examination since fleas spend the majority of their life off the host.[32,39] Owners may also bathe or dip their animals prior to examination and thus remove the evidence.[4] In the cat, fastidious grooming may remove fleas and their excreta.

Careful examination for fleas is essential, particularly in long-coated dogs. Examination of the ventrum and perineal area for the fast moving flea may be rewarding. Flea excreta can easily be identified by moistening any dark-colored foreign particles collected from the coat on a white piece of paper or placing them on moist cotton to obtain the characteristic reddish-brown color of digested blood. The use of a fine-toothed metal comb, a flea comb, or louse comb (32 teeth/inch), can help pick fleas out of a coat or aid in harvesting the flea excreta particles.[40] Additionally, examination of debris left on the examination table with a hand-held magnifying lens may reveal the ovoid, white egg of the flea, some of which adhere to the animal's coat, and fall off during the examination or combing process. Positive identification of fleas, eggs, and excreta using these methods will help overcome the reluctance of owners to accept the diagnosis of a flea-related dermatitis.

Differentiating between the flea-bite dermatitis case and the animal who is truly allergic to the bite of a single flea requires good historical information and the use of intradermal skin testing with aqueous flea antigen. Skin testing should be considered an aid in diagnosis. A positive skin test alone does not justify a diagnosis of FAD. Clinical signs compatible with such a diagnosis and history or presence of flea exposure are necessary to corroborate the presence of disease. Conversely, negative skin test results to intradermal injection of flea antigen in a patient with signs supportive of a diagnosis of FAD may suggest that one should pursue other differentials more vigorously, but does not absolutely rule out the diagnosis of FAD.[3,4]

Reported results of intradermal skin testing for the diagnosis of FAD in dogs and cats have been contradictory and inconclusive.[2,3,12,41–43] In interpreting these results, the clinician must consider that the formulation and concentration of flea antigen used in testing varied from study to study. In 1971, Baker reported nearly 81 percent positive reactions in dogs with clinical FAD, while normal dogs rarely showed positive reactions.[41] In 1978, Kristensen and Kieffer performed intradermal testing with a flea antigen preparation similar to that used by Baker. Testing produced 81 percent specificity and 87 percent sensitivity in 37 dogs clinically diagnosed as having FAD.[42] Halliwell is a strong proponent of the value of intradermal tests with flea antigen and feels that a 1:1,000 wt/vol aqueous solution of antigen extract (Flea Extract 1:100, Greer Laboratories, Lenoir, NC) is a potent and highly specific antigen for diagnostic purposes. He reported that intradermal skin testing with flea antigen was positive in about 98 percent of the dogs with FAD (80 percent immediate reaction, 10 percent immediate and delayed reactions, and 10 percent delayed reactions).[2,3] Another recent study used four commercial flea antigens for intradermal testing in four dogs with FAD and 10 normal dogs.[43] This study concluded that glycerinated antigens gave invalid results (false-positives due to irritative phenomenon), a finding documented in earlier studies.[2,12] Additionally, Van Winkle stated that nonglycerinated antigens need further evaluation as diagnostic aids for flea allergy due to false positive results in a small number of selected normal dogs tested.[43]

Published experience with skin testing in cats is meager. Baker stated that cats with miliary eczema did not uniformly give positive reactions to intradermal injection of flea extracts.[34] This observation may reflect the myriad of causes of miliary dermatitis in the cat.[9] However, Kristensen and Kieffer reported skin test sensitivity of only 35 percent after testing 17 cats with histories and clinical signs consistent with flea allergy, also suggesting that the use of this diagnostic aid in the cat is unreliable.[42]

In a recent study evaluating hyposensitization for the treatment of FAD, 25 carefully screened cats with histories and clinical signs compatible with a diagnosis of FAD and extensive diagnostics to rule out other causes of miliary dermatitis, were skin tested intradermally with flea antigen.[44] All of the highly suspect FAD cats skin tested positive with Halliwell's protocol.[2] This study, although not specifically addressing the skin testing question, suggests that the use of intradermal skin testing in cats with flea antigen may be more useful than previously believed.

Current protocols for skin testing for flea hypersensitivity in the dog and cat involve an intradermal injection of diluent and a 1:100,000 wt/vol solution of histamine phosphate (Eli Lilly and Co., Indianapolis, IN) used as negative and positive controls respectively. A 1:1000 wt/vol aqueous solution of flea antigen extract is used for the diagnosis. A positive immediate hypersensitivity reaction will produce a cutaneous "wheal and flare" within 15 minutes. Sites of flea antigen injections should be reexamined at 24 and 48 hours for a delayed reaction.[2] Animals to be tested should be taken off glucocorticoids, antihistamines, and phenothiazine tranquilizers for appropriate time intervals before testing.[45]

Another diagnostic aid may be the presence of *Dipylidium caninum* segments around the anal area. It has also been reported that blood eosinophilia is present in 13 to 20 percent of dogs and cats with FAD but this finding does not correlate with tissue eosinophilia nor the outcome of intradermal skin testing.[38,42,46]

Skin biopsy is nondiagnostic and reveals a perivascular dermatitis with eosinophils seen as the predominant cell type. Other findings include intraepidermal eosinophilic microabscesses and pathology consistent with secondary pyoderma.[16,32,38]

Differential diagnoses for flea-bite dermatitis and FAD include allergic inhalant dermatitis, food hypersensitivity, drug hypersensitivity, intestinal parasite hypersensitivity, and folliculitis. In the cat, differential diagnoses include cheyletiellosis, dermatophytosis, food hypersensitivity, trombiculidiasis, parasite hypersensitivity, drug hypersensitivity, bacterial folliculitis, allergic inhalant dermatitis, and idiopathic miliary dermatitis.[9]

Although the clinical signs of allergic inhalant dermatitis are somewhat different from those of FAD, atopy can only be conclusively eliminated from the list of differentials by intradermal skin testing.[3] Both allergic conditions may occur in the same animal. More than 70 percent of the atopic animals in Florida were positive to skin testing with a commercial aqueous flea antigen.[47] In another large study of atopic dogs, 90.6 percent were skin test positive for flea antigen.[48] Unfortunately, in the second study glycerinated flea antigen was used for testing which is known to cause false-positive reactions. In studies of insect allergic people, 33 to 40 percent of people who experienced an anaphylactic reaction to an insect were also atopic.[49] Only 0.5 to 0.8 percent of the general population develops an anaphylactic reaction after an insect sting.[49]

TREATMENT

Effective treatment of flea infestation or FAD requires a three-pronged attack: (1) flea eradication from the indoor and outdoor environments, (2) elimination of fleas on all affected animals, and (3) treatment of the existing dermatitis.

In cases of simple flea infestation, eradication is attempted because of the unaesthetic qualities of an insect infested pet and for prevention of clinical signs in the pet and human infestation. In the flea-allergic pet, the animal's discomfort and dermatitis are of paramount concern to the owner. The veterinarian is in the best position to advise owners of the necessity and means of implementing the three-pronged approach to flea control. The practitioner should design a flea control program for each client's needs.

In general, failure to control fleas results from a lapse in client communication or compliance, not from failure of flea control products.[50] Also, the level of knowledge of the veterinarian regarding basic flea biology and new developments in flea control products determines whether the safest, most efficacious flea control program is prescribed. In the last 5 years, this field has changed dramatically. New insecticides have entered the market while older, less effective, more toxic products are being removed. New methods of formulation have been developed which are superior to older standard formulations.[51] In the following sections, principles of flea control, methods of application of pesticides, insecticide groups, and specific products and toxicities will be covered.

Flea Control in the Environment

Outdoor

Environmental flea control has two objectives: to eliminate fleas from both the home and yard. Clients who reside on several acres are not going to be able to spray the entire area, but it is practical to spray parts of the yard where the pet spends the majority of its time. Local spraying reduces the pet's flea exposure and, done frequently, it can decrease the flea population. An enclosed

Table 2-3. Indoor and Outdoor Synchronized 30-Day Flea Control Program

Day of Program	Indoor Treatment	Outdoor Treatment
1	General sanitation[a] followed by an adulticide-methoprene spray[b] followed by adulticide-methoprene foggers[c]	General environmental clean-up[d] followed by an insecticidal dust or spray[e]
2–14	Do not vacuum or mop carpets or floors	
15	As for day 1	As for day 1
16–29	Do not vacuum or mop carpets or floors	
30	As for day 1	As for day 1
	Continue Program Once Monthly or as Necessary	

[a] Thorough vacuum cleaning (discard vacuum bag immediately or add a flea adulticide such as naphlene crystals or a flea collar); mop floors; discard mop and animal bedding or wash and dry at high heat.

[b] Spray along baseboards, in corners, in closets, and under furniture including cushions and mattresses prior to fogging.

[c] Foggers will effectively cover the remaining exposed areas; not necessary if entire house is sprayed.

[d] Mow lawn; rake up all organic debris and discard.

[e] Dust with fertilizer spreader; spray with hand-held spray tank or garden hose spray bottle attachment.

(Adapted from Schick MP, Schick RO: Understanding and implementing safe and effective flea control. J Am Anim Hosp Assoc 22:421, 1986)

yard is more easily treated.[50] For successful outdoor flea control, sanitation of the outdoor premises is of paramount importance. Removal of organic debris by raking or mowing the yard or kennel area should be done prior to insecticidal treatment. In smaller yards, hand-held spray tanks can effectively deliver emulsifiable concentrates. Another method, especially when larger areas must be covered, is a lawn and garden hose sprayer attachment that utilizes water as a pressurized insecticide dispersing medium.[11] Dust may be used in fertilizer spreaders or directly from packages with sprinkle applicator tops.

An optimal integrated flea control program including outdoor and indoor control is presented in Table 2-3.

Indoor

Synchronized sanitation and insecticide treatment which removes the flea eggs, eliminates immature larval forms, and kills adult fleas is necessary for effective control in the inside environment.[11]

An effective flea control program must include thorough sanitation and insecticide application that provides both instant and residual killing activity in the house.[50,52] Indoor sanitation can physically remove flea eggs and larvae from the environment. Vacuuming removes the eggs and larvae from the carpeting or furniture. To prevent completion of the life cycle of the flea within the vacuum bag, one should vacuum up crushed napthalene crystals (moth balls) or place pieces of flea collar within the bag. A more expensive alternative is to discard the vacuum bag after each use. Floors should be mopped, with particular attention paid to cracks and crevices where organic debris and flea eggs accumulate. With severe infestation, steam cleaning of the carpeting is highly effective in removing and killing larvae and eggs. Insecticides can be used in the water of the steam cleaning machine (carbaryl products may cause staining of carpeting). All animal and human bedding frequented by pets must be washed and dried on the maximal heat setting to ensure flea death.[11,50]

Environmental clean-up should be completed before insecticide use begins. The entire floor surface including baseboards, closets, and underneath furniture must be sprayed or dusted with an insecticide. This can be most easily accomplished by using a hand-held spray tank or with the package applicator. Following this surface spraying, fogger canisters (bombs) should be placed in the environment.

Prior to aerosol fogging, air conditioning systems should be turned off and all windows closed. Pets and plants should be removed or handled according to the insecticide manufacturer's label directions. Birds and fish are especially sensitive to insecticides. An adequate number of foggers must be used to get good penetration of all rooms in the house.[11,50] Square footage recommendations on foggers fail to take into account walls and other barriers to circulation of the mist.

No single insecticide treatment can kill all the fleas in the home. Repeated house cleaning must be continued with insecticide applications at 10 to 14 day intervals for 3 consecutive treatments followed by monthly sanitation and insecticide use for optimal results.[50,53]

Some clients will prefer the services provided by a professional exterminator. This method may be more expensive but has the advantages of thorough application with little inconvenience to the client.

Insecticides

Increased public awareness regarding the effects of insecticides on human health and environment has prompted the desire to use safe, effective flea control. Knowledge of the commonly used groups of insecticides allows the veterinarian to make appropriate choices of chemicals for individual pet and premise treatment. The commonly used groups of insecticides include natural pyrethrins, synthetic pyrethroids, rotenone, other organic insecticides, carbamates, chlorinated hydrocarbons, organophosphates, and the insect growth regulator, methoprene.

Organic Insecticides

Natural pyrethrins are relatively nontoxic botanical insecticides isolated from *Chrysanthemum cinerarie-folium* floral parts.[54,55] Historically, the plant materials have been in use longer than other insecticides. Pyrethrin is now the only commonly used botanical insecticide. It is typically found in rapid knockdown sprays in combination with synergists, and one or more synthetic organic insecticides, that contribute to its efficacy.[56] The fast-kill action of synergized pyrethrins combined with low mammalian toxicity are the advantages of these products. The most serious problem with pyrethrins is their rapid biodegradation by oxidation and hydrolysis, especially when exposed to ultraviolet light. They are, therefore, very labile in the environment and lack residual activity.[57]

Synthetic pyrethroids are more stable than pyrethrins upon exposure to ultraviolet light and, therefore, exhibit greater residual activity. Cost of these products is generally less than natural pyrethrin. They may also be safer in mammals.[56] Four synthetic pyrethroids are available for indoor use against fleas; d-transallethrin, resmethrin, d-phenothrin and tetramethrin. A synthetic pyrethroid dip is now available for animals (Table 2-4).

Rotenone, another botanical, is derived from the root of the plants *Derris elliptica* and *Lonchcarpus utilis*.[58] It causes a slower, but more certain insect death as compared to pyrethrin. Rotenone breaks down quickly in the environment, leaving no harmful residue.[56] It may cause a contact dermatitis in man.[54]

Organic insecticides containing citrus extracts are commercially available for flea control. One extract, d-Limonene, exudes a citrus scent and is approved in the United States as an insecticide for use on dogs and cats. d-Limonene causes desiccation and death of the flea by stripping the outer cuticle layer from the exoskeleton and also affects the central nervous system.[56,59] No toxicities have been reported in dogs, but d-Limonene has caused feline toxicities including ataxia, muscle tremors, and hypersalivation.[60]

Dried brewer's yeast (*Saccharomyces cerevisiae*) in various oral formulations has been advocated for flea control on small animals.[61] The efficacy of this substance is questionable. One study reported that brewer's yeast supplementation resulted in significantly reduced flea numbers as compared to non-treated control dogs.[61] The majority of other well conducted and controlled experimental trials in dogs and people have concluded that brewer's yeast and its major component, thiamine HCl (vitamin B_1), is ineffective as a flea repellent or insecticide for dogs or humans.[62–64]

Nonorganic Insecticides

Carbamates are anticholinesterase insecticides. In contrast to organophosphates, carbamate action produces a less stable acetylcholinesterase-inhibitor complex. It is possible that insects may detoxify the unstable complex after prolonged periods of paralysis and then completely recover.[65] Carbamates are found in outdoor and indoor preparations and in shampoo, powder, and dip formulations for dogs and cats. Under certain circumstances, the application of carbaryl to a carpet may lead to staining. This could occur when using

Table 2-4. Prescription Flea Control Products for the Animal[a]

Formulation	Product Name (Manufacturer)	Insecticide	Percent of Active Ingredient	Approved Usage
Shampoos	Adams Flea Off Shampoo (Adams Veterinary Research Labs)	Synergized pyrethrin	0.15	Dogs & cats
	Mycodex Shampoo with Pyrethrins (Beecham Labs)	Synergized pyrethrin	0.05	Dogs & cats
	Duocide Shampoo (Allerderm)	Synthetic pyrethroid	0.08	Dogs & cats
	Mycodex Shampoo with Carbaryl (Beecham Labs)	Carbamate	0.50	Dogs & cats
	Sendran Shampoo (Haver)	Carbamate	0.125	Dogs & cats
	Mycodex Shampoo with Lindane (Beecham Labs)	Lindane	0.30	Dogs
	Thionium Shampoo with Lindane (Coopers Animal Health)	Lindane	0.25	Dogs
	VIP Flea and Tick Shampoo (Hill's Pet Chemicals)	d-Limonene	5.00	Dogs & cats
Collars	Vet-Kem Dursban Flea and Tick Collar for Large Dogs (Vet-Kem)	Chlorpyrifos	8.0	Dogs
	Vet-Kem Flea and Tick Collar with Propoxur (Vet-Kem)	Carbamate	9.4	Dogs
	Vet-Kem Breakaway Flea and Tick Collar for Cats (Vet-Kem)	Carbamate	9.4	Cats
Powders	Wellcome Flea Powder for Cats (Coopers Animal Health)	Carbamate	3.00	Cats
	Diryl Flea Powder for Dogs and Cats (Pitman-Moore)	Synergized pyrethrin/carbamate	0.1/5.0	Dogs & cats
	Adams Flea Off Dust (Adams Veterinary Research Labs)	Synergized pyrethrin/carbamate	0.1/12.5	Dogs & cats
	Dermaton Dust (Coopers Animal Health)	Organophosphate (clorfenvinphos)	0.5	Dogs
	Paramite Powder (Vet-Kem)	Organophosphate (phosmet)		Dogs & Cats

Sprays	Adams Flea-Off Mist (Adams Veterinary Research Labs)	Synergized pyrethrin (alcohol base)	0.15	Dogs & cats
	Mycodex Aquaspray (Beecham Labs)	Synergized pyrethrin	0.20	Dogs & cats
	Sectrol Pet Spray (Animal Care Products/3M)	Microencapsulated synergized pyrethrin	0.11	Dogs & cats
	Sectrol Pet Foam (Animal Care Products/3M)	Microencapsulated synergized pyrethrin	0.15	Dogs & cats
Dips	Expar 3.2% EC (Coopers Animal Health)	Synthetic pyrethroid permethrin	3.2	Dogs
	Paradip (Haver)	Carbaryl/lindane	8.0/3.9	Dogs
	Adams Flea Off Dip (Adams Veterinary Research Labs)	Malathion	52.0	Dogs
	Dermaton III (Coopers Animal Health)	Organophosphate (chlorfenvinphos)	12.25	Dogs
	Ectoral (Pitman-Moore)	Organophosphate (ronnel)	33.34	Dogs & cats
	Paramite (Vet-Kem)	Organophosphate (phosmet)	11.60	Dogs & cats
	VIP Flea & Tick Dip (Hill's Pet Chemicals)	d-Limonene	78.00	
	Durakyl Dip (DVM)	Synergized pyrethrin/rotenone	0.8/1.1	
Systemic–Topical	Pro-Spot (Bayvet Division, Miles Laboratory)	Organophosphate (fenthion)	5.6 and 13.8	Dogs
Systemic–Oral	Proban (Bayvet Division, Miles Laboratory)	Organophosphate (cythioate)	30 mg (tablets)	Dogs

[a] For a more complete list see MacDonald JM, Miller TA: Parasiticide therapy in small animal dermatology. p. 571. In Kirk RW (ed): Current Veterinary Therapy—IX. WB Saunders, Philadelphia, 1986.

an alkaline carpet shampoo or when steam cleaning and then applying a carbamate insecticide.[51,66]

Chlorinated hydrocarbons are highly toxic residual insecticides whose usage has recently declined in the United States.[54] *C. felis* has developed resistance to DDT and chlordane in various parts of the world. Lindane is currently on the market for limited use in flea control. From 1977 through 1980, an Environmental Protection Agency (EPA) review of environmental, animal (neurotoxicity, fetotoxicity, and oncogenicity), and human (aplastic anemia) health hazards related to lindane use was undertaken.[67,68] In June 1984, the use of lindane-containing dips on dogs was restricted by the EPA and lindane-containing powders and shampoos now have strict use requirements including wearing hoods, boots, and protective clothing and shoulder length gloves for application.[67] Chlorinated hydrocarbons are contraindicated for use on the cat.[69]

Organophosphates are cholinesterase inhibitors which are generally much more toxic to vertebrates than are the chlorinated hydrocarbons. They are chemically unstable and thus nonpersistent in the environment.[56] Insect resistance to organophosphates has not been as widespread as that which has developed to chlorinated hydrocarbon insecticides.[54] Like the chlorinated hydrocarbons, organophosphates may cause serious toxicities in the cat with the notable exception being malathion.[16] Malathion is converted by insects to a highly toxic metabolite, maloxon, as compared to mammalian conversion to harmless metabolites that are eliminated from the body.[70]

One of the newer approaches towards pest control has been the development of insect growth regulators. Currently, methoprene is the only insect growth regulator on the market for flea control.[56] Methoprene has been incorporated into several over-the-counter indoor flea-control products available at pet and department stores.

Methoprene acts on the fourth instar larvae. As these larvae pupate they are unable to undergo complete metamorphosis into adults and, therefore, die. The residual action of methoprene foggers is 75 days, and for general application, 90 days. Since it has no action on adult fleas, methoprene should be used in conjunction with a fast-acting insecticide that kills adults. It is reported that the flea cycle can be broken with correct use of this combination.[71] Methoprene undergoes rapid degradation to harmless metabolites and is one of the safest indoor insecticides. It is inactivated by sunlight and, therefore, is not useful on pets or in outdoor environmental control. Toxicity is difficult to produce in mammals.[72] To date, methoprene is the safest insecticide for use where crawling infants are exposed to the treated area or where there is high risk of exposure to insecticides.[51]

Inert insecticides are products that control fleas by mechanical, rather than chemical means. Two are used indoors: silica aerogel and diatomaceous earth. These kill fleas by absorbing waxes from the insect cuticle which results in desiccation and death. Both of these products can be mixed with other insecticides for use as dusts.[56]

Flea Control on the Pet

Experiences with conventional pesticides approved for use in veterinary medicine differ widely from one part of the country and from one country to another. This results from regional variation in the resistance of the flea population.[3]

Keeping this in mind, the clinician should adhere to one of the basic principles of topical therapy: choose and become familiar with a few representative, effective products from each insecticide and formulation category and know all their characteristics.[73] Insecticides for flea control have been compounded into shampoos, powders, sprays (including microcapsules), dips, oral tablets, oral liquids, and plastic collars. In addition to the number of products available from the veterinarian, there is a wide variety of over-the-counter topical flea control products. Many of these have lower concentrations of insecticides than prescription products. Also, the purchase of this type of product does not allow the owner to gain exposure to the concept of simultaneous indoor, outdoor, and pet flea control through discussion with their veterinarian.[11,50]

Some of the more popular over-the-counter and veterinary products are flea shampoos containing synergized pyrethrin insecticides. Pet owners commonly are under the misconception that flea shampoos have residual insecticidal capabilities.[50] These products, along with the physical flushing action of the water, may reduce the animal's flea load during bathing, but there are essentially no active ingredients left on the animal after rinsing.

Flea collars are another form of flea control in which owners place misguided faith. Their convenience makes them attractive to pet owners. Despite the fact that flea collars still have demonstrable efficacy against laboratory-reared fleas, clinical trials with some popular brands have shown them to be of little or no therapeutic value against native fleas in some geographical areas.[74] Their efficacy is questionable, especially in the southern regions of the United States where year-round breeding of the flea has created some extremely resistant strains. Flea collars have produced numerous cases of contact irritant dermatitis and systemic organophosphate intoxication in the past 15 years.[75–77] There appears to be better premarket testing and fewer problems associated with collars currently on the market. These statements are true for both the over-the-counter collars and those available through veterinarians. These products are best thought of as an adjunctive form of flea control along with other treatments.[78]

The use of oral organic products such as garlic, brewer's yeast, thiamine (vitamin B_1), and elemental sulfur are touted as "natural" flea control agents for pets. As mentioned previously, they have proven to be essentially worthless in confirmed problem flea control situations.[62,63]

Flea powder is available over-the-counter and from the veterinarian. Several pyrethrin, carbamate, and organophosphate insecticide powders are commercially available (Table 2-4). These products normally contain 0.10 percent pyrethrin and 3 to 12.5 percent carbamate compounds in a silica powder base. The maximum carbamate concentration should not exceed 5.0 percent for cats and 10.0 percent for dogs.[11] Mixing the 5.0 percent powder with an equal quantity of talcum powder produces a 2.5 percent product which can be safely used on young puppies and kittens. Again, these products have varying efficacy depending on the native flea population's resistance to pyrethrins and carbaryl.

One organophosphate flea powder (Dermaton Dust, Coopers Animal Health, Kansas City, MO) for use on dogs was evaluated under controlled conditions to determine efficacy against *C. felis* infestation. This study reported freedom from flea infestation on dogs for 12 days following a single dusting. No undesirable side effects resulted.[79]

Powders are probably best used between flea dips for additional killing effects as well as offering some repellent activity. Powders are somewhat drying to the skin. The powder must be worked thoroughly into the coat to the level of the skin to be effective. It should be applied once or twice weekly. Some owners will object to the feel, smell, and "aerosol" qualities of flea powder. Powders should not be applied to areas of moist dermatitis.[73]

Insecticide sprays containing pyrethrins, synthetic pyrethroids, carbamates, and organophosphates are sold over-the-counter and as prescription products (Table 2-4). In general, they should not be used on puppies and kittens under the age of 3 months unless otherwise specified on the product label.[11] Many of the currently available products are in an alcohol base. In cases of severe FAD, this can be irritating to the skin. Aqueous based sprays (Mycodex Aquaspray, Beecham Laboratories, Bristol, TN; Marmaduke Flea and Tick Spray, Norden Laboratories, Lincoln, NB) are less irritating and can be used in these cases.

Frequency of application is variable among flea spray preparations. Some of the pyrethrin products are labeled for one or more daily applications due to rapid biodegradation. Because of this short residual activity, these products can be used safely between dip applications on cats and dogs.[55] Another product (Adams Flea Off 14 Day Residual Mist, Adams Veterinary Research Laboratories, Miami, FL) which contains a repellent in addition to synergized pyrethrin, provides more than 99 percent efficacy against flea reinfestation for 21 days.

Sprays must be applied correctly. The entire coat of the animal should be lightly misted while brushed in the direction opposite to the lay of the hair. The coat should be moistened but not soaked. Sprays are convenient but can be messy and difficult to apply correctly.[73] They may also become costly if used on a large, long-coated dog. The elegance of more recently developed products has increased their acceptability to owners.

Microencapsulated insecticides are part of the growing arsenal of slow release insecticide products that have become available. This group is a welcome addition as the process of microencapsulation allows for stabilization and controlled release of active ingredients, and thus have greater residual activity.[56,80] The toxicity of the encapsulated insecticide is decreased over the native chemical. Small nylon or polyurea capsules are used to encapsulate the insecticide. To date, this process has been perfected for pyrethrins and diazinon. The microcapsules are suspended in liquid which is sprayed in the environment.

Small amounts of insecticide diffuse through the wall of the microcapsules and are either absorbed by the insect or pet, or break down from exposure to light and air. More insecticide diffuses through the shell wall to replace the loss. Thus, when a capsule becomes lodged in the integument of the flea, the flea is exposed to the insecticide until it dies.[51,56]

Microencapsulation of synergized natural pyrethrins extends their effective life from a few hours to more than 30 days. There is, however, the disadvantage in losing the quick-kill property common to pyrethrins. In one study the initial kill rate was found to be only 52 percent at 24 hours, but reached 95.6 percent at 30 days.[80] Encapsulation, therefore, allows long-term control of emerging adults.[51] The development of combination products (microencapsulated insecticide plus native pyrethrins) has overcome this disadvantage (Table 2-5).

Microencapsulated insecticidal spray and foam products are now available for use on pets. These products come as combinations of natural and microencapsulated pyrethrins in a low odor, water-based formula. They must be applied while the pet is damp and not toweled or brushed off. Following use of one of these products, an average of 5 minutes is required for "knock-down" of the fleas. Immediate and residual action on the animal provides 83 percent reduction in the number of fleas for 8 days.[81] These products contain significant amounts of free pyrethrin and should be used sparingly on puppies and kittens.[11]

Insecticidal dips are solutions prepared from several different insecticide groups. Their residual activity varies according to the active insecticide and area of the United States.[4,11,12] Dips are routinely applied every 5 to 7 days. Pyrethrin and malathion dips may be used on dogs and cats. Other organophosphate dips are contraindicated for use on cats.[69] Specific age recommendations for use appear on individual product labels. In general, insecticidal dips should not be used on animals less than 3 months of age.

Oral systemic insecticides can be of value in cases where owners object to other forms of flea control or in an animal who has sensitivity to topically applied products. Oral cythioate (Proban, Bayvet Division, Miles Laboratories, Shawnee, KS) at a dosage of 3.3 mg/kg twice weekly, is the only approved oral medication for flea control in the dog. The flea must bite the dog before it can be killed, so in the severely flea-allergic pet the cascade of hypersensitivity (and thus the dermatitis) still occurs with the use of this product. Cythioate does not replace effective environmental flea control. It should be made clear to clients that this drug is an ancillary aid in a total flea control program.[82]

One study evaluated six dogs which were administered cythioate at three times the recommended dosage for 1 year and showed no clinical signs of toxicosis.[83] Another field study of 67 dogs on cythioate for periods varying from 3 to 33 months, measured alanine aminotransferase and blood urea nitrogen (BUN) levels and found no elevation of enzymes nor signs of organophosphate toxicity.[82]

Halliwell recommends a negative heartworm status prior to commencing therapy with cythioate, although this is not listed as a requirement by the manufacturer.[3] Until researchers establish whether cythioate has the potential

Table 2-5. Insecticide Groups and Formulations for Indoor and Outdoor Environmental Flea Control

Common Name	Formulation[a]	Generally Marketed to[b]	May be Used by[b]	Comments
		Indoor Environment		
Methoprene	F, ST	E, V	E, GP, V	Used as sole product, effective on immatures, up to 90 day residual activity; in combination with other insecticides, 75 day residual activity, provides fast kill with good residual activity; ultra-violet light destroys in 24–48 hours; safest insecticides for use with infants present
Methoprene + synergized pyrethrins	A	E, V	E, GP, V	
Methoprene + carbamates + dichlorvos	A, F	E, GP, V	E, GP, V	
Pyrethrins	F, ST	GP	GP	Used as sole product, fast kill action; greater residual activity in combination with carbamates or organophosphates; microencapsulated pyrethrin has slower insecticidal activity (52% kill at 24 hours) but longer residual activity (95.6% kill at 30 days)
Microencapsulated pyrethrins	A, ST	E, V	E, GP, V	
Pyrethrins + chlorpyrifos	A	GP	GP	
Pyrethrins + carbamates	A	GP	GP	
Pyrethrins + carbamate + dichlorvos	F	GP	GP	
Diazinon	ST	E	E, GP, V	Microencapsulated, excellent residual activity with low acute oral and cutaneous toxicity; avoid vacuuming or mopping for sustained periods after application for increased effectiveness
Microencapsulated diazinon				
Synthetic pyrethroids	A, ST	E	E, GP, V	Greater residual activity than natural pyrethrins due to greater stability upon exposure to ultra-violet light
Pyrethroid + chlorpyrifos	A	E, V	E, GP, V	

Ronnel	A, ST	E, GP, V	E, GP, V	Pre-RPAR Investigation (pending EPA approval)
Malathion	D, ST	E, GP, V	E, GP, V	Relatively safe organophosphate; may be odoriferous when used indoors
Chlorpyrifos Chlorpyrifos + dichlorvos	ST A	E, GP, V GP	E, GP, V GP	Available in many formulations for indoor flea control; acts as a residual insecticide
Carbaryl	A, D, ST	E, GP, V	E, GP, V	May stain carpeting; used outdoors more frequently
Bendiocarb	D, ST	E	E, GP, V	Good efficacy for fleas; odorless; 95.9% kill at 24 hours and 100% kill at 30 days
Propoxur	A, ST	E, GP, V	E, GP, V	New, highly effective; highly toxic
Propetamphos	ST	E	E	Most toxic indoor insecticide
DDVP, dichlorovos	A, ST	E	E	Short residual action; quick kill
Outdoor Environment				
Malathion	D, ST	GP	GP	
Diazinon	ST	GP	GP	
Chlorpyrifos	A, ST	GP, V	GP, V	

[a] A, Aerosol spray; D, Dust; F, Fogger; ST, Hand-held spray tank.
[b] E, Exterminator; GP, general public; V, Veterinarian.

to cause heartworm cases to become occult, and whether additive hepatic and nephrotoxicity occur with active microfilaremia and organophosphate administration, this is a prudent recommendation.

Cythioate is not approved for use in cats, but it has been reported to be effective when used at half the canine dosage.[3]

Fenthion is a concentrated organophosphate which has been widely used for flea control on pets in the United States and Australia in the form of a cattle insecticide pour-on (Spotton-20% Fenthion Solution, Cutter Labs, Inc. Shawnee, KS). This product has been registered by the Food and Drug Administration (FDA) Bureau of Veterinary Medicine as a drug for use on livestock. When the registered product is used on dogs or cats, it is a violation of federal law. The EPA has received reports of serious adverse effects, including animal deaths, when fenthion has been used on pets. Peripheral neuropathies have been reported in veterinarians and technicians following exposure to the insecticide.[84,85,86]

Special mention should be made of cases of chronic systemic toxicity seen with fenthion. A clinical syndrome consisting of weight loss, anorexia, depression, and muscular tremors of the head and neck has been noted to occur especially in small dogs (weight less than 7.0 kg) on chronic fenthion treatment. These signs disappeared within 6 to 8 weeks of discontinuation of the drug but would recur if fenthion treatment was reinstituted.[84]

A recent study on fenthion's effect on cholinesterase levels in serum revealed that administration of one dose significantly depressed the activity of this enzyme, with a 2 or 3 week period necessary for reactivity.[85] Efficacy of the product was also monitored in this study and a dose-response curve demonstrated that the optimum effect was obtained at 20 mg/kg and that an increase in dosage gave no significant improvement in efficacy.[85]

Another more extensive study investigated the effects of repeated applications of 33 mg/kg and 44 mg/kg fenthion on canine plasma, red blood cell, muscle, and brain cholinesterase activity.[86] Four doses at weekly intervals decreased plasma cholinesterase by 80 percent, muscle cholinesterase by 55 percent, and brain cholinesterase by 67 percent of control. Red blood cell cholinesterase activity was not apparently depressed by fenthion at either dose level. Despite the dramatic suppression of cholinesterase values in plasma, brain, and muscle, no clinical signs of intoxication were noted. This study suggests that assigning diagnostic significance to blood cholinesterase activity level may be misleading, depending on whether plasma or red blood cell cholinesterase is measured. Also, a precipitous drop in plasma cholinesterase may not be accompanied by clinical signs of toxicity.[86]

The drug has significant potential for toxicity and should be used after other methods of flea control have proved to be ineffective. For the animal unrestricted in the external environment, or animals walked through heavily infested areas, it may be the only effective alternative. This drug has spared the life of many animals in whom owners were considering euthanasia due to failure of other flea control methods.[3]

Fenthion has recently undergone reformulation and packaging for FDA approved use in dogs only. This product (Pro-Spot, Bayvet Division, Miles Laboratories, Shawnee, KS) was anticipated to satisfy the legal requirements for FDA usage and at the same time be an effective method of flea control. The approved recommended dose of Pro-Spot is 4 to 8 mg/kg which is significantly lower than the previously demonstrated optimal effective dose of fenthion at 20 mg/kg.[85] The clinical efficacy of Pro-Spot at this lower dosage is yet to be determined. The manufacturer strongly emphasizes the need for concurrent environmental treatment as part of a total flea control program.

Flea Repellents

Topical preparations produced for mosquito control are probably effective against fleas but have significant limitations. They require application several times daily (depending on temperature, humidity, wind speed, and moisture), feel oily, irritate mucous membranes, stain clothes, and fail against some species.[73] The practical and aesthetic considerations on fully haired species prevent their routine use.[3,73] The product of choice is n,n Diethyl-m-toluamide (D.M.T. Insect Repellent; Maurry Biologic Company, Los Angeles, CA).

Another product which has achieved some popularity in the southern United States as a mosquito and flea repellent is dilute Avon Skin-So-Soft (Avon Products, Inc., New York, NY). A limited study showed that a mixture of 1.5 oz/gallon of water used as a dip statistically decreased the mean average number of fleas on treated animals.[87] Used at a higher concentration (4 oz/gallon) this product was more effective but left the animals with greasy coats. The mechanism of Skin-So-Soft's repellancy is unknown. Certainly, an alternative or adjunctive therapy to currently used insecticides would be welcome after the repellent ingredient of Skin-So-Soft is determined and studied.[87]

Adjunctive and Antiinflammatory Therapy

Despite rigorous flea control, certain cases will require adjunctive dermatologic therapy in the form of shampoos, oil rinses, antibiotics, and antiinflammatory therapy.

Antiseborrheic shampoos may be helpful to reduce scales and crusts (Allerseb-T, Allerderm Inc., Hurst, TX; Sebbafon, Winthrop Laboratories, New York, NY: Clear Tar, Veterinary Dermatology Products, Inc., West Lake Village, CA). Animals with significant amounts of pyoderma may benefit from products containing benzoyl peroxide (Pyoben, Allerderm Inc., Hurst, TX; Oxydex, Dermatologics for Veterinary Medicine, Miami, FL). For routine cleansing of the animal with normal or irritated skin, a mild detergent-free shampoo may be used (Allergroom, Allerderm, Inc., Hurst, TX).

Emollient rinses may be used after shampooing (Alpha-Keri, Westwood Pharmaceuticals, Buffalo, NY; Humilac, Allerderm Inc., Hurst, TX). These can be added to prepared flea dip or used alone on animals with other flea control preparations. These products help to counteract the drying effects of the dips and sprays.

Treatment of the pyoderma which accompanies some cases of FAD with systemic antibiotics may decrease the odor and pruritus of the animal. Bacterial lesions will quickly recur without concurrent flea control.

Antiinflammatory therapy must be used in conjunction with other therapy rather than in lieu of other measures. Owners must understand that these medications provide symptomatic relief for the pet and that the problem will persist and return swiftly once the medication is stopped if definitive flea control measures are not employed.

Glucocorticoids are the most effective drugs available to control pruritus in the dog and cat. Oral steroids should be used whenever possible to minimize side effects and give better control over the medication. The short-acting glucocorticoids such as prednisolone, prednisone, or methylprednisolone should be used, since these can be given on an alternate day basis. Every other day steroid administration minimizes the hypothalmic-pituitary-adrenal suppression. Before an animal is placed on an alternate-day regimen, daily therapy will be necessary to initiate the healing process.[88] Generally, the authors start animals on 0.5 mg/kg of prednisolone every 12 hours for 7 to 14 days then 0.5 to 1.0 mg/kg once every other morning. After the dog is on the alternate day regimen, the dosage should be decreased until the dog is mildly pruritic. Cats often require slightly higher doses than dogs.[88] The judicious use of corticosteroid therapy can help prevent occurrence of secondary changes in the skin and the pruritus which accompanies the development of this stage.

Hyposensitization

The efficacy of hyposensitization in canine and feline FAD is controversial. As is the case with intradermal skin testing for the diagnosis of flea hypersensitivity, studies on flea hyposensitization have used different preparations of flea antigen (vaccine), varying dosage schedules and routes of administration, and differing criteria for admission of animals to the studies and interpretation of response[12,21,39,44,89–93] (Table 2-6 and 2-7).

In a recent double-blind, well controlled study in the dog, it was reported that three commercial whole flea antigens were ineffective in the treatment of canine FAD.[93] Dogs in the study received six weekly injections via the intradermal route. Another excellent double-blind study using 25 cats evaluated intradermal and subcutaneous administration of flea antigen weekly over 20 weeks.[44] Statistically, there was no difference between response in groups receiving the flea vaccine and the control group. However, the clinical status in two cats improved markedly.

At this time, flea hyposensitization cannot be strongly recommended except as a "last ditch" therapeutic effort having little chance of success.[9,44,93]

Table 2-6. Studies Supporting Hyposensitization for Treatment of Flea Allergy Dermatitis in the Dog and Cat

Investigators	Year Study Published	Number of Dogs	Number of Cats	Vaccine and Protocol	Results	Comments
Feingold and Benjamini[21]	1961	Unknown		Flea saliva; protocol unknown	Successful protection; percentage unknown	Research protocol involved inducing hypersensitivity in non-flea-allergic animals; success monitored by lack of response to massive flea bite exposure and intradermal skin test unresponsiveness
Keep and Taylor[89]	1967	160		1:5000 wt/vol suspension of ground flea (*C. canis*) in phenol glycerol saline; 0.5 cc once weekly for 3–4 weeks	98% showed improvement	No skin testing for diagnosis; no control animals; no corticosteroids given; no change in environmental flea control
Michaeli and Goldfarb[90]	1968	61 Total: No breakdown of dogs/cats		10 mg flea saliva plus sodium alginate; 2 cc given SC or ID every 7–14 days for 3–4 injections	47/61 (77%) rendered clinically hyposensitive for periods exceeding 4 weeks; average duration of hyposensitive state 5–6 weeks	No skin testing for diagnosis, although some animals (unknown number) pretested by controlled flea exposure and observation of reactions; no controls; no corticosteroids given; no environmental flea control done during study
Reedy[91]	1975		20	1:5000 wt/vol phenolized glycerine-buffered saline extract of fleas;[a] 3 doses, protocol unknown	15/20 (75%) good to excellent response; 4/20 (20%) fair response; 1/20 (5%) poor response	No skin testing for diagnosis; no control group of animals in study; no corticosteroids given; rigorous environmental flea control used in 18/20 cases (90%); cats were flea-powdered twice weekly

table continues

Table 2-6. Studies Supporting Hyposensitization for Treatment of Flea Allergy Dermatitis in the Dog and Cat (*continued*)

Investigators	Year Study Published	Number of Dogs	Number of Cats	Vaccine and Protocol	Results	Comments
Saunders[92]	1977		Unknown	1:5000 wt/vol phenolized glycerine-buffered saline extract of fleas; 0.5 cc given ID in flank or part ID and part SC weekly until arthus-like reaction occured (usually 5–7 injections)	Significant response (no statistics given)	Skin testing used in diagnosis; vaccine used in combination with environmental flea control; no control animals in study
Nesbitt and Schmitz[12]	1978	118		1:5000 wt/vol phenolized glycerine-buffered saline suspension of ground fleas;[b] 0.5 cc given ID weekly for 3 weeks	101/118 (85.6%) good response; 14/118 (11.9%) fair response; 3/118 (2.5%) poor response	Diagnosis made by skin testing with glycerinated antigen; no control group of animals; corticosteroids given to small percentage (number unknown); rigorous environmental and animal flea control used in this same study; 21/25 (84%) of the dogs on flea control *only* showed good clinical response; 40% of 70 dogs that didn't respond to flea control responded better after hyposensitization initiated

[a] Haver-Lockhart Flea Antigen; Kansas City, MO
[b] Hollister-Stier Flea Antigen; Spokane, WA

Table 2-7. Studies Not Supporting Hyposensitization for Treatment of Flea Allergy Dermatitis in the Dog and Cat

Investigators	Year Study Published	Number of Dogs	Number of Cats	Vaccine and Protocol	Results	Comments
Lorenz[39]	1980	Unknown		Various whole flea extracts	25% received some relief but signs recurred quickly after discontinuing vaccine	Did not comment on use of skin testing for diagnosis, environmental treatment, or corticosteroid use
Halliwell[93]	1981	52		1/100 wt/vol aqueous whole flea extract[a] or 1/5000 wt/vol phenolized glycerine buffered saline suspension of fleas;[b] 1 cc ID (4 sites) weekly for 6 weeks	14.83% overall improvement 29.29% overall improvement	Diagnosis confirmed by intradermal skin testing with aqueous antigen;[b] numerical grading of animals pre and post treatment protocol; double-blind study; no change in environmental or animal flea control; minimal corticosteroid use (3/52) and withdrawn 2 weeks before grading
Kunkle and Milcarsky[44]	1985		18	1/100 wt/vol aqueous whole flea extract[b] given 1 cc ID (8 cats) or 1 cc SC (10 cats) weekly for 20 wks	1/8 (13%) improved markedly 1/10 (10%) improved markedly	Diagnosis confirmed by intradermal skin testing with aqueous antigen;[b] numerical grading of animals pre and post treatment protocol; double-blind study; no change in environmental or animal flea control; minimal corticosteroid use (7/25) and withdrawn 2 weeks before grading

[a] Hollister-Stier Flea Antigen; Spokane, WA.
[b] Greer Flea Antigen; Lenoir, NC

Table 2-8. Clinical Signs and Treatment of Insecticide Toxicity

Insecticide Group	Clinical Signs	Treatment[a]
Carbamates	Abdominal cramping, vomiting, diarrhea, miosis, dyspnea, cyanosis, muscle twitching, seizures; rarely tetany followed by weakness and paralysis	Atropine sulfate: .2–.5 mg/kg to effect (mydriasis and reduced salivation) usually $\frac{1}{4}$ dose IV and $\frac{3}{4}$ SC; may need to repeat at 3–6 hours for 1–2 days depending upon response; 2-PAM (pralidoxime) is *contraindicated*
Chlorinated hydrocarbons	Onset can be minutes to days after exposure, usually several hours; signs include apprehension, exaggerated response to stimuli, vomiting, muscle twitching of face and head that progresses posteriorly to severe fasiculations and tremors, clonic and tonic seizures, elevated body temperature; these compounds are stored in fat and the clinical course may be protracted	Emesis (may induce seizures), gastric lavage; no specific antidote; seizures may be controlled with diazepam (Valium) at 2.5–20 mg IV as needed; barbiturate to effect; do *not* use phenothiazines as they lower seizure threshold; calcium gluconate 10% at 2–10 ml given slowly IV and vitamin B complex IM to protect liver function; critical period is 24–36 hours
d-Limonene	Cats: hypersalivation, ataxia and muscle tremors	Supportive; no specific therapy
Methoprene	No toxic effects have been described; there were no deaths recorded at the highest oral dose tested	If ingested, remove by gastric lavage; do not induce vomiting; treat symptomatically; if eye or skin exposure occurs wash directly with stream of water for 15 minutes
Organophosphates	Muscarinic: salivation, lacrimation, diarrhea, abdominal cramping, miosis, pallor, cyanosis, dyspnea, emesis	Atropine as for carbamates
	Nicotinic: twitching of facial and tongue muscles progressing to generalized twitching followed by paralysis	2-PAM (pralidoxime): 20 mg/kg IV, twice per day; give over 5 minute duration; if poisoned for less than 24 hours treatment is necessary for 1–2 days; if longer may require therapy for several days
	Central nervous system: depression, tonic-clonic seizures; death is due to hypoxia from respiratory muscle paralysis, bronchoconstriction, excessive pulmonary secretions, pulmonary edema and bradycardia	Diphenhydramine hydrochloride (Benadryl): 4 mg/kg IV (dogs) or IM (dogs or cats) every 8 hours until asymptomatic; if animal becomes depressed decrease dose to 1–2 mg/kg
Pyrethrins and synthetic pyrethroids	Usually observed only with very high dosages; vomiting and diarrhea, ataxia, CNS excitation and seizures; paralysis	Supportive; as for chlorinated hydrocarbons
Rotenone	Vomiting, nausea, diarrhea, respiratory stimulation, convulsions, followed by respiratory depression, coma, respiratory failure and death; in man causes irritant dermatitis	Emesis, gastric lavage before convulsive state, warmth, quiet, assist respiration; diazepam (Valium), calcium gluconate and B complex as for chlorinated hydrocarbons

[a] Bathing with a noninsecticide-containing shampoo should be done in all cases where poisoning resulted from a topically applied product.

Insecticide Toxicity in the Animal

In order to institute appropriate therapy in cases of systemic insecticide toxicity, it is imperative to know the brand name and chemical ingredient of the product and the time of exposure.

A general principle of treatment for animals showing signs of intoxication secondary to insecticide exposure involves thorough shampooing of the animal with a noninsecticidal shampoo. Other specific measures to limit the chemical's systemic effects are listed in Table 2-8.

CONCLUSION

Since FAD is the most common veterinary dermatologic entity in the world,[2,3] the importance of a thorough knowledge of the pathogenesis, clinical signs, diagnostic tests, and therapy cannot be overemphasized. Exciting new discoveries on the immunopathogenesis of canine flea allergy have been made over the last 5 years. Current studies should not only expand this knowledge but offer better methods of diagnosis and means to prevent or control flea-bite hypersensitivity by modulation of the immune system.

The recent advances in therapy such as synthetic pyrethrins, methoprene, and the microencapsulation process have greatly improved the ability to control the ubiquitous flea while ensuring maximum safety to the pet and owner. It should be remembered that each particular flea problem will be different and requires an individually tailored therapeutic approach for successful handling. This requires attention to details of product selection, environmental preparation, and timing of applications. It must also be determined if the pet is simply flea infested or truly flea allergic since different treatment approaches and long-term prognoses are necessary for each.

Finally, insecticides are poisons. If used improperly or without sufficient knowledge of their side effects, they can endanger man and animals. Insecticides are classified as pesticides which fall under the jurisdiction of the EPA in the United States and the Department of the Environment in the United Kingdom. The EPA's regulations regarding the use, repackaging, or mixing of insecticides are stringent due to their potential toxicity and environmental hazards. Veterinarians must be familiar with these regulations (EPA, Federal Register, 1979).

REFERENCES

1. Benton AH: An Atlas of the Fleas of the Eastern United States. Marginal Media, Fredonia, NY, 1980
2. Halliwell REW: Flea bite dermatitis. Comp Cont Ed Pract Vet 1:367, 1979
3. Halliwell REW: Flea allergy dermatitis. p. 496. In Kirk RW (ed): Current Veterinary Therapy VIII. WB Saunders, Philadelphia, 1983

4. MacDonald JM: Ectoparasites. p. 488. In Kirk RW (ed): Current Veterinary Therapy VIII. WB Saunders, Philadelphia, 1983
5. Lever WF, Schaumburg-Lever G: Histopathology of the Skin. 6th Ed. JB Lippincott Co, Philadelphia, 1983
6. Derbes VJ: Arthropod bites and stings. p. 1656. In Fitzpatrick TB, Eisen AZ, Wolff K, et al (eds): Dermatology in General Medicine. 2nd Ed. McGraw-Hill, New York, 1979
7. Reedy L: Ectoparasites. p. 547. In Kirk RW (ed): Current Veterinary Therapy VI. WB Saunders, Philadelphia, 1977
8. Georgi JR: Parasitology for Veterinarians. 2nd Ed. WB Saunders, Philadelphia, 1974
9. Muller GH, Kirk RW, Scott DW: Small Animal Dermatology. 3rd Ed. WB Saunders, Philadelphia, 1983
10. Harwood RF, James MT: Entomology in Human and Animal Health. 7th Ed. MacMillan Publishing Co, New York, 1979
11. Schick MP, Schick RO: Understanding and implementing safe and effective flea control. J Am Anim Hosp Assoc 22:421, 1986
12. Nesbitt GH, Schmitz JA: Fleabite allergic dermatitis: A review and survey of 330 cases. J Am Vet Med Assoc. 173:282, 1978
13. Ihrke PJ: In Pratt PW (ed): Feline Medicine. 1st Ed. American Veterinary Publications, Santa Barbara, CA, 1983
14. Traub R, Wisseman CL, Farhang-Azad A: The ecology of murine typhus—a critical review. Trop Dis Bull 75:237, 1978
15. Pollitzer R: A review of recent literature on plague. Bull WHO 23:397, 1960
16. Scott DW: Feline dermatology 1900–1978: A monograph. J Am Anim Hosp Assoc 16:331, 1980
17. Kalkofen VP, Greenberg J: Public health implications of *Pulex irritans* infestations of dogs. J Am Vet Med Assoc 165:903, 1974
18. Hudson BW, Feingold BF, Kartman L: Allergy to flea bites. II. Investigations of flea bite sensitivity in humans. Exp Parasit 9:264, 1960
19. Benton AH, Lee SY: Sensory reactions of Siphonoptera in relation to host finding. Amer Midl Nat 74:119, 1965
20. Molyneux DH: Feeding behavior of the larval rat flea, *Nosopsyllus fasciatus* (Bosc). Nature 215:779, 1967
21. Feingold BF, Benjamini E: Allergy to flea bites. Clinical and experimental observations. Ann Allerg 19:1275, 1961
22. Hudson BW, Feingold BF, Kartman L: Allergy to flea bites. I. Experimental induction of flea-bite sensitivity in guinea pigs. Exp Parasit 9:18, 1960
23. Benjamini E, Feingold BF, Kartman L: Allergy to flea bites. III. The experimental induction of flea bite sensitivity in guinea pigs by exposure to flea bites and by antigen prepared from whole flea extracts of *Ctenocephalides felis felis*. Exp Parasit 10:214, 1960
24. Benjamini E, Feingold BF, Kartman L: Skin reactivity in guinea pigs sensitized to flea bites: The sequence of reactions. Proc Soc Exp Biol Med 108:700, 1961
25. Benjamini E, Feingold BF, Young JD, et al: Allergy to flea bites. IV. *In vitro* collection and antigenic properties of the oral secretion of the cat flea, *Ctenocephalides felis felis*. Exp Parasit 13:143, 1963
26. Michaeli D, Benjamini E, de Buren FP, et al: The role of collagen in the induction of flea bite hypersensitivity. J Immunol 95:162, 1965
27. Michaeli D, Benjamini E, Miner RC, et al: *In vitro* studies on the role of collagen in the induction of hypersensitivity to flea bites. J Immunol 97:402, 1966

28. Halliwell REW, Longino SJ: IgE and IgG antibodies to flea antigen in differing dog populations. Vet Immunol Immunopathol 8:215, 1985
29. Gross TL, Halliwell REW: Lesions of experimental flea bite hypersensitivity in the dog. Vet Pathol 22:78, 1985
30. Halliwell REW, Schemmer KR: The role of basophils in the immunopathogenesis of hypersensitivity to fleas (*Ctenocephalides felis*) in dogs. Vet Immunol Immunopathol, in press
31. Muller GH: Flea allergy dermatitis. Small Anim Clin 1:185, 1961
32. Baker KP, O'Flanagan J: Hypersensitivity of dog skin to fleas—a clinical report. J Small Animal Pract 16:317, 1975
33. Mackin A, Dunsmore J, Clark WT: Flea bite allergic dermatitis in dogs: A review of 78 cases. Aust Vet Pract 13:5, 1983
34. Baker KP: The hypersensitive response of the skin to fleas with observations on treatment and control. Irish Vet J 10:141, 1977
35. Willemse TA: Crusting dermatoses in cats. p. 469. In Kirk RW (ed): Current Veterinary Therapy VII. WB Saunders, Philadelphia, 1980
36. Kirk RW: Feline alopecias. p. 490. In Kirk RW (ed): Current Veterinary Therapy VII. WB Saunders, Philadelphia, 1980
37. Thoday KL: Canine pruritus: An approach to diagnosis. Stages III and IV. Allergy and idiopathy. J Small Anim Pract 21:483, 1980
38. Baker KP: Observations on allergic reactions to arthropod parasites. Irish Vet J 28:65, 1974
39. Lorenz MD: The management of flea allergy dermatitis. p. 446. In Kirk RW (ed): Current Veterinary Therapy VII. WB Saunders, Philadelphia, 1980
40. Kissileff A: Flea bite dermatitis. Vet Med Sm An Clin 64:580, 1969
41. Baker KP: Intradermal tests as an aid to the diagnosis of skin diseases in dogs. J Small Anim Pract 12:445, 1971
42. Kristensen S, Kieffer M: A study of skin diseases in dogs and cats. V. The intradermal test in the diagnosis of flea allergy in dogs and cats. Nord Vet Med 30:414, 1978
43. Van Winkle KA: An evaluation of flea antigens used in intradermal skin testing for flea allergy in the canine. J Am Anim Hosp Assoc 17:343, 1981
44. Kunkle GA, Milcarsky J: Double-blind flea hyposensitization trial in cats. J Am Vet Med Assoc 186:677, 1985
45. Reedy LM: The diagnosis of canine atopic disease. p. 480. In Kirk RW (ed): Current Veterinary Therapy VII. WB Saunders, Philadelphia, 1980
46. Kieffer M, Kristensen S: Flea hypersensitivity in dogs and cats. Int J Derm 18:707, 1979
47. Halliwell REW: Immunopathogenesis of flea allergy. Vet Med Sm An Clin 79:249, 1984
48. Nesbitt GH: Canine allergic inhalant dermatitis: A review of 230 cases. J Am Vet Med Assoc 172:55, 1978
49. Burkhart CG: Insect allergy. Int J Dermatol 19:388, 1980
50. Fadok VA: Challenge your clients to gain control of fleas in the environment. Vet Med 79:1039, 1984
51. Bledsoe B, Fadok VA, Bledsoe ME: Current therapy and new developments in indoor flea control. J Am Anim Hosp Assoc 18:415, 1982
52. Reese D: Guidelines for flea control. Pest Control. May:19, 1981
53. El-Gassar LM, Milo J, Koehler PG: Relative susceptibilities of two cat flea (*Ctenocephalides felis*) colonies to nine insecticides. Accepted for publication by the J Econ Entomol, 1984

54. Der Marderosian AH: Pesticides. p. 1188. In Osol A (ed): Remington's Pharmaceutical Sciences. 16th Ed. Mack Publishing Co, Easton, PA, 1975
55. Miller TA: Maximizing the potency of nature's own flea and tick insecticide—pyrethrin. Vet Med Sm An Clin 79:1383, 1984
56. Ware GW: Pesticides: Therapy and Application, WH Freeman, San Francisco, 1983
57. Quarishi MS: Biochemical Insect Control; It's Impact on Economy, Environment and Natural Selection. 2nd Ed. John Wiley and Sons, New York, 1977
58. Soloway SB: Naturally occurring insecticides. Environ Health Perspect 14:109, 1976
59. Technical Data, Hills VIP Organic Formula Dip and Organic Formula Shampoos. Pet Chemicals, Inc. Miami Springs, FL, 1984
60. Hooser SB: Letter to the editor: Citrus insecticide hazardous to cats. J Am Vet Med Assoc 184:236, 1984
61. Bradley RE: Brewer's yeast for flea control: fact or fiction? Vet Med Sm An Clin 78:1042, 1983
62. Baker NF, Farver TB: Failure of brewer's yeast as a repellent to fleas on dogs. J Am Vet Med Assoc 183:212, 1983
63. Halliwell REW: Ineffectiveness of thiamine (vitamin B_1) as a flea repellent in dogs. J Am Anim Hosp Assoc 18:423, 1982
64. Kahn AA, Maibach HI, Strauss WG, et al: Vitamin B_1 is not a systemic mosquito repellent in man. Trans St Johns Hosp Derm Soc 55:99, 1969
65. Kuhr RJ, Dorough HW: Carbamate Insecticides: Chemistry, Biochemistry, and Toxicology. CRC Press, Cleveland, OH, 1976
66. Windholz MM: Merck Index: An Encyclopedia of Chemicals and Drugs. 9th Ed. Merck and Co, Rahway, NJ, 1977
67. Federal Register of June 1984. Environmental Protection Agency Published Rulings
68. Kramer MS: Operational criteria for adverse drug reactions: An updated evaluation of 1% gamma benzene hexachloride. Drug Info J July/Sept: 140, 1982
69. Atkins CE, Johnson RK: Clinical toxicities of cats. Vet Clin N Am 5:623, 1975
70. Derache R: Organophosphorous Pesticides. Pergamon Press. New York, NY, 1977
71. Technical Release ESPC 061401: New Pesticide Precor-5E, National Pest Control Association, Inc., Vienna, VA, 1980
72. Wright JE: Environmental and toxicological aspects of insect growth regulators. Environ Health Perspect 24:127, 1976
73. Scott DW: Topical cutaneous medicine. Proceedings of the 79th Annual Meeting of the American Animal Hospital Association, New Orleans, 1979
74. Randell WF, Bradley RE, Brown DL: Field evaluation of anti-flea collars for initial and residual efficacy on dogs. Vet Med Sm An Clin 75:606, 1980
75. Muller GH: Flea collar dermatitis in animals. J Am Vet Med Assoc 157:1616, 1970
76. Fisch H, Angerhofer RA, Nelson JH: Evaluation of a carbamate-impregnated flea and tick collar for dogs. J Am Vet Med Assoc 171:269, 1977
77. Bell TG, Farrell RK, Padgett GA, et al: Ataxia, depression and dermatitis associated with the use of dichlorvos-impregnated collars in the laboratory cat. J Am Vet Med Assoc 167:579, 1975
78. Miller JE, Baker NF, Colburn EL: Insecticide activity of propoxur- and carbaryl-impregnated flea collars against *Ctenocephalides felis*. Am J Vet Res 38:923, 1977
79. Technical Data File 155. Dermaton Dust. Coopers Animal Health, Inc., Kansas City, MO, 1975
80. Bennett GW, Lund RD: Evaluation of encapsulated pyrethrins (Sectrol Insecticide) for German cockroach and cat flea control. Pest Contr Mag Reprint. Sept. 1977

81. Fridinger TL: Designing the ultimate weapon against fleas. Vet Med 79:1151, 1984
82. Fenster P: Designing a long term flea control program. Vet Med 80:45, 1985
83. Schmidl JA, Kohlenberg ML, Johnson GL, et al: Assessing the safety of long-term cythioate therapy. Vet Med Sm An Clin 79:1159, 1984
84. Lorenz M: Should you use systemic therapy to control flea allergy dermatitis? Vet Med 79:1148, 1984
85. Mason KV, Ring J, Duggan J: Fenthion for flea control on dogs under field conditions: Dose response efficacy studies and effect on cholinesterase activity. J Am Anim Hosp Assoc 20:591, 1984
86. Sundlof SF, Clemmons RM, Meyer DJ, et al: Cholinesterase activity in plasma, red blood cells, muscle and brain of dogs following repeated exposure to Spotton (fenthion). Vet Human Toxicol 26:112, 1984
87. Fehrer SL: The efficacy of Skin-So-Soft as a flea repellent. In: Proceedings, Annual Member's Meeting of the American Academy of Veterinary Dermatology and American College of Veterinary Dermatology, 1985
88. Miller WH: The pruritic dog. p. 499. In Kirk RW (ed): Current Veterinary Therapy VIII. WB Saunders, Philadelphia, 1983
89. Keep JM, Taylor JH: Whole flea extract as a densentizing agent in canine summer dermatitis. Aust Vet J 43:4125, 1967
90. Michaeli D, Goldfarb S: Clinical studies on the hyposensitization of dogs and cats to flea bites. Aust Vet J 44:161, 1968
91. Reedy LM: Use of flea antigen in treatment of feline flea allergy dermatitis. Vet Med Sm An Clin 70:703, 1975
92. Saunders EB: Hyposensitization for flea bite hypersensitivity. Vet Med Sm An Clin 72:879, 1977
93. Halliwell REW: Hyposensitization in the treatment of flea-bite hypersensitivity: Results of a double-blind study. J Am Anim Hosp Assoc 17:249, 1981

3 Atopic Dermatitis

Ton A. Willemse

In dogs, atopy is considered to be a hereditary clinical hypersensitivity state[1] or a hereditary, reagin-mediated hypersensitivity to inhalant allergens.[2–4] As early as 1941 Wittich described a dog with hay-fever–like symptoms and he was able to passively transfer immediate skin test reactivity to recipient dogs.[5] However, it was not until the late 1960s and early 1970s that further information became available about the immunologic background of canine atopy.

PATHOPHYSIOLOGY

Four types of hypersensitivity reactions are distinguished according to the classification of Gell and Coombs.[6] In particular, anaphylactic or type I reactions are of importance in relation to atopy. In its simplest form the sequence of events in this type of reaction is as follows: in animals with a hereditary basis for atopic disease, contact with inhalant allergens initiates the formation of a reagin isotype. Subsequently, these homocytotropic antibodies are fixed to the surfaces of basophil granulocytes and mast cells. On reexposure to the allergen, vasoactive mediators are released from these cells and result in the clinical manifestation of atopic disease.

Regulatory Mechanisms of Antibody Formation

The regulation of the immune response is determined by interactions between T- and B-lymphocytes and macrophages. Initially, antigen is processed by macrophages and presented to the B-cell while fixed to the macrophage surface. In addition, the macrophages promote the T-cell response by releasing interleukin 1, which activates the T-helper cells (Fig. 3-1). Subsequently, T-

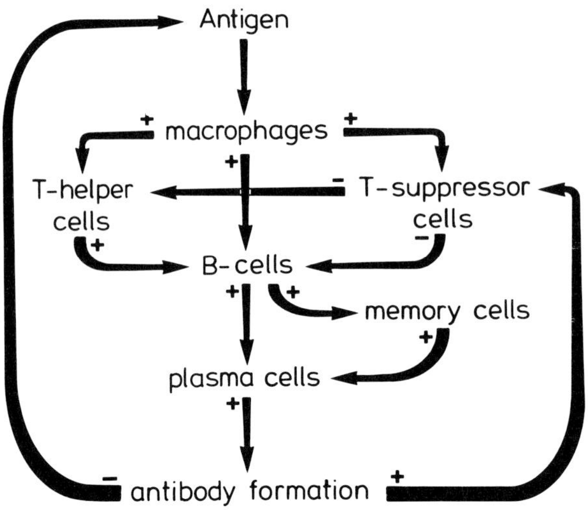

Fig. 3-1. Postulated regulation of the immune response.

helper cells secrete substances such as interleukin 2, which enhances the response of B-cells. As the result of these interactions two types of cells are formed: (1) plasma cells, which are able to produce large quantities of antibodies, and (2) memory cells, which are small lymphocytes able to memorize the first exposure to the particular antigen and stimulate the production of numerous antigen-sensitive cells after reexposure.

In contrast, subpopulation of T-cells, known as suppressor cells, inhibit the B-cell response to antigen by releasing soluble suppressor factors. These factors act directly on the antigen-sensitive B-cells or inhibit T-helper cells. Once antibody formation has been initiated, a negative feedback on B-cells is observed.

Immunoglobulins

IgE

In 1921 Prausnitz and Küstner performed their classic experiment of passively sensitizing human skin with serum from an allergic individual.[7] The substance present in the serum and capable of mediating immediate hypersensitivity reactions in response to antigenic challenge was called reagin (IgE). As in humans, reagin in the dog is a homocytotropic antibody and is inactivated by 56°C heat for 2 to 4 hours. Conclusive evidence for antigenic similarities between canine and human IgE have been found.[8] In healthy dogs serum IgE in canine skin showed the antibody to be associated exclusively with mast cells and to be located in the cytoplasm of the mast cell.

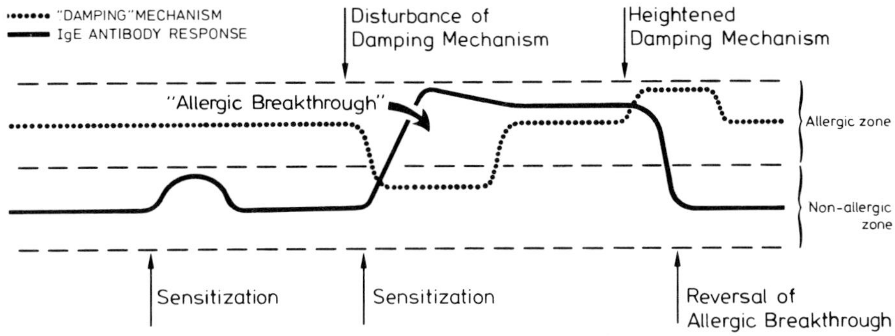

Fig. 3-2. Possible pathogenesis of 'allergic breakthrough'.

IgGd

Recently, anaphylactic antibodies other than IgE were found in dogs with spontaneous atopic disease.[9,10] The IgGd antibodies had properties similar to short-term sensitizing antibodies in humans (IgG S-ST).[11] These antibodies have been found in association with food allergy, asthma, and atopic dermatitis in man. IgGd is not inactivated by heating at 56°C for 2 hours, is not reduced by 2-mercaptoethanol, and is able to elicit Prausnitz-Küstner (P-K) activity in recipient skin after sensitization of 3 to 4 hours.

T-Cell Disorders in Relation to Atopy

The pathogenesis of reagin-mediated allergic disorders in man has been explained by means of the "allergic breakthrough" and an imbalance in normal "damping" of IgE[12] (Fig. 3-2). It is postulated that the normal damping is regulated by antigen-specific helper and suppressor T-cells, but also by non-specific "suppressor factors of allergy." If the threshold of the damping mechanism is lowered to a level insufficient to control the magnitude of IgE antibody synthesis and exposure to an allergen then occurs, an "allergic breakthrough" might result. Evidence of a comparable phenomenon in dogs has been provided.[13] Attenuated live virus vaccines may selectively deplete suppressor T-lymphoctyes, thereby leading to a naturally occurring "breakthrough."

Cellular Mechanisms and Mediator Release

Mast cells have receptors for the Fc portion of IgE (and most likely also of IgGd) and hence are able to bind the reagin molecules. When two immunoglobulin molecules, bound to a mast cell, are cross-linked by combining with an antigen, mast cell degranulation occurs. Mast cells release preformed granule-associated mediators, including histamine, neutral proteases, exoglycosidases and the eosinophilic chemotactic factor of anaphylaxis (ECF-A), and membrane-derived mediators such as prostaglandins, thromboxanes, and leukotrienes. Histamine and leukotrienes are most important in dogs.

The major actions of histamine include smooth muscle contraction, increased vascular permeability, and increased exocrine secretion, these effects being mediated by H_1 and H_2 receptors. The leukotrienes are potent bronchoconstrictors and also increase vascular permeability. It has been shown that the so-called slow reacting substance of anaphylaxis (SRS-A) consists of several subtypes of leukotrienes.

The release of mast cell mediators is the culmination of a cascade of enzymatic processes. The adenylate cyclase and guanylate cyclase system seems to play a crucial role. Elevation of cyclic adenosine monophosphate AMP(cAMP) or depression of cyclic guanosine monophosphate GMP(cGMP) inhibits mast cell degranulation, while the opposite enhances this phenomenon. It is suggested that the ratio between cAMP and cGMP determines the final effect. In addition, arachidonic acid metabolism is shown to be of great importance in the formation of mediators like leukotrienes.

Disorders of Granulocyte Function

Neutrophilic chemotaxis may be impaired in allergic people. This leukotactic dysfunction might result from an abnormal sensitivity of leukocytes to histamine and could be explained by an increased number of cellular histamine receptors, a higher sensitivity to cAMP, or an increased formation of intracellular cAMP. In dogs with atopic dermatitis, neutrophilic chemotactic movement was found to be normal.[14,15]

DIAGNOSIS

History

There is nothing more important in the evaluation of an allergic patient than a thorough, systematic, and recorded history. The use of a standard form has several advantages: (1) it gives direction and purpose to the questioning, (2) it helps the clinician to have an organized approach to fact finding and prevents overlooking facts that may be of relevance in identifying offending allergens, (3) it tends to restrict the client to pertinent information, and (4) it makes the client aware of allergenic environmental conditions and materials that may correlate with the patient's condition. (See Chapter 1 for a sample history form.)

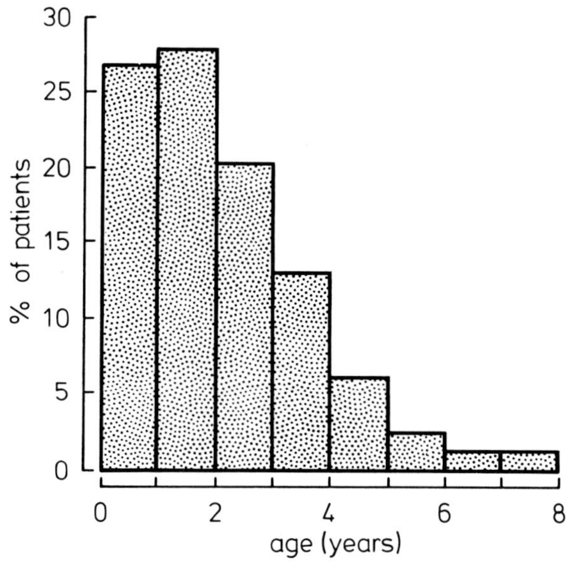

Fig. 3-3. Age of onset in canine atopic dermatitis (n = 208).

Date of Onset

By knowing the date of onset, it is possible to determine if the patient has ever experienced problems that were mild or transient forms of allergy, but were not given much consideration because the patient responded rapidly to treatment or recovered spontaneously with a change of seasons or environmental conditions. In 75 percent of dogs with atopic dermatitis the first symptoms occur before the age of 3 years.[16,17] Dogs under the age of 6 months are rarely affected (Fig. 3-3).

Sex Predilection

In canine atopic disease sex predilection has been suggested with a reported incidence in male dogs of 56,[18] 60,[19] and 71 percent.[3] However, both female and male dogs were equally represented in other studies.[17,19]

Family Nature

Although the family nature of atopic dermatitis is well known in humans,[20] no genetic markers have been found for canine atopy.[21] An attempt to establish a colony of atopic dogs from two lines of dogs with a seaonal dermatitis and positive skin tests to airborne allergens has been unsuccessful.[22]

Breed Predisposition

Certain breeds have been reported to be predisposed to atopic disease including Lhasa apsos, miniature schnauzers, poodles, terriers (West Highland white terriers and fox terriers in particular), dalmatians, setters,[16,23] and boxers and German shepherds.[17]

Seasonal Incidence

It is helpful to know what time of the year the signs initially occur and when they subside. This information must be modified according to the types of vegetation in the area where the dog lives. If there is a seasonal incidence, then pollen from grasses, trees, flowering plants, or mold spores are the most likely cause. The signs of canine atopy are usually seasonal in the beginning, often becoming nonseasonal with time, and occasionally are nonseasonal from the beginning. Halliwell and Schwartzman[3] found that 53 percent of 60 cases of canine atopy were seasonal, whereas Scott[16] reported a seasonal incidence of 42 percent and a nonseasonal occurrence in 55 percent and of the first group 15 percent of the dogs progressed from seasonal to nonseasonal. The seasonal incidence in dogs with atopic dermatitis and immediate skin test reactivity to single allergens has been evaluated.[17] A seasonal occurrence was observed in all dogs reacting to pollen allergens whereas animal danders always resulted in perennial problems. Although reaction to human dander tends to be seasonal in humans, this observation could not be confirmed in dogs. House dust allergies in humans usually result in winter and autumn exacerbations, but in dogs, house dust allergies were usually perennial (Fig. 3-4).

In the case of perennial problems, the clinician's attention must be focused on house dust, household materials like wool, kapok, and feathers, indoor plants, and other animals. Continuous exposure to any of these allergens may cause a persistent pruritic dermatitis. Although the concomitant occurrence of

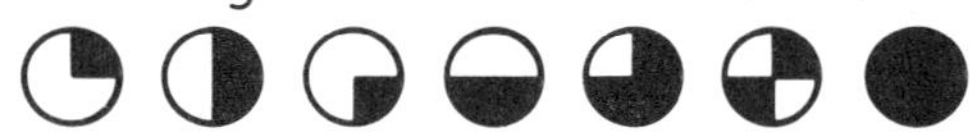

allergen	Nr of dogs with seasonal exacerbations						
house dust	1	-	1	-	-	-	5
human dander	-	-	2	1	-	-	7
animal danders	-	-	-	-	-	-	15
pollens	-	4	3	-	1	2	-

: spring : summer : autumn : winter

Fig. 3-4. Seasonal exacerbations of atopic dermatitis in dogs with immediate type skin test reactivity to single allergens (n = 42).

food intolerance has been reported,[2] a study by the author did not establish a food allergy in any of 208 dogs with atopic dermatitis.[17]

Physical Examination and Clinical Manifestations

In addition to a thorough case history, a systematically performed physical examination is essential to evaluate the patient properly. Allergy diagnostic tests are indicated only after other diseases are ruled out. It is essential to describe the distribution of the lesions, the type of efflorescencies, and their configuration. In this respect one has to realize that the initial skin changes may not be present at the moment of examination. The frequency of signs and symptoms expected in atopic dogs are listed in Table 3-1.

Although symptoms similar to hay fever and canine asthma have been reported occasionally,[24] the predominant sign in canine atopy is pruritus. Most commonly, the pruritus is manifested by face rubbing and feet licking. Other signs including bilateral conjunctivitis, reversed sneezing, and discoloration of the coat may be observed.

Table 3-1. Frequency of Signs and Symptoms as Observed in 208 Dogs Having Atopic Dermatitis by Clinical Definition

	Number of Dogs With Immediate Skin Test Reactivity (n = 170)		Number of Dogs Without Immediate Skin Test Reactivity (n = 38)	
Symptoms				
Pruritus, face rubbing, paw-and-feet licking	170	(100.0%)	38	(100.0%)
Bilateral conjunctivitis	51	(30.0%)	11	(28.9%)
Sweating	41	(24.1%)	9	(23.7%)
Sneezing	38	(22.4%)	9	(23.7%)
Discoloration of coat	13	(7.6%)	3	(7.9%)
Cutaneous involvement	161	(94.7%)	37	(97.4%)
Lichenification	143	(84.1%)	33	(86.8%)
Superficial pyoderma	45	(26.5%)	4	(10.5%)
Seborrhea	39	(22.9%)	9	(23.7%)
Affected skin regions				
Digits	124	(72.9%)	28	(73.7%)
Head	101	(59.4%)	24	(63.2%)
Extensor side carpal joint	70	(41.2%)	0	(0)
Axillae	60	(35.3%)	7	(18.4%)
Flexural side tarsal joint	52	(30.6%)	0	(0)
Groin	31	(18.2%)	7	(18.4%)
Ear pinnae	29	(17.1%)	6	(15.8%)
Abdomen	27	(15.9%)	6	(15.8%)
Flexural side elbows	12	(7.1%)	2	(5.3%)

(Adapted from Willemse A, van den Brom WE: Investigations of the symptomology and the significance of immediate skin test reactivity in canine atopic dermatitis. Res Vet Sci 34:261, 1983.)

In a study by the author only 5 percent of dogs with atopic signs but without cutaneous involvement manifested a discoloration of the coat, bilateral conjunctivitis, and/or reversed sneezing.[17] Although it is known from the case history that patients show feet licking and face rubbing, approximately 60 to 70 percent of them also have visible skin lesions in these areas. The aspect of the lesions may vary between erythema, papules, pustules, and scales to hyperkeratosis and lichenification, depending on the duration of the disease. In 30 percent of 45 atopic dogs the pyoderma was associated only with seborrhea, while 55 percent of them had a coexistent seborrhea as well as skin sweating. This skin sweating (hyperhydrosis) is likely due to excessive apocrine sweat gland secretion.

Besides the involvement of the digits and the head, other parts of the body may be affected: axillae (35 percent), groin (20 percent), ears (17 percent), and abdomen (15 percent). Lichenification was noticed in 85 percent of dogs on the flexor and extensor surfaces of joints as well as in the axillary and inguinal regions and on digits. It must be emphasized that in dogs with atopic signs, but without immediate skin test reactivity, involvement of the extensor surface of the carpal joint and the flexural surface of the tarsal joint was significantly less common as was the occurrence of a superficial pyoderma.

Differential Diagnosis

Following the case history and physical examination, it is essential to rule out other diseases before starting additional tests to confirm the diagnosis of atopy. In this respect the most common differential diagnoses include demodicosis, dermatophytosis, food allergy, contact dermatoses, idiopathic pododermatitis, hookworm infestation, and trombiculiasis. The latter disease is caused by several species of chigger mites. *Neotrombicula autumnalis*, which is pinhead-sized and orange-colored, live in grassland areas of Europe which have a moderate climate from April/May through September/October. *Neotrombicula alfreddugesi* (North American Chigger) is a summer and fall seasonal problem especially common in the central United States. Therefore, as in atopic disease, trombiculiasis sometimes gives rise to seasonal symptoms. The larvae of *Neotrombicula* most commonly hatch on the skin of interdigital spaces and initiate a severe pruritus, thus mimicking a "characteristic" atopic sign such as feet licking. *N. alfreddugesi* are usually found in ground-skin contact areas.

Skin scrapings, bacterial and fungal cultures, and fecal analysis are essential as are elimination and provocation dietary tests. Only if these examinations are negative is it indicated to do additional allergy tests for atopic disease.

Diagnostic Tests

Intradermal Allergy Test

Intradermal (ID) testing is the most commonly used and most reliable method for identifying inhalent allergens. Prior to testing, all steroids, sedatives, immunosuppressants, antihistamines, and tranquilizers must be discontinued for at least 14 days. The duration of the therapy, the type of drug, the dose, and the frequency of administration will determine whether the period of 14 days is sufficient.

The skin test is performed on the ventral part of the thoracic wall after gentle shaving and clipping. The injection sites are marked with a felt-tipped pen, leaving 2.0 to 2.5 cm between subsequent sites, and 0.05 ml of each allergen or control solution is injected intradermally with a tuberculin syringe and a 26 gauge needle.

Control solutions consist of isotonic phosphate buffered saline as a diluent (negative) control and 0.01 percent histamine diphosphate solution as a positive control. Aqueous solutions of allergens are most commonly used. It is essential to use standardized allergens, with a preference for standardization by the determination of skin threshold concentrations.[25] It must be emphasized that there are great differences according to geographic distribution. Therefore, it is most helpful to consult a local allergist about the allergens for that particular area. The characteristics of aeroallergens have been reviewed.[26] Most of the time the following allergens will be included in the testing: house dust, *Dermatophagoides pteronysisinus* and *D. farinae* (house dust mites), human dander, mixed feathers, mixed molds, mixed epidermals (horse, cow, sheep, goat), dog dander, cat dander, pollens of grasses, trees and weeds, mixed insects, and flea antigen.

The intradermal test must be read 15 to 20 minutes after injection. Interpretation of intradermal reactions is not standardized.[27] Both subjective and objective criteria have been used. This author considers a reaction site positive if the wheal diameter exceeds the diluent control by 5 mm or more. Table 3-2 lists the various methods used for interpreting the reaction. It is essential to exclude all types of non-relevant or false-positive reactions. Reasons for false-positive skin reactions include the following:[28]

1. Excessive concentration of test allergen
2. Too high a dose of test allergen
3. Irritant test allergens, in particular those containing glycerine and bacterial vaccines
4. Contaminated allergens
5. Poor technique including traumatic placement of needle, dulled or burred needle
6. Harbinger of future sensitivity or remnant of past sensitivity

Table 3-2. Criteria for Grading Intradermal Skin Test Reactions

I. Subjective
   1. Compare size and color of wheal and steepness of wall.
   2. Compare positive and negative controls to allergen reaction.
   3. Grade individual reactions 0 through 4:
      a. Negative control = 0
      b. Postive control = 4
      c. 2 × size of negative control = 1
      d. 3 × size of negative control = 2
      e. 4 × size of negative control = 3
      f. Equal to size of positive control = 4
   4. Increased erythema and/or steep walls has positive influence on the grade.
   5. Known mild irritant reaction of allergen has negative influence on grade.

II. Objective
   1. Measure diameter of negative control.
   2. Measure diameter of individual reactions.
   3. Grading:
      a. Negative reaction = $<$ 3 mm or $<$ 5 mm larger than negative control.
      b. Positive reaction = $>$ 3 mm or $>$ 5 mm larger than negative control.
         or
      c. Average the diameter of negative and positive controls. Any wheal greater than the above average is a positive reaction.

(Adapted from Nesbitt GH: Canine and Feline Dermatology: A systematic approach. Lea & Febiger, Philadelphia, p 49, 1983.)

7. Use of substances which cause nonimmunologic histamine release including narcotics (morphine derivatives) and foods such as cheese
8. Non-specific enhancement through axon reflex from nearby strong reaction
9. Dermographism: large reaction to all injected substances including diluent (negative) control.

False-negative reactions should also be eliminated. Specific reasons for these type of skin test reactions may be the following:[28]

1. Improper technique, including subcutaneous injection of test allergen and the injection of air ("splash")
2. Insufficient allergen caused by mixes or group testing of antigenic nonrelated allergens, old or outdated test extract, poor initial potency, lack of stability, and over-diluted allergens
3. Drug interference including glucocorticoids, antihistamines, tranquilizers, sedatives, progesterone compounds, cromoglycate (a mast cell membrane stabilizing drug), and any drug that lowers blood pressure
4. Inherent host factors including chronic systemic disease, estrus or false pregnancy, severe stress, excessive fright or struggling, immunosuppression, and very young or old age
5. Not including the offending allergen
6. Prolonged allergy
7. Late off-season allergy testing (low allergen-specific antibodies).

Significance and Relevance of Skin Test. In addition to characteristic symptoms such as facial and pedal pruritus, the intradermal allergy test is generally considered to be especially helpful in the final diagnosis of canine atopic dermatitis.[23,27,29] Positive reactions have been reported for house dust (35 to 71 percent), molds (8 to 88 percent), grasses (19 to 85 percent), trees (17 to 64 percent), and weeds (23 to 86 percent).[2,3,16,18] The author found 82 percent of 208 dogs with atopic symptoms exhibited immediate skin test reactivity.[17] Multisensitivity was noticed in 59 percent, with house dust (30 percent), human dander (40 percent), dog dander (25 percent), cat dander (30 percent), and grasses (21 percent) most common. Among these dogs no specific pattern of multisensitivity could be recognized. *Alopecurus pratensis* (fox tail grass) and *Phleum pratense* (timothy grass) contributed the most to the total number of grass pollen mixture reactions. The number of positive reactions to allergens, in relation to the age of the dogs, showed a significantly lowered frequency of immediate skin test reactions in dogs older than 6 years. Studies of Nesbitt did not identify any significant differences in the number of positive reactions for either individual or mixed allergens when compared to age of testing.[27] The age of onset of the clinical symptoms did not influence the frequency distribution of positive reactions to the tested allergens except for the reactions to animal danders that were more frequent in dogs between 3 and 4 years of age (Fig. 3-5).

When evaluating the skin test results, not only the wheal configuration

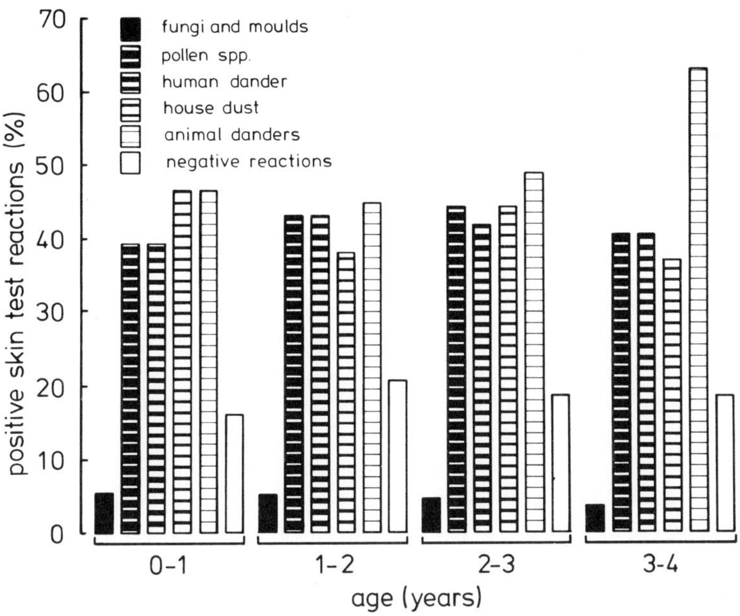

Fig. 3-5. Frequency distribution of immediate skin test reactions to different allergens in relation to age of onset.

and size are important, but it is most essential to correlate the skin reactions with a history of exposure: In other words determine whether the reactions are relevant or not. Animal danders often result in nonrelevant skin reactions. A peak incidence in these nonrelevant (false-positive) skin reactions was observed between 2 and 3 years after the onset of clinical symptoms.[17] False-positive skin reactions were observed to danders of guinea pigs (72 percent), rabbits (47 percent), poultry (48 percent), horses (70 percent), and cats (27 percent). Other false-positive reactions reported include tobacco (22 percent), human dander (10 percent), house dust and wool (8 percent), mixed epidermals (8 percent), and mixed feathers (3 percent).[16] However, it must be realized that nonrelevant reactions might indicate future atopic reactions, as they only reflect the presence of skin sensitizing antibodies at the moment of testing. In addition, these reactions might be the result of cross-reactivity among similar dander proteins.

Prausnitz-Küstner Test

In 1921 Prausnitz and Küstner performed their classical experiment of passively sensitizing human skin with serum from an allergic individual.[7] The Prausnitz-Küstner (P-K) test is still used to determine the presence of anaphylactic antibodies mediating immediate type hypersensitivity reactions in humans. It is not routinely used in veterinary clinical practice. A 24- to 48-hour period of sensitization prior to antigen challenge is characteristic for an IgE-mediated reaction. However, in atopic disease in dogs contradictory figures regarding the presence of positive P-K tests are reported.[22,30,33] This observation might indicate that not only IgE-mediated reactions occur in canine atopic dermatitis, but that, for example, IgGd-mediated reactions might play a role in the pathogenesis of the disease.

Histopathology and Eosinophilia

In humans, eosinophilia is considered to be highly characteristic, although not conclusive, of IgE-dependent diseases and some related conditions. However, it must be realized that eosinophilic granulocytes are not involved in the allergic reactions themselves, but are especially important in postallergic phenomena. Subsequent to mast cell degranulation, eosinophilic granulocytes are attracted to the site of action by leukotriene B and by the so-called eosinophil chemotactic factor of anaphylaxis (ECF-A). In addition, by its H_1 action, histamine enhances migration of leucocytes and is, itself, a weak chemotactic factor for eosinophils. Hereafter, eosinophilic enzymes are released: Histaminase breaks down histamine directly, while arylsulfatase-B exerts the same effect through inactivation of leukotrienes. In addition, eosinophils promote the production of prostaglandin E_1, which through an increase of cAMP inhibits the release of vasoactive mediators from the mast cells. In dogs with atopic dermatitis, eosinophilic granulocytes play a minor role in postallergic reactions.

Histopathologic examination of lesional skin from atopic dogs reveals varying degrees of chronic nonsuppurative dermatitis. Although not diagnostic of canine atopy, the observed changes are consistent and supportive. Angiocentric accumulations of inflammatory cells are confined to the superficial dermal blood vessels. Mononuclear cells and neutrophils, in varying proportions, are the predominant inflammatory cells seen. Eosinophils are seen in only 15 percent of the cases, and then only in very small numbers (one to three cells per skin section). Mast cell numbers are increased in 35 percent of the cases.[16] These dermatologic findings are virtually identical to those described in human atopic dermatitis.[32]

The number of circulating eosinophilic granulocytes is within reference limits in dogs with atopic disease.[16,33] Occasionally a mild absolute eosinophilia is observed.[18]

Eosinophilia in nasal smears of atopic dogs has been studied.[33] However, eosinophilic granulocytes were not found in nasal smears of any of 46 dogs with symptoms of atopic disease and skin test reactivity to one or more inhalant allergens. This important observation is even more significant, as half of the dogs had additional signs of reversed sneezing and bilateral conjunctivitis, comparable to hay fever symptoms in man.

Nasal Provocation Test

Isolated respiratory allergies are seen only occasionally, but reversed sneezing and conjunctivitis may be observed in conjunction with atopic dermatitis. However, the allergic nature of these symptoms has been the subject of discussion. The author performed nasal provocation tests with inhalant allergens in atopic dogs and measured nasal airway resistance by means of passive anterior rhinomanometry.[33] Compared to the values found in healthy dogs, only in 3 out of 46 atopic dogs could a positive nasal provocation test be observed. These three dogs had, in addition to characteristic atopic symptoms, signs of sneezing and conjunctivitis, a positive 24-hour P-K test to the particular allergens, and seasonal exacerbations related to the pollination season. Increased nasal airway resistance was only observed after provocation with extracts of grass pollens and summer weed pollens. It is concluded in this study that only pollen allergies are associated with allergic rhinitis. However, in the majority of cases reversed sneezing is most likely not a symptom caused by an allergic reaction in the nasal cavity.

In vitro Diagnostic Tests

Two methods are available for the determination of allergen-specific anaphylactic antibodies (reagins: IgE or IgGd).

The Radio Allergosorbent Test (RAST). The RAST has become the most common in vitro test for measuring IgE specific antibodies in man. IgE antibodies to many different allergens can be determined by the RAST test, including antibodies to some pollens, molds, dust, *Dermatophagoides* sp, animal danders, and stinging insects. The RAST test offers some advantages over the skin test in the diagnosis of allergic disease: there is no patient risk, the results are quantitative, it is convenient for most patients, results are not influenced by drugs, the allergen is stable and in a solid-phase state, and it is preferable to skin testing in excited dogs, animals with dermographism, and those with diffuse, widespread dermatitis.

The RAST test is expensive and difficult to perform because it involves radioactive material. A canine RAST test has recently become available in the United States.

The agreement between positive RAST scores and skin test results in atopic dogs ranged from 82 percent for ragweed to 42 percent for *D. farinae* and only 12.5 percent for dandelion. RAST tests using whole house dust extract as antigen were invariably negative despite the fact that sera of the dogs gave positive P-K tests with the same extract.[34] It is not yet certain whether these variable findings are due to the presence of other immunoglobulin classes interfering with the binding of IgE antibodies to solid-phase antigens in RAST.

Therefore, there is much evidence that the RAST test cannot be used as the sole diagnostic test in canine atopy. It must be used concomitantly with other tests, e.g., the intradermal allergy test.

The Enzyme-Linked Immunosorbent Assay (ELISA). The ELISA is a specific and highly sensitive immunoassay with certain advantages over the RAST test in terms of simplicity, cost and reagents. The most important advantage is the use of enzymes for labeling instead of radioactive materials. The advantages of the ELISA over skin testing are similar to those noted for the RAST test. So far, the ELISA is only used for the determination of allergen-specific reagins of the IgGd subclass. However, the essentials of the test are equal for other reaginic antibodies. In the ELISA system, reaginic antibodies to many different allergens can be determined including house dust, human dander, animal danders, flea antigen, and different pollen extracts. In a group of 62 dogs with clinical symptoms of atopic dermatitis and immediate skin test reactivity to one or more inhalant allergens, 89 percent of them had specific IgGd antibodies against inhalants. In addition, 11 of 20 dogs (55 percent) with atopic signs, but without immediate skin test reactivity also had elevated titers. The agreement between the presence of skin test reactivity and allergen-specific IgGd titers in atopic dogs ranged from 66 percent for house dust to 50 percent for summer weeds, 58 percent for grasses, and 7 percent for cat dander.[10] Although the discrepancies may be explained in part by the difference in sensitivity of the two tests or by the use of crude mixed-antigen preparations, it may also be seen as supporting the idea that both immediate skin test reactivity and the presence of allergen-specific antibodies are no more than secondary features of atopic dermatitis.

Presently, the ELISA test is in the developmental stage. However, it does show much promise as a concomitant test for the diagnosis of atopy in dogs.

The canine ELISA test has recently become commercially available in the United States.

Reconsideration of Diagnostic Criteria

In an attempt to provide consistency in the diagnosis of atopic dermatitis in man, the concept of major and minor diagnostic features was proposed.[35,36] According to the criteria for the diagnosis of human atopic dermatitis, at least three of the following major features must be present: pruritus, a typical morphology and distribution including flexural lichenification in adults and facial and extensor involvement in infants and children, a tendency towards chronic or chronically-relapsing dermatitis, and a personal or family history of atopy (asthma, allergic rhinitis, atopic dermatitis).

In addition, three or more of the following minor features must be present: early age of onset; immediate (type I) skin test reactivity; elevated serum IgE concentrations; xerosis; tendency towards cutaneous infections; impaired cell-mediated immunity; recurrent conjunctivitis; cheilitis; tendency towards non-specific hand or foot dermatitis; facial pallor, facial erythema, and orbital darkening; food intolerance or intolerance to wool and lipid solvents; itch when sweating; course influenced by environmental or emotional factors; and white dermographism and delayed blanch.

Striking similarities are observed between atopic dogs and the disease in humans. These similarities include initiation of the disease at a young age; a family nature of the disease; absence of genetic markers; variable clinical manifestations, but lichenification of flexor and extensor surfaces being highly characteristic; immediate skin test reactivity in 80 percent of dogs with concomitant atopic symptoms; indications for the presence of reaginic allergen-specific antibodies other than IgE; and discrepancies between the results of different diagnostic tests (RAST/ELISA vs. immediate skin test reactivity). It is apparent

Table 3-3. Criteria for the Definitive Diagnosis of Canine Atopic Dermatitis

Basic Features (at least three)
Pruritus
A typical morphology and distribution:
Facial and/or digital involvement
Lichenification of the flexor surface of the tarsal joint and/or the extensor surface of carpal joint
Chronic or chronic-relapsing dermatitis
An individual or family history of atopy and/or the presence of a breed predispostion
Minor Features (at least three)
Onset of symptoms before the age of 3 years
Facial erythema and cheilitis
Bilateral conjunctivitis
Superficial Staphylococcal pyoderma
Hyperhydrosis
Immediate skin test reactivity to inhalants
Elevated allergen-specific IgGd
Elevated allergen-specific IgE

that most of the diagnostic criteria suggested for humans[35] may be used in dogs including both basic features such as pruritus, typical morphology, and distribution and several other minor features. Criteria for the definitive diagnosis of canine atopic dermatitis are listed in Table 3-3.

TREATMENT

Avoidance Therapy

Elimination of the identified allergen(s), whether done through an extensive case history and provocation tests or by skin testing, results in the most successful therapy. However, it is often impractical to consider and it is restricted to a few antigens such as feathers, kapok, wool and occasionally animal danders. Air conditioning or electrostatic air filtration may be helpful in lessening airborne allergens, but most of the time it will be insufficient to keep the allergic condition under control.

Medical Therapy

Many different pharmacologic agents are available for use in canine atopic disease. Antihistamines, although effective in the treatment of human atopic disease, are usually ineffective in dogs. It appears that in addition to the release of histamine from mast cells, other mediators such as proteolytic enzymes and leukotrienes are released and that these mediators are responsible for the majority of the resulting pruritus.

Disodiumcromoglycate is a membrane stabilizing agent. It acts to inhibit mediator release from the mast cells. Although efficacious in man, their effect in dogs has not been evaluated properly.

Treatment with corticosteroids is the most effective medical therapy in atopic dogs. Corticosteroids act in many ways, resulting in a decreased or blocked release of mediators from the mast cells. They potentiate cAMP activity and inhibit cGMP by an enhanced antiphosphodiesterase activity and inhibition of ATP-ase and guanylate cyclase. They have a direct inhibiting effect on mediator release by membrane stabilization. They diminish the production of arachidonic acid, thereby resulting in decreased formation of prostaglandins, via the cyclooxygenase pathway, and of leukotrienes via the lipoxygenase pathway. In addition, corticosteroids have a negative effect on vascular permeability, neutrophil chemotaxis and the production of interleukin 2.

To avoid long-term side effects of corticosteroids, it is preferable to administer these drugs in an alternate-day therapeutic regimen, either every other day or once every 3 to 4 days, depending on the final individual effect. As a wide variability exists in atopic dogs in keeping the atopic condition under control, an initial dose of 1.0 to 2.0 mg/kg body weight of prednisone, every other day, is recommended. After 14 days this dosage is lowered to a maintenance level. This type of medical therapy is favored in dogs with a short-term seasonal atopy, for example 2 months a year. Corticosteroid therapy is also indicated in dogs with a sensitivity to many allergens, making hyposensitization impossible; the very old dog; and the dog with an atopic constitution with unidentified causative allergens.

Hyposensitization

Immunotherapy or hyposensitization is a therapy which, by injecting causative allergens in increasing doses and gradually longer intervals between subsequent injections, is administered to make the animal tolerant to the allergens.

Several theories have been proposed to explain the immunologic background mechanisms of hyposensitization, ranging from an increased T-suppressor cell activity and a gradual decrease of IgE, via a direct effect on mast cell degranulation, to the widely accepted "blocking antibody" theory. These blocking antibodies, belonging to the IgG immunoglobulins, are directed against the specific antigens and are the result of the administration of implicated antigen parenterally. It is suggested that the antigens bind directly with the IgG antibody before it reaches the tissue-fixed IgE, or that the IgG antibodies block the mast cell receptors thereby preventing mast cell release. The entire mechanism is still rather vague, but the theory about enhanced T-suppressor cell activity is rapidly gaining ground.

There are two main approaches to hyposensitization using aqueous or alum-precipitated extracts. Alum-precipitated extracts are absorbed slowly and therefore require fewer injections spaced at greater intervals. In contrast, aqueous extracts are rapidly absorbed and require a large number of injections. The selection of antigens in both mixed and individual forms is limited and the cost may be higher for alum-precipitated antigens compared to the aqueous type. Aqueous antigens are the most widely used type in the United States.

Hyposensitization is usually indicated in dogs with symptoms more than 3 to 4 months a year, have an allergy caused by a restricted number of allergens, and are not older than 10 years. The treatment vaccine is usually restricted to a maximum of ten allergens. Increasing the number can result in either administering an allergic load so heavy as to be potentially dangerous or diluting each one to such an extent that it may not be therapeutic. A study that compared the total antigen load administered and the clinical response clearly supported the recommendation that a maximum of 20,000 protein nitrogen units (PNUs) should be administered per maintenance injection.[37] This finding is consistent with the prior recommendation to limit the number of allergens to 10, since 20,000 PNUs of each allergen is generally used to make 10 ml of maintenance vaccine.

It is important to realize that hyposensitization usually is a lifelong treatment and that in case of a seasonal allergy the schedule should commence in time to permit the dose to reach the optimal maintenance level at least 1 month before the clinical symptoms are due to start.

Table 3-4. Injection Schedule for Hyposensitization With Aqueous Extracts

		Vial 1 (100–200 PNU/ml)	Vial 2 (1000–2000 PNU/ml)	Vial 3 (10,000–20,000 PNU/ml)
Day	0	0.1 ml		
	2	0.2		
	4	0.4		
	6	0.8		
	8	1.0		
	10		0.1 ml	
	12		0.2	
	14		0.4	
	16		0.8	
	18		1.0	
	20			0.1 ml
	22			0.2
	24			0.4
	26			0.8
	28			1.0
	38			1.0
	48[a]			1.0

[a] Thereafter, repeat injections (1.0 ml) every 20 to 40 days for the next 18 months.
(Kunkle GA: The treatment of canine atopic disease p. 456. In Kirk RW (ed): Current Veterinary Therapy VII. WB Saunders, Philadelphia, 1980.)

Table 3-4 shows the injection schedule for hyposensitization with aqueous extracts.[38] The injections are given subcutaneously. Approximately 60 to 70 percent of the dogs treated with aqueous extracts obtain clinical improvement of more than 50 percent.[31,37,39]

Rush hyposensitization with aqueous extracts is a new approach. Injections are given at 2 to 6 hour intervals for the first 4 to 6 days, enabling a maintenance level to be reached within that period of time. Although studies have shown that this appears to be a safe and efficacious technique,[39] the risk of such a rush therapy for systemic reactions may be higher than with other methods.

Tables 3-5 and 3-6 show the injection schedule for hyposensitization with alum-precipitated extracts currently used. The injections are given subcutaneously.

Hyposensitization in atopic dogs was evaluated for the first time in a double-blind study conducted by the author.[31] When comparing the treatment results, a significant difference in clinical improvement was established in favor of the allergen-treated dogs. A significant improvement of more than 50 percent was observed in approximately 60 percent of the allergen-treated dogs. This figure is in agreement with the results of Baker,[40] but lower than those reported by Halliwell (75 percent)[39] and Nesbitt (80 percent)[18] and higher than those found by Kunkle (40 percent).[38]

The final interval at which booster injections are administered to dogs on immunotherapy varies. Alum-precipitated allergens require a booster an average of every 2 to 3 months. The majority of dogs on aqueous immunotherapy require boosters every 1 to 4 weeks. It has been reported that some affected

Table 3-5. Kunkle's Injection Schedule for Hyposensitization with Alum-precipitated Extracts

		Vial 1 (100–200 PNU/ml)	Vial 2 (10,000–20,000 PNU/ml)
Week	1	0.1 ml	
	2	0.2	
	3	0.4	
	4	0.8	
	5		0.1 ml
	6		0.2
	7		0.4
	8		0.8
	9		1.0
	12		1.0
	16		1.0
	20		1.0
	24		1.0
	28		1.0
	32		1.0

(Kunkle GA: The treatment of canine atopic disease. p. 457 In Kirk RW (ed): Current Veterinary Therapy VII. WB Saunders, Philadelphia, 1980.)

animals may not need further hyposensitization treatment after 1 to 2 years.[39] In most dogs, however, this degree of control is not obtained.

The concurrent use of short-acting glucocorticosteroids with hyposensitization is controversial, yet such a therapy is widely accepted in the United States. As the clinical response from hyposensitization improves, the dosage for alternate day steroid therapy decreases. Similar clinical responses are reported in long-term follow-up studies for dogs hyposensitized with and without concurrent glucocorticoids.[37]

Immediate skin test reactivity during hyposensitization disappeared in

Table 3-6. The Willemse, van den Brom and Rijnberk Injection Schedule for Hyposensitization with Alum-precipitated Extracts

Injection Number	Interval (weeks)	Vial Number	Consecutive Dose(s) (ml)
1–3	1	1[a]	0.2–0.6–1.0
4–6	1	2[b]	0.2–0.6–1.0
7–9	1	3[b]	0.2–0.6–1.0
10–12	2	3	1.0
13–15	3	3	1.0
16–18	4	3	1.0
19	To effect	3	1.0

[a]1 The concentration of allergens in vial 1 are 100 Noon Units of pollen/ml, 0.05% of danders, and/or 0.5% of house dust.

[b] Vials 2 and 3 contain a 10-fold and 100-fold concentrated solution, respectively.

(Adapted from Willemse A, van den Brom WE, Rijnberk A: Effect of hyposensitization on atopic dermatitis in dogs. J Am Vet Med Assoc 184, 1277, 1984.)

those dogs with a good clinical response.[31] Therefore, in some dogs immediate skin test reactivity may be used as a parameter for the evaluation of the effect of hyposensitization.

Side effects from injections of allergen(s) are extremely rare and usually consist merely of short-term pruritus (1 to 2 days) following injection.[31,39]

It is concluded that hyposensitization is an effective and safe method of therapy in a selected number of dogs with atopic dermatitis.

REFERENCES

1. Muller GH, Kirk RW, Scott DW: Small Animal Dermatology. 3rd Ed. WB Saunders, Philadelphia, 1983
2. Chamberlain KW: Basic immunologic principles of allergic disease. Vet Clin North Am 4:3, 1974
3. Halliwell REW, Schwartzman RM: Atopic disease in the dog. Vet Rec 89:209, 1971
4. Patterson R: Laboratory models of reaginic allergy. Progr Allergy 13:332, 1969
5. Wittich FW: Spontaneous allergy (atopy) in the lower animal. J Allergy 12:247, 1941
6. Gell PGC, Coombs RRA (ed): Clinical aspects of immunology. 3rd Ed. Blackwell Sci Publ, Oxford, 1975
7. Prausnitz C, Kustner H: Studien uber die Ueberempfindlichkeit. Centralbl Bakt 86:160, 1921
8. Halliwell REW, Schwartzman RM, Rockey JH: Antigenic relationship between human IgE and canine IgE. Clin Exp Immunol 10:399, 1972
9. Willemse A, Noordzij A, Rutten VPMG, Bernadina WE: Induction of non-IgE anaphylactic antibodies in dogs. Clin Exp Immunol 59:351, 1985
10. Willemse A, Noordzij A, van den Brom WE, Rutten VPMG: Allergen-specific IgGd antibodies in dogs with atopic dermatitis. Clin Exp Immunol 59:359, 1985
11. Parish WE: Short-term anaphylactic IgG antibodies in human sera. Lancet ii:591, 1970
12. Katz DH: The allergic phenotype: manifestation of 'allergic breakthrough' and imbalance in normal 'damping' of IgE antibody production. Immunol Rev 41:77, 1978
13. Frick OL, Brooks DL: Immunoglobulin E antibodies to pollens augmented in dogs by virus vaccines. Am J Vet Res 44:440, 1983
14. Kroese FGM, Willemse A, Slappendel RJ: Granulocyte function tests in canine infectious diseases. Methods and preliminary results. Vet Immunol Immunopathol 2:455, 1981
15. Latimer KS, Prasse KW, Mahaffey DL, et al.: Neutrophil movement in selected canine skin diseases. Am J Vet Res 44:601, 1983
16. Scott DW: Observations on canine atopy. J Am Anim Hosp Assoc 17:91, 1981
17. Willemse A, van den Brom WE: Investigations of the symptomatology and the significance of immediate skin test reactivity in canine atopic dermatitis. Res Vet Sci 34:261, 1983
18. Nesbitt GH: Canine allergic inhalant dermatitis: a review of 230 cases. J Am Vet Med Assoc 172:55, 1978
19. Edmonds MJ: Preliminary investigations into the use of allergy skin testing solutions and desensitizing vaccines in dogs. J Small Anim Pract 21:153, 1980
20. Hanifin JM: Atopic dermatitis. J Am Acad Dermatol 6:1, 1982

21. Vriesendorp HM, Smid-Mercx BMJ, Visser TP, et al.: Serological DL-A typing of normal and atopic dogs. Transpl Proc 7:375, 1975
22. Schwartzman RM, Massicot JG, Sogn DD, Cohen SG: The atopic dog model: report of an attempt to establish a colony. Int Archs Allergy Appl Immunol 72:97, 1983
23. Reedy LM: The diagnosis of canine atopic disease. In Kirk RW (ed): Current Veterinary Therapy VII. WB Saunders, Philadelphia, 1980
24. Patterson R, Pruzansky JJ, Chang WWY: Spontaneous canine hypersensitivity to ragweed. Characterization of the serum factor transferring skin, bronchial and anaphylactic sensitivity. J Immunol 90:35, 1963
25. Willemse A, van den Brom WE: Evaluation of the intradermal allergy test in normal dogs. Res Vet Sci 32:57, 1982
26. Nesbitt GH, Kedan GS, Caciolo P: Aeroallergens. Compend Cont Educ Pract Vet 6:63, 1984
27. Nesbitt GH, Kedan GS, Caciolo P: Canine atopy. Part I. Etiology and diagnosis. Compend Cont Educ Pract Vet 6:73, 1984
28. Reedy LM: Canine and feline atopy-diagnosis. Proc Am Anim Hosp Assoc 105, 1985
29. Baker E: Allergy skin testing in the dog. J Am Vet Med Assoc 148:1160, 1966
30. Halliwell REW: Studies on canine IgE. Thesis, Cambridge, 1973
31. Willemse A, van den Brom WE, Rijnberk A: Effect of hyposensitization on atopic dermatitis in dogs. J Am Vet Med Assoc 184:1277, 1984
32. Lever WF, Schaumberg-Lever G (ed): Histopathology of the Skin. 5th Ed. JB Lippincott Co., New York, 1975
33. Willemse A: Canine atopic disease: Investigations of eosinophils and the nasal mucosa. Am J Vet Res 45:1867, 1984
34. Halliwell REW, Kunkle GA: The radioallergosorbent test in the diagnosis of canine atopic disease. J Allergy Clin Immunol 62:236, 1978
35. Hanifin JM, Rajka G: Diagnostic features of atopic dermatitis. Acta Derm Venereol 92:44, 1980
36. Hanifin JM, Lobitz WC: Newer concepts of atopic dermatitis. Arch Dermatol 113:663, 1977
37. Nesbitt GH, Kedan GS, Caciolo P: Canine atopy. Part II. Management. Compend Cont Educ Pract Vet 6:264, 1984
38. Kunkle GA: The treatment of canine atopic disease. In Kirk RW (ed): Current Veterinary Therapy VII. WB Saunders, Philadelphia, 1980
39. Halliwell REW: Hyposensitization in the treatment of atopic disease. In Kirk RW (ed): Current Veterinary Therapy VI, WB Saunders, Philadelphia, 1977
40. Baker E: Management of allergic disease by hyposensitization. J Am Vet Med Assoc 154:491, 1969

4 Autoimmune Dermatoses

Donna Walton Angarano

The autoimmune dermatoses are a group of skin diseases in which the body develops antibodies directed against its own tissue. There has been tremendous progress during the last 5 to 10 years in the classification and understanding of these disorders. Presently, there are many dermatoses which may be grouped under the heading of immune-mediated diseases. These include vasculitis, toxic epidermal necrolysis, erythema multiforme, alopecia areata, and linear IgA dermatosis. Graft-versus-host disease, cold agglutinin disease, and dermatitis herpetiformis have also been classified as autoimmune or immune-mediated dermatoses. This chapter includes a discussion of pemphigus, bullous pemphigoid, and lupus erythematosus. These diseases are rare to uncommon in a small animal practice yet they represent the most frequently recognized autoimmune dermatoses.

The cutaneous signs of the autoimmune diseases differ depending on the depth of the lesion in the epidermis or dermoepidermal junction. This discussion begins with the most superficial disease (pemphigus foliaceus) and progresses down through the epidermis.

PEMPHIGUS

Pemphigus, the Greek word for blister, was originally used to describe any blistering dermatosis. Pemphigus was reported in humans in the nineteenth century and thought to represent a cutaneous manifestation of an internal disorder. Pemphigus vulgaris was the first variant reported in domestic animals and was described in two dogs in 1975. Today the term pemphigus is used to describe a group of chronic, blistering skin disorders which are characterized by the presence of circulating and/or tissue-bound autoantibodies directed against an intercellular epidermal substance. This results in acantholysis or the rounding up and separation of epidermal cells and eventually intraepidermal cleft formation. Four variants of pemphigus have been reported in domestic animals. There does not appear to be any age, breed, or sex predilection.

Pemphigus Foliaceus

The most common form of pemphigus is pemphigus foliaceus. It has been reported in both dogs and cats. Clinically, pemphigus foliaceus is a blistering disease with pustules and/or vesicles. The blisters, however, are often short-lived due to the superficial location in the epidermis and this commonly results in an animal that is presented with a scaling or crusting dermatosis.

Lesions of pemphigus foliaceus may occur at any location on the body. In many cases, vesicles, crusts, epidermal collarettes, oozing, and alopecia will be found predominantly on the muzzle, pinna, and periocular areas. The nasal planum may be depigmented and/or ulcerated (Fig. 4-1). Oral lesions are uncommon. Other animals will be presented for seborrheic skin disorders (Fig. 4-2). These cases may or may not have facial lesions as well. A less common presenting complaint for pemphigus foliaceus is footpad hyperkeratosis which may result in fissuring, ulceration, and/or lameness (Fig. 4-3). These various

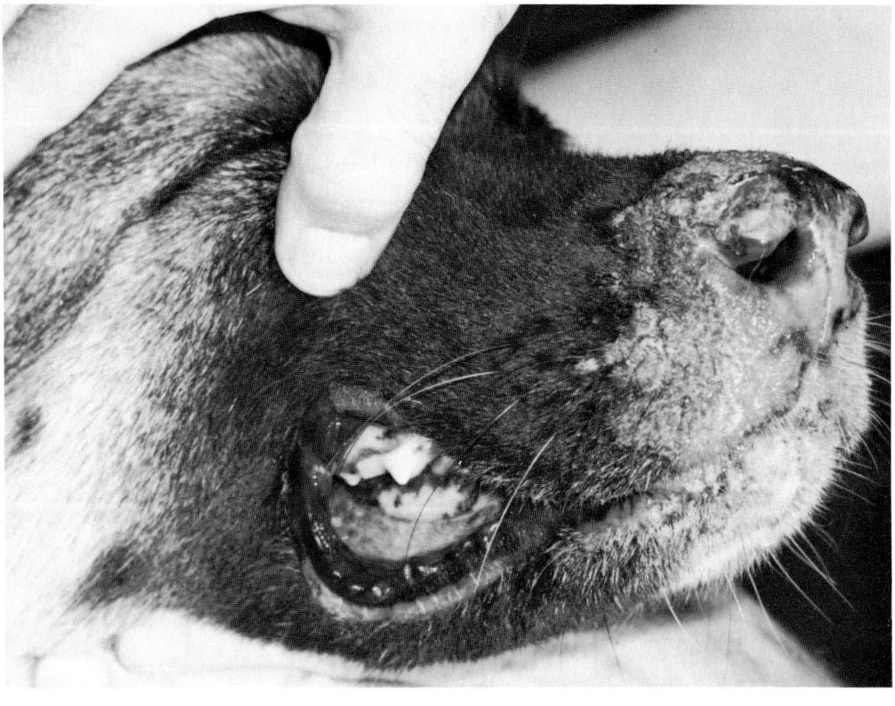

Fig. 4-1. Facial lesions of pemphigus foliaceus in a dog.

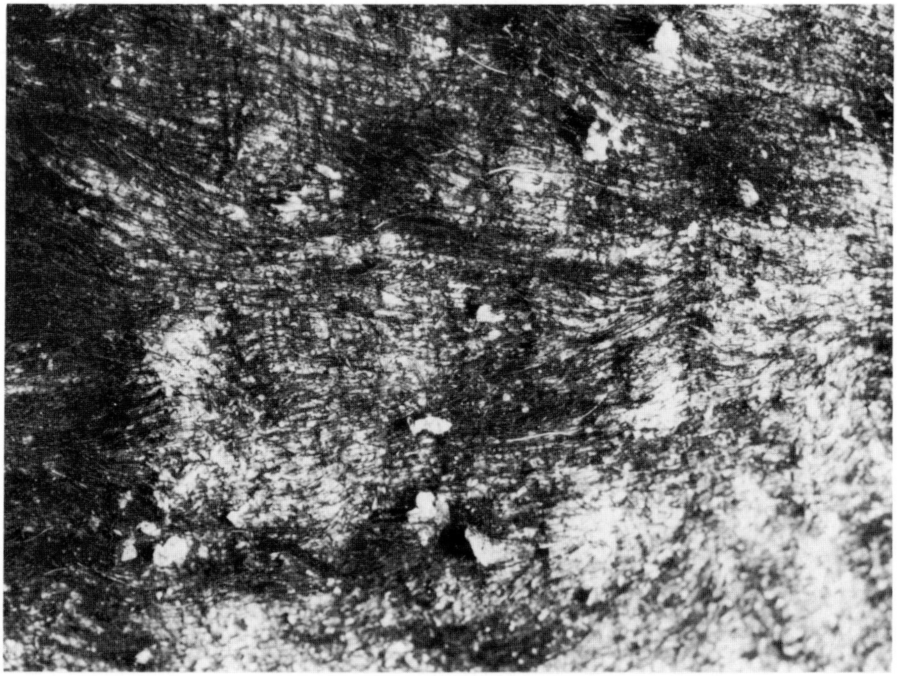

Fig. 4-2. Crusty lesions of pemphigus foliaceus in a dog.

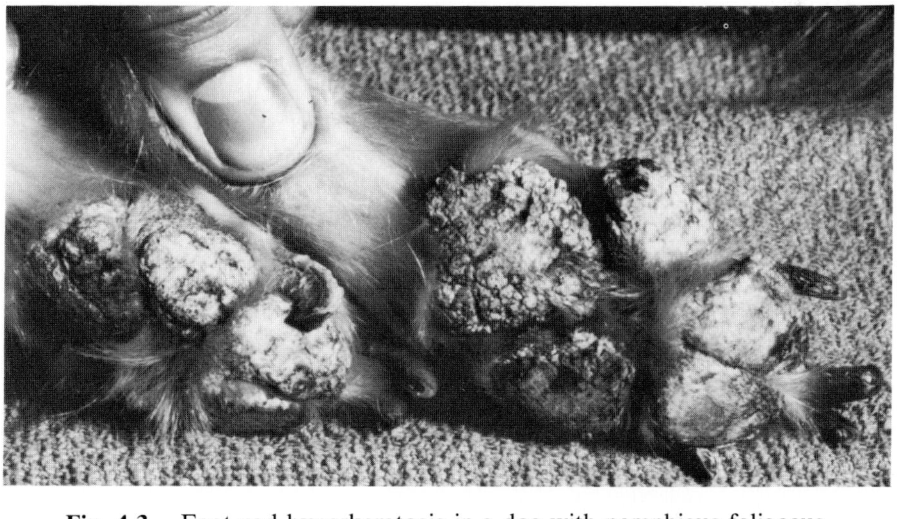

Fig. 4-3. Foot pad hyperkeratosis in a dog with pemphigus foliaceus.

lesions may be seen independently or as a group in any individual dog or cat. Dogs with pemphigus foliaceus are usually in otherwise good general health. The animal may be pruritic or in pain, particularly after ulceration and crust formation. Cats are frequently febrile, depressed, and anorexic.

Histologically, the intraepidermal cleft of pemphigus foliaceus is found below the stratum corneum, the most superficial layer of the epidermis, and is either subcorneal or intragranular in location. This results in a very superficial lesion and thus the superficial erosive, scaling, and crusting dermatosis previously described.

Immunologically, pemphigus foliaceus is characterized by tissue-bound autoantibodies directed at the intercellular epidermal spaces. Circulating autoantibodies are not typically present.

Pemphigus Erythematosus

Described in both dogs and cats, pemphigus erythematosus is considered by many to represent a benign or abortive form of pemphigus foliaceus. Clinically, there are strong similarities between these two diseases. A patient with pemphigus erythematosus may present with pustules, vesicles, crusts, erosions, epidermal collarettes, and/or alopecia. The lesions are limited to the ears and face. Nasal depigmentation and ulceration is common. Because of this facial distribution, pemphigus erythematosus is one of the diseases which in many cases was previously referred to as nasal solar dermatitis or "collie nose." It has been demonstrated that the facial lesions of autoimmune diseases tend to exacerbate with sun exposure. The histologic lesions of pemphigus erythematosus are identical to those of pemphigus foliaceus with subcorneal or intragranular acantholysis and cleft formation.

While pemphigus erythematosus and pemphigus foliaceus share many characteristics, pemphigus erythematosus also resembles lupus erythematosus particularly in regards to its immunologic characteristics. This has caused pemphigus erythematosus to be regarded as a cross-over syndrome between pemphigus and lupus erythematosus. In pemphigus erythematosus, there are tissue-bound autoantibodies directed at an interepidermal cell antigen, just as in all pemphigus variants. In addition, many cases also have autoantibodies present at the basement membrane zone. An antinuclear antibody test (ANA) is usually positive. These later two findings are characteristics found in cases of lupus erythematosus.

Pemphigus Vulgaris

The second major type of pemphigus is pemphigus vulgaris. It was the first form described in domestic animals and has been reported in dogs and cats. Clinically, patients may present with vesicles, bulla, crusts, or ulcers which affect the mucocutaneous junctions (eyelids, lips, nostrils, vulva, pre-

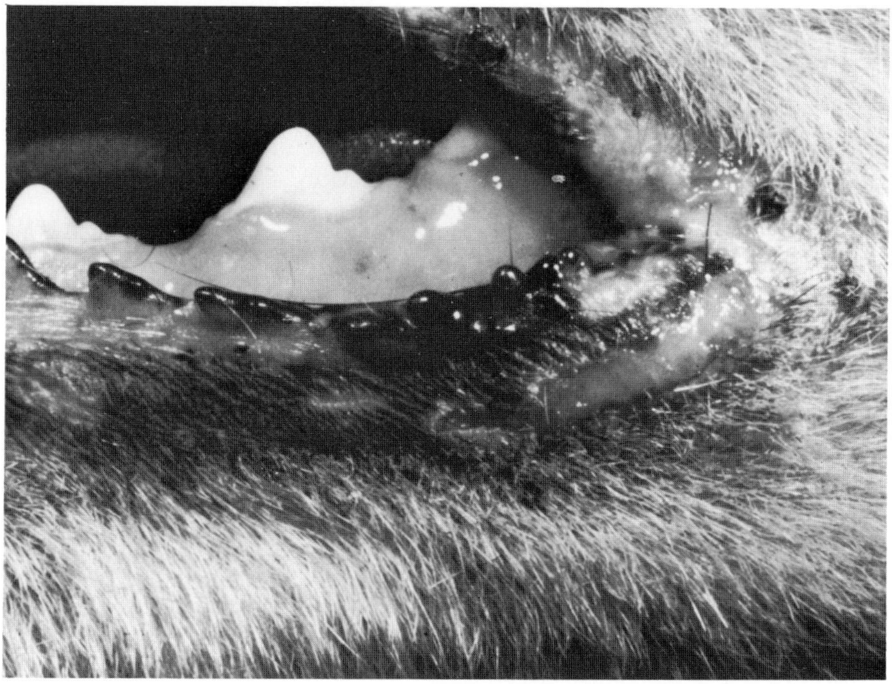

Fig. 4-4. Mucocutaneous ulcers in a dog with pemphigus vulgaris.

puce, and anus), oral cavity, and skin (Fig. 4-4). These lesions may occur in any combination. Oral ulceration is found in the majority of cases and frequently is the initial sign of the disease. When skin lesions are present, they tend to affect the axillary and inguinal areas.

On histologic examination, the intraepidermal cleft of pemphigus vulgaris is found to occur above the basal cell layer of the epidermis. This is two to three cell layers deeper than the lesion of pemphigus foliaceus and this difference in depth may be appreciated when examining the clinical lesions. As the lesions are deeper, secondary pyoderma is common and severely affected patients may be febrile, depressed, and anorexic. This is especially true when extensive oral ulceration is present. Results of immunofluorescence tests for pemphigus vulgaris are identical to those of pemphigus foliaceus.

Pemphigus Vegetans

Pemphigus vegetans has been reported in the dog and is thought to represent a benign or abortive form of pemphigus vulgaris. This is the least common of the autoimmune dermatoses discussed in this chapter. The clinical lesion begins as a vesicular or pustular eruption which progresses to a vegetative or papillomatous proliferation. Too few cases have been described to adequately predict the clinical appearance. Oral lesions have not been reported.

Histopathologically, pemphigus vegetans is characterized by intraepidermal abscesses which may occur anywhere between the stratum corneum or stratum basale. They typically are filled with eosinophils and acantholytic cells. Papillomatosis is also prominent. Immunofluorescence testing is identical to that of pemphigus foliaceus.

BULLOUS PEMPHIGOID

Bullous pemphigoid is a rare autoimmune dermatosis which may affect the skin and oral mucosa. While the exact etiology is unknown, the pathogenesis is thought to involve the deposition of pemphigoid autoantibody at the basement membrane zone. There is eventual dermoepidermal separation and cleft formation. Since the epidermis is lifted off intact from the dermis, there is no acantholysis.

Bullous pemphigoid has been reported in the dog. There is no sex or age predilection. However, the collie appears to be over-represented in those cases which have been described. The clinical signs are very similar to those of pemphigus vulgaris. Vesicles, bulla, crusts, and ulceration are common and

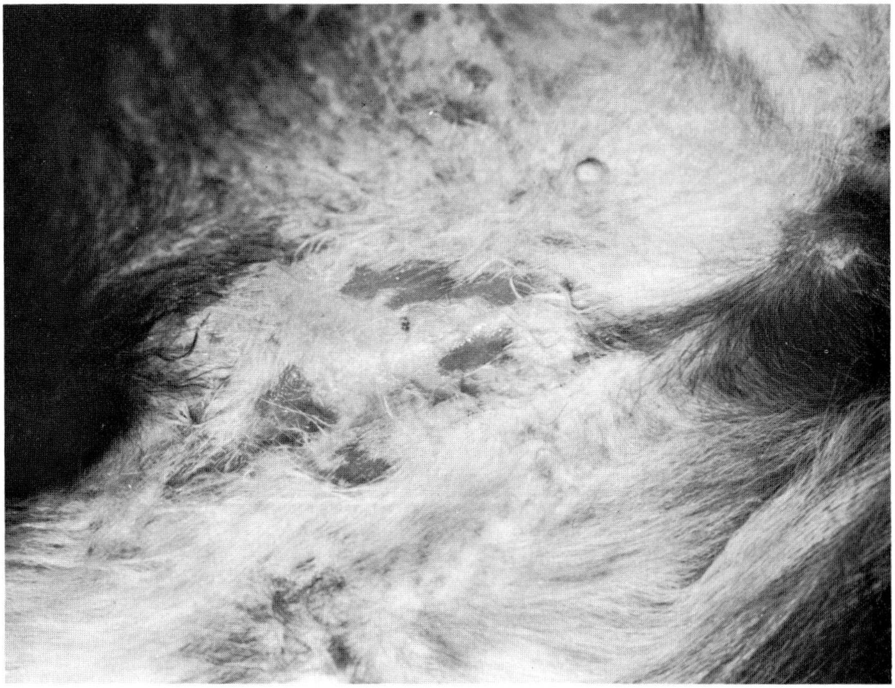

Fig. 4-5. Ulceration in a dog with bullous pemphigoid.

may occur at the mucocutaneous junction, skin, and oral mucosa. Oral ulceration is very common and the inguinal and axillary skin is also frequently affected (Fig. 4-5).

Histologic examination reveals a subepidermal cleft. In early lesions, subepidermal vacuolization may be a feature. Acantholytic cells are not seen. Direct immunofluorescence testing may demonstrate the presence of immunoglobulin and usually complement at the basement membrane zone.

DIAGNOSIS AND THERAPY OF PEMPHIGUS AND PEMPHIGOID

The diagnosis of pemphigus and bullous pemphigoid is based primarily on clinical signs coupled with histopathologic and direct immunofluorescent findings. Results of routine laboratory tests (hemogram, serum biochemical panel, and urinalysis) are usually nonspecific. This data, however, should be obtained, particularly as long-term medical therapy is usually required. Cytology is often helpful in establishing the suspicion of pemphigus. Impression smears from ulcers or the under surface of crusts may be examined along with aspirates from pustules or vesicles (if present in sufficient numbers). These smears may be stained with Diff-Quik (Harleco) or new methylene blue and examined for the presence of acantholytic cells (Fig. 4-6). While this finding does not establish a diagnosis of pemphigus, it should increase suspicion to a level to warrant further diagnostic tests.

Several early lesions should be selected for skin biopsy and histopathologic examination. Intact vesicles and bulla are the most rewarding to biopsy although perilesional areas are also helpful at times. The leading edge of an ulcer may reveal diagnostic characteristics; however, ulcers themselves are generally not helpful in obtaining a diagnosis. Skin biopsies must be taken with great care and gentleness in an attempt to maintain intact vesicles or bulla. Multiple samples should be collected to increase the likelihood of obtaining diagnostic features. Samples for histopathologic examination should be submitted in 10 percent formalin. The histopathologic differences between the pemphigus variants and bullous pemphigoid are shown in Table 4-1.

Immunofluorescence testing has been considered to be the ultimate diagnostic test for the autoimmune diseases. Unfortunately, there are still problems associated with its use including its limited availability and subsequent expense. Results of immunofluorescence testing are affected by previous corticosteroid administration, the age of the particular lesion along with the lesion itself (bulla versus ulcer) and the media in which the sample is submitted. It has also been recently demonstrated that samples from the same patient may yield differing results from different laboratories.

Intact vesicles, pustules, and their perilesional skin are the ideal lesions to biopsy. These samples should be quick-frozen in isopentane at $-160°C$ and held at $-70°C$ or they should be fixed in a special medium called Michel's solution (Tissue Fixative and Wash Solution, Lews Scientific, Inc., Raritan,

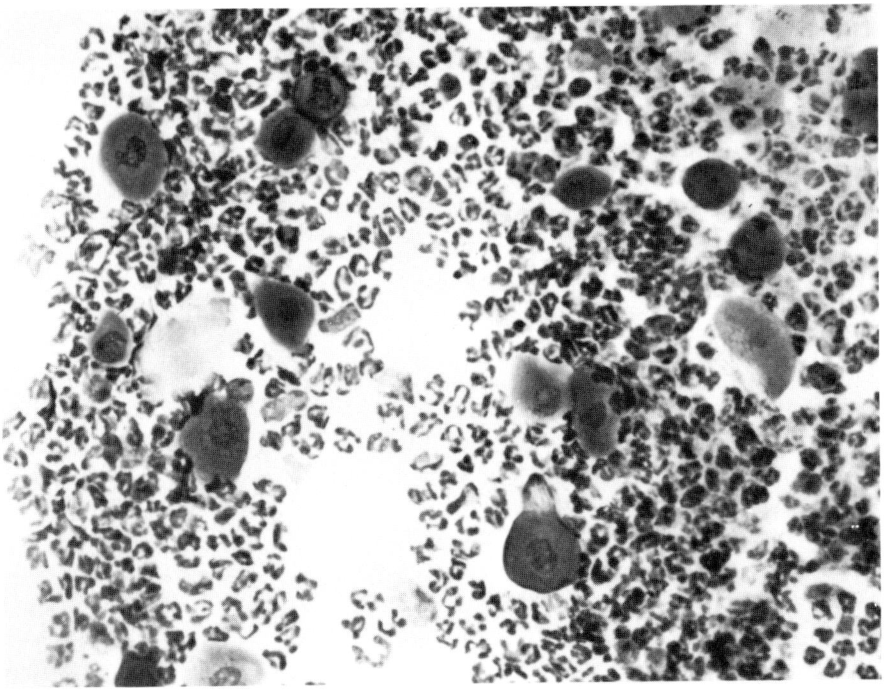

Fig. 4-6. Numerous neutrophils and acantholytic cells from a direct smear (Diff-Quik stain).

NJ). Samples may be preserved in Michel's fixative for 7 to 14 days and still yield reliable results. Unfortunately, the medium must be maintained at a pH of 7.0 for best results. The findings with direct immunofluorescence testing in pemphigus and pemphigoid are shown in Table 4-1.

Indirect immunofluorescence testing in canine and feline patients with pemphigus or pemphigoid is usually negative. Patients with pemphigus erythematosus usually have a positive ANA test.

Therapeutic protocols for pemphigus and pemphigoid are discussed. However, it must be remembered that each individual reacts differently to various drugs and thus each patient must be treated as an individual. Oral glucocorticoids (2.2 to 4.4 mg prednisolone/kg/day) are the initial therapy of choice for pemphigus and pemphigoid. This is divided into a b.i.d. dosage and given until improvement in cutaneous signs is obvious. The dosage is then decreased to s.i.d. and as soon as possible, alternate-day therapy is instituted and a maintenance dosage is reached. Frequently, slight dosage adjustments must be made as the disease tends to wax and wane in severity. Unfortunately, oral corticosteroids either fail to maintain remission or result in intolerable side effects in many cases. In these instances, gold compounds (chrysotherapy), azathioprine (Imuran) or cyclophosphamide (Cytoxan) may be added to the protocol or substituted for the corticosteroids altogether. In many cases, the addition

Table 4-1. Histologic and Immunofluorescent Findings in Pemphigus and Pemphigoid

	Histologic Lesion	Direct Immunofluorescene	ANA Tests
Pemphigus foliaceus	Subcorneal cleft with acantholysis	Immunoglobulin and/or complement deposited at the intercellular epidermal spaces	Usually negative
Pemphigus erythematosus	Subcorneal cleft with acantholysis	Immunoglobulin and/or complement deposited at the intercellular epidermal spaces *and* immunoglobulin and/or complement at the basement membrane zone	Usually positive
Pemphigus vulgaris	Suprabasilar cleft with acantholysis	Immunoglobulin and/or complement deposited at the intercellular epidermal spaces	Usually negative
Pemphigus vegetans	Intraepidermal pustule with eosinophils and acantholysis. Papillomatosis	Immunoglobulin and/or complement deposited at the intercellular epidermal spaces	Usually negative
Bullous pemphigoid	Subepidermal cleft	Linear deposition of immunoglobulin and/or complement at the basement membrane zone	Usually negative

of these immunomodulating drugs allows the corticosteroid dosage to be reduced to a level that is tolerated by the animal. Azathioprine (Imuran) has produced satisfactory results when given orally at 2.2 mg/kg s.i.d. or every other day.

Many cases of pemphigus and pemphigoid at the New York State College of Veterinary Medicine are treated with a combination of oral corticosteroids which are eventually reduced to an alternate-day maintenance therapy and chrysotherapy (gold compounds). Aurothioglucose (Solganol) is administered as an intramuscular injection once weekly for 6 to 10 weeks. The first 2 weeks a test dose is given (1 and 2 mg for cats and small dogs; and 5 and 10 mg for dogs over 25 pounds). Thereafter the dosage is 1 mg/kg/week. Chrysotherapy does tend to have a lag-phase and it may be 6 to 8 weeks before response is seen. During this time, the corticosteroid dosage is gradually decreased to the lowest possible maintenance dosage. After 6 to 10 weekly injections, the gold is administered every other week for 1 to 2 months, then once monthly. In a few cases, gold therapy has been stopped with the animal going into a prolonged remission. It is recommended that a hemogram and urinalysis be monitored periodically during induction and maintenance therapy.

In patients with nasal depigmentation and ulceration, exacerbation is common with sun exposure. In these cases, the avoidance of direct sunlight or the use of sunscreens containing paraaminobenzoic acid (PABA) is very helpful. Symptomatic and supportive therapy using wet soaks and antibiotics may also be helpful, particularly during early induction therapy.

The prognosis for pemphigus and pemphigoid in domestic animals is somewhat variable. Pemphigus vulgaris appears to be a severe disease which is often fatal unless treated. Pemphigus foliaceus is less severe, but may also be fatal. In both cases, death is probably due to secondary infections rather than the autoimmune disease itself. Pemphigus erythematosus and pemphigus vegetans are less likely to result in systemic signs and are more of a chronic dermatosis. Bullous pemphigoid is usually a severe disease with control being difficult. However, cases have been seen where maintenance was achieved at a low therapeutic dose of corticosteroids.

LUPUS ERYTHEMATOSUS

The name *lupus erythematosus* was derived from the Latin word for wolf (lupus) because humans with cutaneous lesions of the disease had an appearance as if they had been gnarled by a wolf. The true etiology of the disease is unknown; however, it is characterized by the presence of numerous autoantibodies and multisystemic involvement. Several factors have been considered in regards to the etiology including genetic predilection, viral infection, ultraviolet light, and immunologic disorders. A number of drugs have been shown to produce or exacerbate systemic lupus erythematosus in humans.

Systemic Lupus Erythematosus

In the canine, systemic lupus erythematosus (SLE) is most commonly recognized in collies, Shetland sheepdogs, German shepherds, beagles, and poodles, although any breed may be affected. Females are represented with a slightly higher frequency than males and there does not appear to be any age predilection. Feline SLE is a very uncommon disorder and in the limited number of cases, there does not appear to be any age, breed, or sex predilection. SLE has been termed the *great impersonator* because of the variety of clinical manifestations it may possess. The traditional case has involved some combination of glomerulonephritis (proteinuria), polyarthritis, autoimmune hemolytic anemia, and thrombocytopenia. Other clinical signs may include fever, peripheral lymphadenopathy, skin disease, oral ulceration, pericarditis, polymyositis, myocarditis, pneumonitis, splenomegaly, pleuritis, neurologic disorders, and lymphedema.

The cutaneous lesions which may be present in approximately one-third of the cases are also very diverse. The classic case is presented with facial and mucocutaneous lesions of alopecia, ulceration, and crust formation. These may be distributed in a butterfly pattern over the muzzle and periocular areas (Fig. 4-7). There is frequently depigmentation and ulceration of the nasal planum and nostrils. Oral ulceration is a common finding as is stomatitis (Fig. 4-8). This may be the only clinical manifestation in some cases. The pinna may have erosions or alopecia. The footpads are often hyperkeratotic. In other cases the footpads may be ulcerated and appear as if they are going to slough. The trunk and extremities may be seborrheic, erythemic, alopecic, or ulcerated. All of

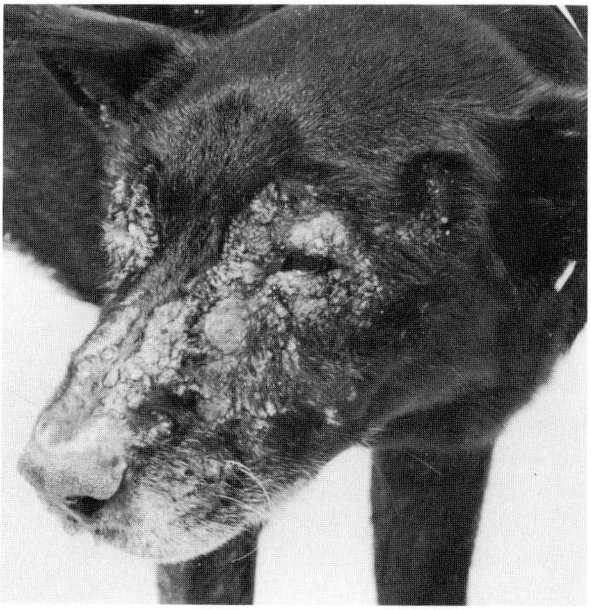

Fig. 4-7. Butterfly pattern of lesions in canine systemic lupus erythematosus.

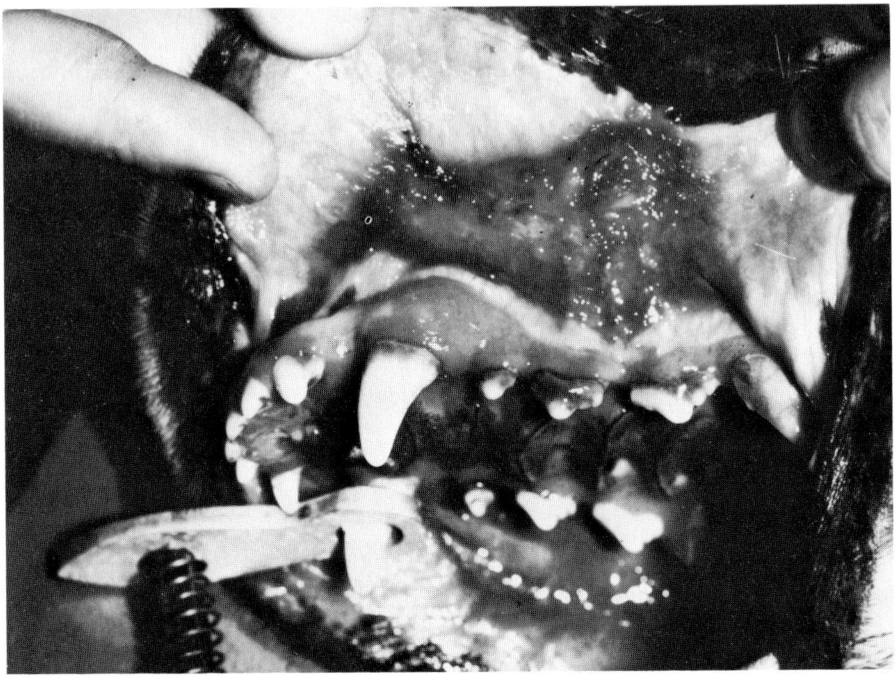

Fig. 4-8. Stomatitis in a dog with systemic lupus erythematosus.

these signs may occur alone or in combination. When the lesions have a seborrheic appearance and are erythematous affecting the trunk, pinna, and extremities, they are often quite pruritic.

SLE is a very challenging definitive diagnosis to make in the majority of cases. Patients which are presented with obvious multisystemic involvement and mucocutaneous and facial lesions are more likely to be suspected of having SLE and thus are pursued diagnostically.

Unfortunately, in many instances, the signs are subtle (mild proteinuria, pruritic, seborrheic skin lesions, etc.) and the history is vague. The disease does tend to wax and wane regardless of medical therapy, so previous apparent response to therapy may not be extremely helpful. Equally unfortunate is the fact that previous therapy (particularly the use of corticosteroids) may interfere with the results of diagnostic tests making the definitive diagnosis even more elusive.

The definitive diagnosis must be based on a combination of clinical signs and laboratory findings. The pathologic findings will differ depending upon which organ systems are involved. Patients should be evaluated for anemia (hemolytic or nonregenerative), thrombocytopenia, and proteinuria. The antinuclear antibody test (ANA) is considered to be the most specific and sensitive serologic test for SLE. However, this diagnostic test is not always positive. Unfortunately, even a positive ANA titer does not confirm the diagnosis of

SLE as it may also be positive with other disease processes or in normal patients. Thus, the clinician must be familiar with normal ANA results from each particular laboratory. Also, the pattern of fluorescence is important as the rim pattern is most specific for SLE.

The lupus erythematosus (LE) cell test is another diagnostic aid in some cases of SLE. The results of LE cell tests are known to vary from day to day, are affected by steroids, and lack specificity and sensitivity. Positive test results may help in establishing a diagnosis. Negative results, however, should not be used to eliminate the possibility.

When cutaneous lesions are present, direct immunofluorescence and histopathology of lesional tissue may assist greatly in obtaining a diagnosis. The histologic appearance may be as variable as the cutaneous lesions. The findings which suggest SLE include a thickened basement membrane zone, a lichenoid infiltrate (band of mononuclear cells in the superficial dermis), and hydropic degeneration of the basal cells. Direct immunofluorescence may reveal the deposition of immunoglobulin and complement at the basement membrane zone.

The therapy of SLE is variable. In the vast majority of cases, the initial drug of choice is oral glucocorticoids (2.2 to 4.4 mg of prednisolone/kg divided b.i.d.). As in pemphigus and pemphigoid, this dosage is reduced as the signs come under control and then alternate-day maintenance therapy is continued. In some cases other chemotherapeutic drugs are needed. Those which have been shown to be effective include azathioprine (Imuran) given orally at 2.2 mg/kg s.i.d. or every other day; chlorambucil (Leukeran) given orally at 0.2 mg/kg s.i.d.; and cyclophosphamide (Cytoxan) given orally at 50 mg/m^2 body surface area (BSA) every other day. In some canine cases with joint or muscle disease, aspirin has been effective in controlling signs. As in the other autoimmune dermatoses, facial lesions are exacerbated with sun exposure and thus sun avoidance or the use of sunscreens is recommended.

The prognosis of SLE must be guarded because of its multisystemic nature. Less satisfactory medical management should be anticipated in patients with glomerulonephritis, hemolytic anemia, or thrombocytopenia.

Discoid Lupus Erythematosus

An uncommon autoimmune skin disease, discoid lupus erythematosus (DLE) is probably the most common of the diseases discussed in this chapter. DLE has not been described in the cat. Collies, Shetland sheepdogs, German shepherds, and Siberian huskies account for the majority of cases and females are slightly predisposed. There does not appear to be any age predilection.

Discoid lupus erythematosus is a benign variant of SLE. The lesions of DLE are limited to the skin and in the majority of cases are limited to the face. These cutaneous lesions may consist of a butterfly pattern of erythema, alopecia, and crusting around the eyes, as well as around the lips. The nasal planum is usually depigmented and sometimes ulcerated. This area of depigmentation

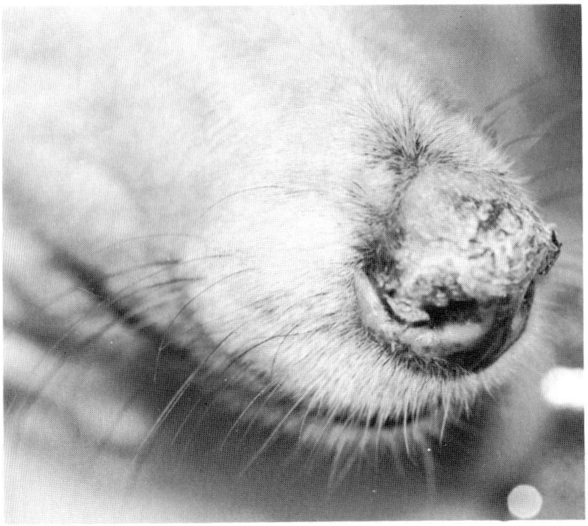

Fig. 4-9. Depigmentation, crusts, and ulceration of the nasal planum in a dog with discoid lupus erythematosus.

may extend up the muzzle as well as into the nares (Fig. 4-9). DLE probably represents the majority of cases which were previously referred to as nasal solar dermatitis or "collie nose." Some cases of DLE will also have alopecia and erythema on the distal margins of the pinna. These are occasionally the only presenting signs. Footpad hyperkeratosis is less frequently seen and oral ulceration is uncommon. As with SLE, scarring is a common sequela.

The diagnosis of DLE is based on clinical signs, histopathology, and direct immunofluorescence findings. Routine laboratory tests are usually normal and ANA and LE cell tests are almost always negative.

The histologic signs of DLE are more consistent than SLE and are usually composed of an interface dermatitis with a lichenoid infiltrate or hydropic degeneration. Thickening of the basement membrane zone, pigmentary incontinence, and Civatte bodies (degenerated basal cells) are frequent findings. The results of direct immunofluorescence testing are identical to those of SLE with immunoglobulin and/or complement deposition at the basement membrane zone.

Therapy for DLE is variable depending on the severity of the lesions. Sunscreens and sun avoidance are helpful. Topical steroids are beneficial in many cases. With more severe lesions, oral glucocorticoids (2.2 mg prednisolone/kg/day initially, then reduced to an alternate-day maintenance dosage) may be necessary. Vitamin E (dl-alpha-tocopherol acetate) has been shown to be helpful in some cases where corticosteroid therapy was unsatisfactory. Vitamin E is given orally at an empirical dosage of 200 to 400 IU b.i.d. It should not be given within 2 hours of a major feeding. Vitamin E does have a 1 to 2 month lag effect and thus may be given along with corticosteroids initially.

The prognosis for DLE is good. However, exacerbation with sun exposure is common and this may predispose to squamous cell carcinoma.

SUMMARY

In spite of the rapid advancement in understanding of the autoimmune skin diseases within the last 10 years, many questions remain unanswered. It is likely that as our understanding continues to advance, so will our questions. In particular is the question of why the body suddenly attempts to destroy itself. While we are becoming adept at suppressing the immune system (with corticosteroids and other immunomodulating drugs), it would be better to understand and prevent the initial self-destruction.

The autoimmune diseases discussed in this chapter are uncommon to rare, but they will be seen in a small animal clinic. With the excitement over "new diseases" such as these, the tendency is to overdiagnose them based solely on their unusual clinical appearance. When patients with facial lesions are presented, the autoimmune diseases should be considered. However, prior to an elaborate diagnostic work-up, one must be certain to rule out the possibility of the more common dermatoses such as demodicosis, dermatophytosis, and bacterial pyodermas. Patients with generalized erythema and scale may have pemphigus foliaceus or lupus erythematosus, but they could also have sarcoptic mange, atopy, or mycosis fungoides. Dogs with footpad hyperkeratosis are certainly uncommon and pemphigus foliaceus and lupus erythematosus should be considered along with zinc-responsive dermatosis and contact dermatitis.

The therapy for the autoimmune diseases is vigorous in most cases and potentially harmful if the diagnosis is incorrect. Therefore, the diagnosis should be confirmed by laboratory tests in addition to the suspicion based on clinical signs. Once the diagnosis is established, therapy is usually for life.

The prognosis varies depending on the disease and its severity. However, the seriousness of the autoimmune diseases should be discussed with the client at the onset. The diseases tend to wax and wane even with proper therapy, thus continued veterinary client interaction is extremely important.

With continued advancement in the understanding of the autoimmune dermatoses, we can anticipate that the definitive diagnosis will become less challenging and the outcome of therapy will become more rewarding.

SUGGESTED READINGS

Halliwell REW: Skin diseases associated with autoimmunity. Part 1. The bullous autoimmune skin diseases. Comp Cont Ed Pract Vet 2(12):911, 1980

Halliwell REW: Skin diseases associated with autoimmunity. Part 2. The nonbullous autoimmune skin diseases. Comp Cont Ed Pract Vet 3(2):156, 1981

Hurvitz AI, Feldman E: A disease in dogs resembling human pemphigus vulgaris: Case reports. J Am Vet Med Assoc 166:585, 1975

Ihrke PJ, Stannard AA, Adams AA, et al: Pemphigus foliaceus in dogs: A review of 37 cases. J Am Vet Med Assoc 186:59, 1985

Muller GH, Kirk RW, Scott DW: Small Animal Dermatology 3rd Ed. WB Saunders, Philadelphia, 1983

Scott DW, Walton DK, Manning TO, et al: Canine lupus erythematosus. Part I. Systemic lupus erythematosus. J Am Anim Hosp Assoc 19:461, 1983

Scott DW, Walton DK, Manning TO, et al: Canine lupus erythematosus. Part II. Discoid lupus erythematosus. J Am Anim Hosp Assoc 19:481, 1983

Stannard AA, Gribble DH, Baker BB: A mucocutaneous disease in the dog resembling pemphigus vulgaris in man. J Am Vet Med Assoc 166:575, 1975

5 Pyoderma

Stephen D. White
Peter J. Ihrke

Pyoderma, a pyogenic bacterial infection of the skin, is a common skin disease in the dog and is seen occasionally in the cat. Despite the definition, pus is not always visible grossly nor is the presence of pustules always indicative of a bacterial etiology. The very diversity of clinical syndromes and lesions designated as pyodermas often makes the diagnosis and management of these diseases difficult. Knowledge of the etiology and pathogenesis of pyodermas is still incomplete, especially as regards immune deficiency and other contributory disease mechanisms. Successful recognition and therapy of pyodermas is dependent on an understanding of cutaneous microbiology, identification of the clinical manifestations of pyoderma, ancillary diagnostic tests, and proper use of systemic and topical therapy.

CUTANEOUS MICROBIOLOGY

Microorganisms inhabiting normal skin have been termed residents or transients. Residents are able to multiply within the skin microenvironment, while transients cannot and are presumed to originate from the mucous membranes or the environment.[1] Coagulase-negative micrococci, alpha-hemolytic streptococci, and occasional *Clostridia* sp and diptheroids[2,3] are residents of normal canine skin, and similar bacteria have been reported on normal cat skin.[3] Various cutaneous bacterial transients of both dogs and cats have been identified as *Proteus, Pseudomonas, Corynebacterium* sp, coagulase-positive *Staphylococcus* sp and others.[3]

Both resident and transient bacteria may act as pathogens, though the latter are more commonly implicated. Primary bacterial pathogens initiate disease in normal-appearing skin. Secondary pathogens ordinarily do not initiate the disease, but do contribute to the disease process.[4] In contrast to pathogens, bacterial colonizers' presence on the diseased skin neither contributes significantly to the disease process nor elicits a host response.[5] Differentiation between secondary pathogens and colonizers may be difficult.[4] The primary pathogen of most canine pyodermas are the coagulase-positive *Staphylococcus* sp. Until recently these were identified as *S. aureus*; however newer data has confirmed the majority of these bacteria to be *S. intermedius*.[6] Many of these coagulase-positive *Staphylococcus* species produce enzymes known as beta-lactamases.[7] These enzymes destroy the beta-lactam ring of penicillin and related drugs, thus endowing resistance to bacteria producing such enzymes.

While coagulase-positive staphylococci are not usually cultured from normal dog skin[8], these organisms are found on 90 percent of normal dogs' hair coats:[4] thus a population of potential pathogens exists. Factors such as seborrhea, ectoparasitism, immune incompetence, endocrine imbalance, or trauma predispose the skin to infection. It should be emphasized that not all external or internal host factors which will make the skin environment more conducive to infection are well understood. Other bacteria such as *Proteus* or *Pseudomonas* sp isolated from pyodermas are probably secondary pathogens, enabled to survive in the tissue changes wrought by the *Staphylococcus* infection. Occasionally a coagulase-negative *Staphylococcus* may cause a pyoderma.[3]

Pyodermas are uncommon in cats, with the exception of bite-wound abscesses. *Pasturella multocida* is the usual bacterium isolated from these lesions.[7] Skin infections due to mycobacteria, *Nocardia*, or *Dermatophilus* have been documented in both cats and dogs.[3,9–11] However, disease due to these organisms are uncommon compared to the incidence of *S. intermedius* pyodermas in dogs and *P. multocida* abscesses in cats.

PYODERMA CLASSIFICATION

Classification of pyodermas is important both in recognizing the clinical disease as well as determining therapy and prognosis (Table 5-1). Often the clinical signs alone will suggest the diagnostic tests and therapeutic management needed. In general, the deeper the pyoderma, the longer and more aggressive the therapy required.

Surface Pyoderma

Surface pyoderma refers to two disease entities with ulcers or erosions as their clinical signs. The role of bacteria is probably confined to colonizers or secondary pathogens, and underlying causes need to be identified and controlled.

Table 5-1. Classification of Pyoderma

- Surface Pyoderma
  - Pyotraumatic dermatitis (''hot spots'', acute moist dermatitis)
  - Intertrigo (skin fold pyoderma)
    - Lip fold pyoderma
    - Facial fold pyoderma
    - Vulvar fold pyoderma
    - Tail fold pyoderma
    - Obesity fold pyoderma
- Superficial Pyoderma
  - Impetigo (puppy pyoderma)
  - Superficial folliculitis
- Deep Pyoderma
  - Muzzle folliculitis and furunculosis (''Canine acne'')
  - Nasal pyoderma
  - Interdigital pyoderma
  - Pressure point pyoderma
  - Generalized deep pyoderma
  - Subcutaneous abscess
  - Mycobacterial Infection
    - Cutaneous tuberculosis
    - Feline leprosy
    - Cutaneous atypical mycobacteriosis
- Disease previously classified as pyoderma
  - Juvenile pyoderma (juvenile cellulitis, puppy strangles)

Pyotraumatic Dermatitis

More commonly known as ''hot spots,'' (acute moist dermatitis) pyotraumatic dermatitis is both a frequent and poorly understood disease in the dog. It is typified by pruritic, erythematous, ulcerated, exudative lesions, usually on the dorsal caudal trunk. The lateral limbs, neck, and face may also be involved (Fig. 5-1). Long-haired breeds are more commonly affected, and most observers note a seasonal incidence with more cases seen in the warmer months. The bacteria isolated from the lesions are most likely colonizers, and their role in the disease process is probably minimal. Not surprisingly, antibiotics are seldom effective in treating the condition.

Successful management depends on determining the underlying cause and controlling the pruritus. Allergies, otitis externa, ectoparasites, and poor grooming may all be contributing factors. In the authors' experience, flea allergy dermatitis (FAD) is the most common reason for ''hot spots,'' and flea control should always be considered if no other cause is apparent. Control of pruritus is best affected by systemic, short-term oral corticosteroid therapy, as well as clipping the hair coat around the lesion and gentle cleansing. Topical therapy is optional, but messy, thick, or harsh medications should be avoided as they only serve to mat the hair coat and refocus the dog's attention to the lesion. Clinicians should be aware that both demodicosis and deep pyoderma may occasionally mimic pyotraumatic dermatitis (particularly when it occurs on the head and neck)[12] (Fig. 5-2). Appropriate measures should be taken (skin scrapings, biopsies and/or empiric antibiotic therapy) before using corticosteroids in these dogs.

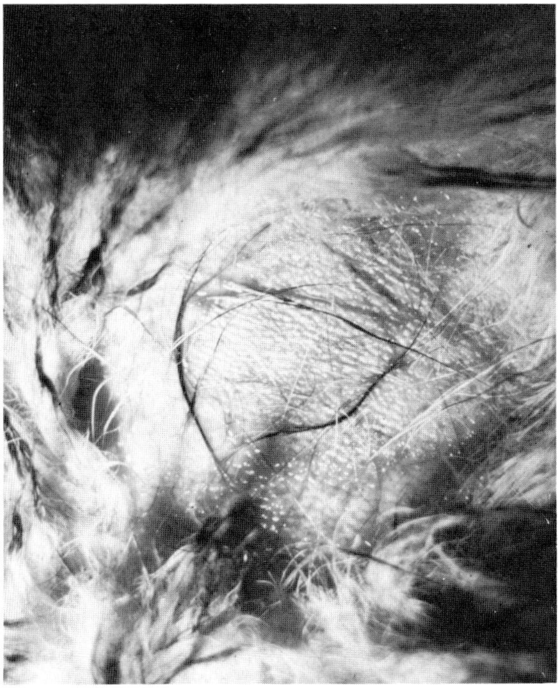

Fig. 5-1. Pyotraumatic dermatitis ("hot spot").

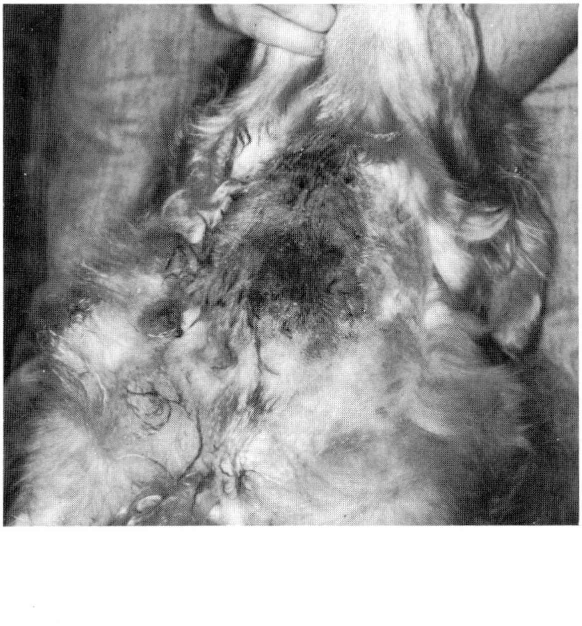

Fig. 5-2. Deep pyoderma on neck, resembling pyotraumatic dermatitis.

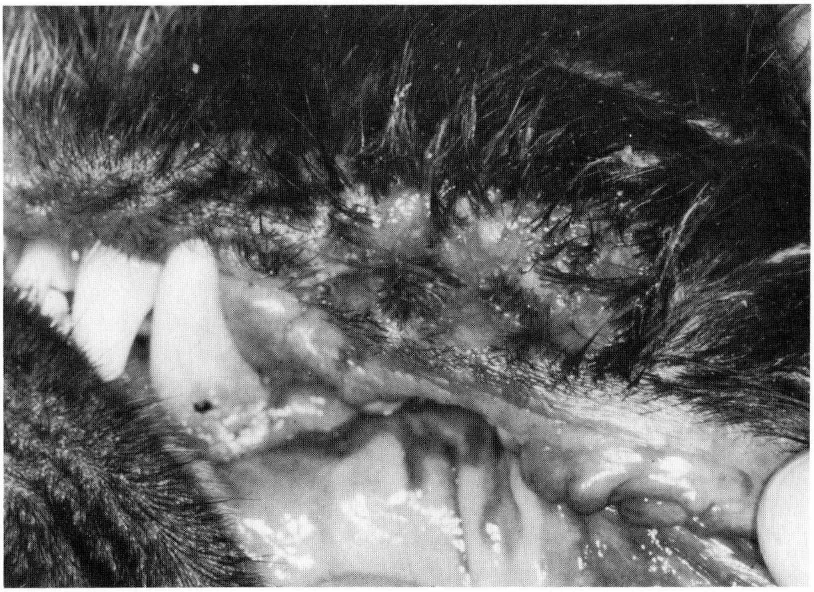

Fig. 5-3. Lip fold pyoderma.

"Hot spots" are uncommon in cats, but the preceeding discussion is applicable to that species as well.

Intertrigo

In intertrigo, or skin fold pyoderma, the underlying cause of the secondary bacterial infection is readily apparent.[2] The dark, moist, warm environment and frictional trauma caused by the skin folds create an ideal place for bacterial growth. The anatomic area affected varies somewhat by breed. Lip fold pyodermas are more common in spaniels and setters (Fig. 5-3). Halitosis is often the owner's initial complaint. If two separate cotton swabs are used to collect exudate from both the lip fold and the mouth, the difference in odor from each swab will convince the owner of the source of the halitosis. Facial fold pyodermas are most common in brachycephalic breeds and Shar Peis. Corneal ulceration may be seen secondary to self-trauma. Vulvar fold pyodermas are seen in obese females spayed before their first estrus. Breeds with corkscrew tails such as bulldogs are most susceptable to tail fold pyodermas (Fig. 5-4). Skin scrapings of all fold pyodermas should be performed, as demodicosis may mimic this disease.

All skin fold pyodermas are similar in clinical appearance. Pruritus is variable, but erythema, ulceration, and exudation are common. The folds may need to be separated to visualize the lesion. Although bacteria do play a secondary role in this disease, systemic antibiotics are rarely needed. Management of skin

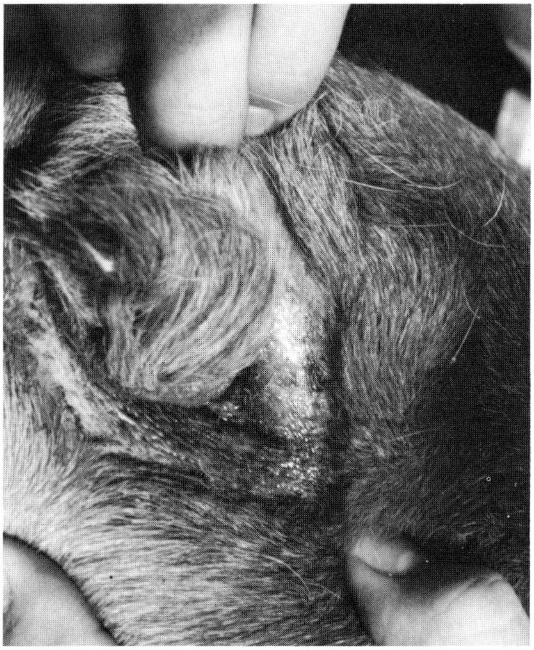

Fig. 5-4. Tail fold pyoderma.

fold pyodermas is usually accomplished using a 2.5 to 3 percent benzoyl peroxide shampoo. Initial application should be daily, with eventual maintenance cleansing two to three times weekly. Tail fold pyodermas may benefit from use of an antibiotic-steroid ointment. Vulvar fold pyodermas, difficult to treat with shampoos, respond best to weight reduction and corrective surgery. The total cure of any skin fold pyoderma is usually possible only with surgical ablation of the folds, which requires some expertise in cutaneous surgery.[2] Since some breeds are judged to be more desirable with skin folds, owners contemplating surgery should be advised that ablation may have adverse consequences in the show ring.

Persian and Himalayan cats will occasionally develop a facial fold dermatitis, characterized by either erythema and erosion, or excessive production of a dark sebaceous excretion.[3] Benzoyl peroxide shampoos (2.5 percent), administered with cotton applicators, may be helpful in controlling this syndrome. Benzoyl peroxide may be irritating to some cats.

Superficial Pyoderma

A superficial pyoderma is a bacterial infection present beneath the stratum corneum or within the superficial portion of the hair follicle. Because of their various clinical signs, superficial pyodermas pose more of a diagnostic challenge than surface or deep pyodermas. In general, superficial pyodermas should be included in the differential diagnosis of any pustular, papular, or crusting disease.[2]

Impetigo

Impetigo, more commonly known as "puppy pyoderma," is a relatively benign condition in which subcorneal pustules are found in the inguinal and axillary areas of prepubescent dogs (Fig. 5-5). The condition may be asymptomatic or mildly pruritic. Smears of the pustules demonstrate variable numbers of cocci and neutrophils. Therapy with antibacterial shampoos such as benzoyl peroxide 2 or 3 times weekly for 1 month is usually effective. Occasionally a short (2- to 3-week) course of empiric antibiotic therapy is necessary. Rarely, a bullous impetigo with large pustules may be seen in dogs with hyperadrenocorticism, or occasionally unassociated with any underlying disease.

An impetigo-like pustular dermatitis has been reported in young kittens.[13] The condition begins on the dorsal neck, with variable involvement of the head, ventral thorax, shoulders, and abdomen. One or all of a litter may be affected. *Pasturella multocida* and/or beta-hemolytic streptococci have been cultured.[13]

It should be stressed that impetigo in dogs and cats is a different disease than impetigo in human beings. The latter is usually caused by a streptococci species, and is frequently very contagious.[14] Owners who may associate the term with the human disease should be reassured that impetigo in small animals is neither contagious nor a zoonosis.

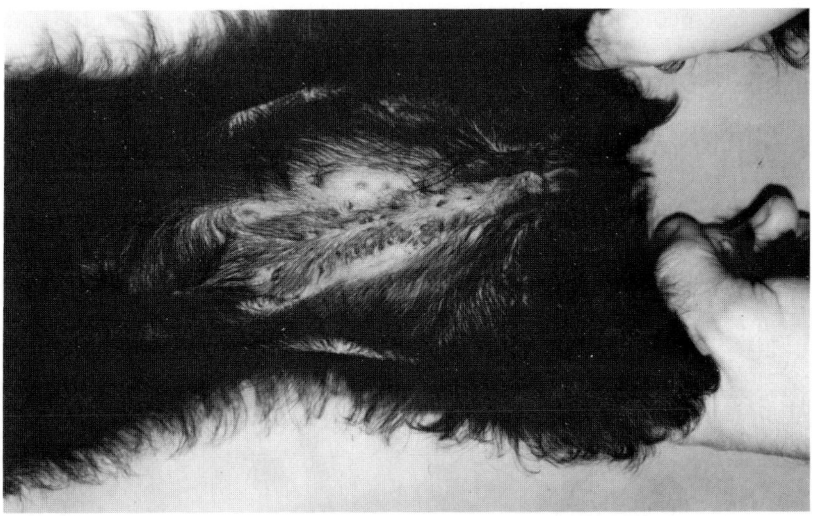

Fig. 5-5. Impetigo ("puppy pyoderma").

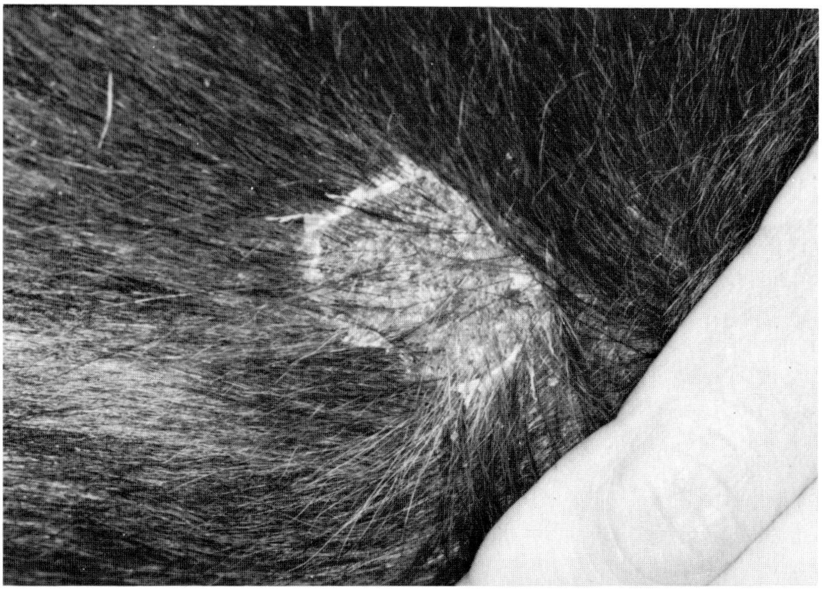

Fig. 5-6. Epidermal collarette.

Superficial Folliculitis

Members of this group of diseases have been termed recurrent pyoderma, pruritic pyoderma, short-haired dog pyoderma, staphylococcal allergy, and bacterial hypersensitivity. The authors prefer to discuss these diseases under one heading due to similarities in clinical signs and therapeutic management. These pyodermas are characterized by a pustular or papular eruption, often in association with expanding circular patches of alopecia, erythema, and subsequent hyperpigmentation. The periphery of these alopecic areas may have a border of peeling stratum corneum, termed an epidermal collarette (Fig. 5-6). Epidermal collarettes may be seen in any inflammatory disease with an initial pustule or vesicle which eventually ruptures. They have been reported in dogs with pemphigus foliaceus,[15] drug eruptions,[3] and food allergy.[16] They may also be seen with impetigo (P.J. Ihrke, unpublished data). However, the vast majority of epidermal collarettes are seen in association with superficial folliculitis. These lesions may occur anywhere on the dog's body, though perhaps most frequently in the inguinal and axillary regions. When present, residual hyperpigmentation may be dramatic (Fig. 5-7). A more papular, less expansive variant of this disease occurs in short-haired dogs and often gives a moth-eaten appearance to the coat, especially the lateral thighs and dorsum of the animal (Fig. 5-8).

Initial diagnosis is made by clinical signs. Papules examined under magnification are follicular in their orientation. A smear of any pustules present shows neutrophils and moderate numbers of cocci. Epidermal collarettes are

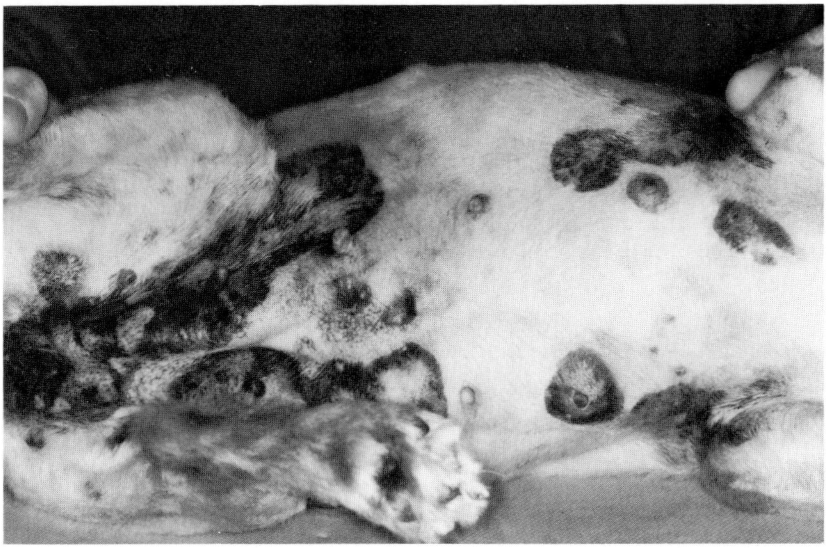

Fig. 5-7. Residual hyperpigmentation following superficial pyoderma.

usually present. Systemic antibiotics for at least 2 to 4 weeks is appropriate therapy. The antibiotic chosen should have a known efficacy against penicillinase (beta-lactamase)-positive *Staphylococcus*. Bacterial cultures and sensitivities are usually unnecessary. However, any pustular eruption not responding to conventional therapy should be biopsied and cultured.

In most superficial pyodermas, antibiotics will generally improve or eliminate the clinical signs. However, recurrence is common, and the owner should be informed that persistent or recurring folliculitis necessitates a search for

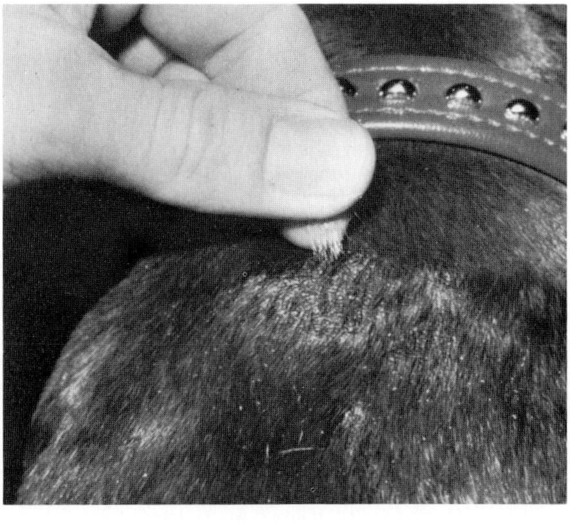

Fig. 5-8. Superficial pyoderma in short-haired dog.

predisposing factors. In the dog with nonpruritic superficial pyoderma, hypothyroidism and less commonly hyperadrenocorticism and other poorly understood immune incompetence syndromes should be suspected. Because bacterial infection of the skin can itself be pruritic, the presence of pruritus does not eliminate the aforementioned diseases as underlying causes. In pruritic superficial folliculitis, particulary in those dogs where antibiotics improve the appearance of the dog but not the pruritus, allergies, ectoparasites, and idiopathic seborrhea must also be considered as contributory factors. Of 100 dogs with superficial folliculitis seen at the Angell Memorial Animal Hospital in Massachusetts, 43 had flea allergy or flea infestation as a concurrent problem. (S.D. White, unpublished data.) Once the flea problem was controlled, the superficial folliculitis (having been treated with antibiotics) no longer recurred. Forty-six dogs had no determined underlying cause, while a small number of cases were attributable to hypothyroidism, hyperadrenocorticism, atopy, food allergy, and scabies. While not all 46 dogs without apparent underlying cause had all diagnostic procedures performed (such as intradermal skin testing) the uncomfortable fact remains that there is a significant number of dogs with recurrent superficial pyodermas in which an underlying etiology is not known. In these cases clinicians are left with the option of life-long antibiotic therapy, or the use of bacterins and other immune stimulants. It should be pointed out that even in those cases where an underlying cause is determined, the mechanisms predisposing to pyoderma are not well understood.

Superficial folliculitis is uncommon in cats.[13] Willemse has reported a syndrome in short-haired cats in the Netherlands similar to short-haired dog pyoderma.[17] One of the authors (SDW) has seen two cats with epidermal collarettes which responded dramatically to antibiotics. Staphylococci or streptococci are most commonly isolated from the lesions.[13] It would seem that cats with folliculitis respond to a short course of antibiotics with little tendency for relapse.

Deep Pyoderma

Deep pyodermas are serious bacterial infections of the skin involving not only the hair follicles but surrounding tissues as well.[2] Frequently the follicle wall weakens and ruptures, with the released bacteria and hair shaft keratin initiating an inflammatory, pyogranulomatous dermal reaction termed a furuncle. Less commonly, deep pyoderma may occur when the bacteria is introduced directly into the deeper tissues, as in a bite wound. Deep pyodermas may be either localized or generalized. Regions involved most often are the face, feet, and pressure points, though any area may be affected. Deep pyoderma in the dog and the cat, with the exception of the "acne" syndromes, should always be biopsied and cultured. Underlying causes should be investigated. *Deep pyoderma in the dog should always be considered secondary to demodicosis until proven otherwise.* Other possible contributory factors include hypothyroidism, hyperadrenocorticism (endogenous or iatrogenic), tumor-associated immunosuppression, and idiopathic immunodeficiency.

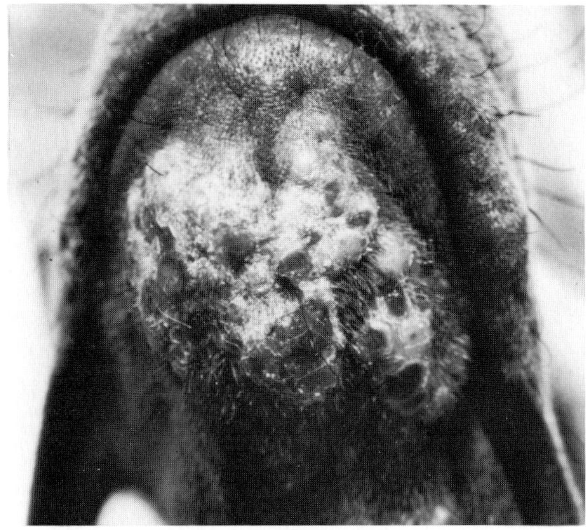

Fig. 5-9. Chin and muzzle folliculitis ("canine acne").

"Acne" (Muzzle and Chin Folliculitis and Furunculosis)

While muzzle-chin folliculitis-furunculosis is a more accurate name for this disease, the term acne is commonly used to underscore the potential chronicity of the condition.[2] Histologic differences and the lack of a definitive etiology make exact analogy to human acne controversial. The role of bacteria in canine and feline acne has not been determined. Some authors consider these diseases to be disorders of follicular keratinization with bacterial infection playing a secondary role.[3] Acne is generally seen in the adolescent dog, with a period of involvement of a few months. However, in English bulldogs, boxers, Great Danes, Doberman pinschers, and occasionally other breeds, the condition may persist for the life of the dog. In cats, acne may occur at any age and is frequently a life-long problem.

In both species, a papulopustular eruption with occasional comedones is noted on physical examination (Fig. 5-9). Animals with more severe disease have firm or fluctuant furuncles with erythema and draining tracts, particularly in mature dogs. Despite serious appearance, acne is rarely symptomatic. Therapy in both dogs and cats includes use of benzoyl peroxide, usually a 2.5 to 3 percent shampoo. A 5 percent gel may be used in dogs. Medication is applied once daily until clinical improvement is noted, then two to three times weekly as needed for maintenance therapy. In mild cases, treatment may not be necessary. In severe cases, antistaphylococcal antibiotics and warm water soaks should be used.

Nasal Pyoderma

Nasal pyoderma, an uncommon, poorly understood disease, is characterized by painful, swollen areas on the dorsum of the nose, occasionally associated with erythema and alopecia (Fig. 5-10). The onset is rapid, with a severe

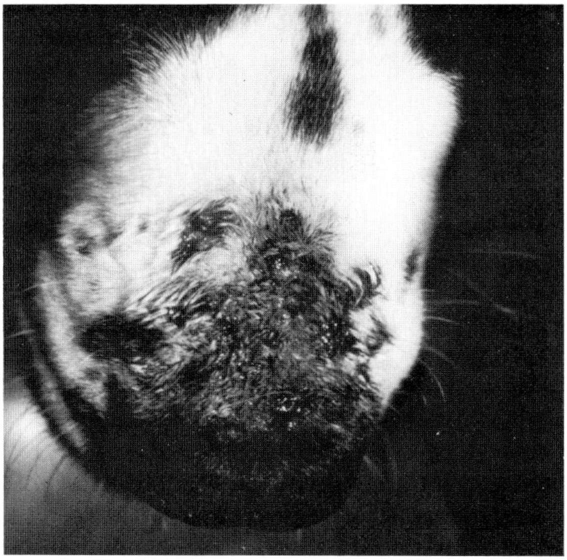

Fig. 5-10. Nasal pyoderma.

furunculosis seen on biopsy.[2,3] The differential diagnosis for nasal pyoderma includes demodicosis, dermatophytosis, trauma, drug eruption, pemphigus foliaceus, pemphigus vulgaris, and lupus erythematosus. Skin scrapings, exudate smears, fungal culture, and bacterial culture and sensitivity should be performed. Appropriate antibiotics should be given for at least 3 weeks, with frequent wet soaks. Because of the painful nature of the disease, any topical therapy should be applied gently, and sedatives may be helpful until clinical improvement is seen. Failure to respond to antibiotic therapy indicates the need for biopsy and immunologic tests.

Interdigital Pyoderma

Like all interdigital disease in the dog, interdigital pyoderma is frequently clinically frustrating. The disease is most commonly characterized by swelling, alopecia, erythema, pruritus, and thinning of the skin over areas of pus accumulation (Fig. 5-11). These latter entities have the misnomer of "interdigital cysts," though no cystic structures are present. Because of the potentially chronic nature of interdigital pyoderma, a thorough search for underlying causes is essential. Demodicosis, dermatophytosis, hypothyroidism, food allergy, sterile pyogranulomas, and foreign bodies such as plant awns should all be considered.[18,19] In severe cases of demodectic pododermatitis, the thickening and scarring of the paws may be so extensive that clinicians may not be able to scrape deep enough to demonstrate the mites and biopsy may be necessary to establish the diagnosis.[20] All cases of interdigital pyoderma require skin scraping and bacterial culture and sensitivity. If no underlying cause is

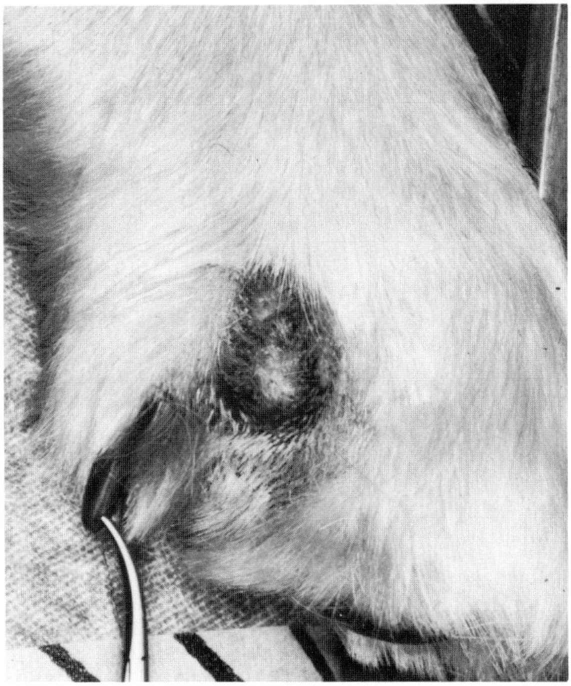

Fig. 5-11. Interdigital pyoderma.

determined for persistent interdigital pyoderma, life-long antibiotics, with or without immunostimulants, in combination with topical chlorhexidine or povidone-iodine soaks, will usually effect control if not clinical cure.

Pressure Point Pyoderma

Pressure point pyodermas are deep bacterial infections commonly affecting mature large breed dogs. Areas involved may be the lateral stifles, elbows, hocks, and digits. Ulceration and draining tracts may be present but concealed by matting and crusting. Hypothyroidism is felt to be a common cause,[2] though other less well-understood immunoincompetency conditions may also be at fault. Clipping the hair coat of the affected areas, whirlpool baths of povidone iodine or chlorohexidine, and appropriate antibiotics are the indicated therapies. Providing the dog with soft bedding may also be helpful.

Generalized Deep Pyoderma

Generalized deep pyoderma is a very severe folliculitis and furunculosis involving the entire body. Feet, lateral thighs, pressure points, and the dorsum may be most affected. The lesions may be erythematous, exudative, alopecic

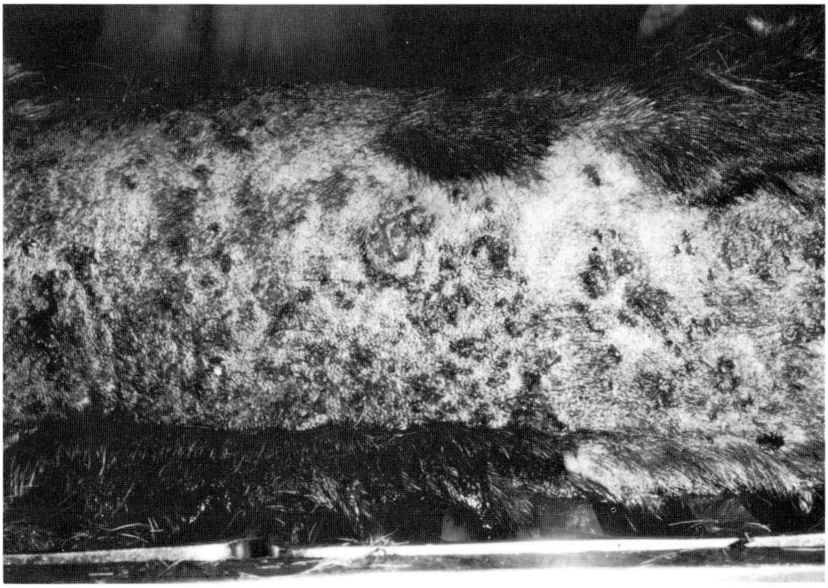

Fig. 5-12. Generalized deep pyoderma.

areas, or frank draining tracts with a "punched-out" appearance (Fig. 5-12). The surrounding skin may be quite friable. The animals are frequently febrile and depressed. A complete blood count often shows a leukocytosis. If the infection becomes very suppurative and dissects through tissue planes, it is termed a cellulitis. Demodicosis and hypothyroidism are the two most important potential underlying causes. Unfortunately, many of these cases are idiopathic. German shepherds are the most commonly observed breed with this disease.[3] (S. D. White, unpublished data.) A biopsy and bacterial culture and sensitivity should be done in all cases. Therapy is as noted for pressure point pyodermas. Clipping the hair coat may require general anesthesia. Antibiotic therapy is usually long term (6 to 8 months) or lifelong if no underlying cause is determined. Bacterins[21] and levamisole[3] have been effective in some cases.

Subcutaneous Abscesses

Most frequently seen in cats, subcutaneous abscesses usually follow bite wounds. A firm to fluctuant subcutaneous swelling is usually noted, though in some cases the abscess has already burst and a draining tract is present. On closer examination teeth marks may be seen. The involved area is warm and usually painful to the touch. In areas of minimal subcutaneous tissue, such as the distal limbs, the infection may present as a poorly defined area of swelling. Diagnosis is usually made by history and physical examination.

Therapy consists of lancing and draining the abscess and flushing it with chlorohexidine or povidine-iodine solution. The latter may be irritating to some cats. Drainage should be maintained by frequent (three to four times daily) warm compresses of the area involved. Antibiotics such as ampicillin or amoxicillin are generally effective against the bacteria that are part of the normal flora of a cat's mouth (*Pasturella multocida* especially) and should be given for 7 to 10 days.[7,13] Areas of swelling but not gross purulence (as on the distal limbs) may be treated with antibiotics and warm compresses only. Recurrent or poorly healing cat abscesses may be due to feline leukemia virus (FeLV) infections or other causes of immunosuppression, or infection with potentially resistent organisms such as *Nocardia*, mycobacteria, or mycoses.[3]

Mycobacterial Infections

Mycobacteria are uncommon pathogens of skin disease in small animals.[9,10,22] Cutaneous mycobacteriosis should be suspected in the dog or cat presenting with nodular skin disease and/or draining tracts. Biopsy samples should be taken for impression smears, histopathology, and culture and sensitivity. The impression smears and histopathology samples should be stained and examined for acid-fast organisms. Animal innoculation should be performed if tuberculosis is suspected. Therapy is dependent on which mycobacteria is the etiologic agent, and should proceed as outlined below. Categories of cutaneous mycobacteriosis are cutaneous tuberculosis, feline leprosy, and cutaneous atypical mycobacteriosis.

Cutaneous Tuberculosis

In small animals, tuberculosis has decreased along with the decreased incidence of the disease in humans and cattle. The causative agent is either *M. bovis* or *M. tuberculosis*. The former may be contracted from humans via airborne infection; the latter is usually ingested through infected milk. Cutaneous tuberculosis occurs either by hematogenous spread from the intestinal or respiratory tracts, or from infected skin wounds. Lesions may be nodules, ulcers, or abscesses. Tubercular animals often have systemic signs such as weight loss, anorexia, fever, and/or lymphadenopathy.[23]

Histopathology of lesions shows a pyogranulomatous response with or without caseation necrosis. Variable numbers of bacilli are seen on acid-fast stains. Diagnosis is by culture and animal innoculation tests. Tuberculosis bacilli generally take 6 to 8 weeks to grow in special media, and a similar length of time to cause death in innoculated guinea pigs.

Therapy is not recommended, due to the public health hazard tubercular animals represent. The animal should be euthanized and the public health authorities notified.

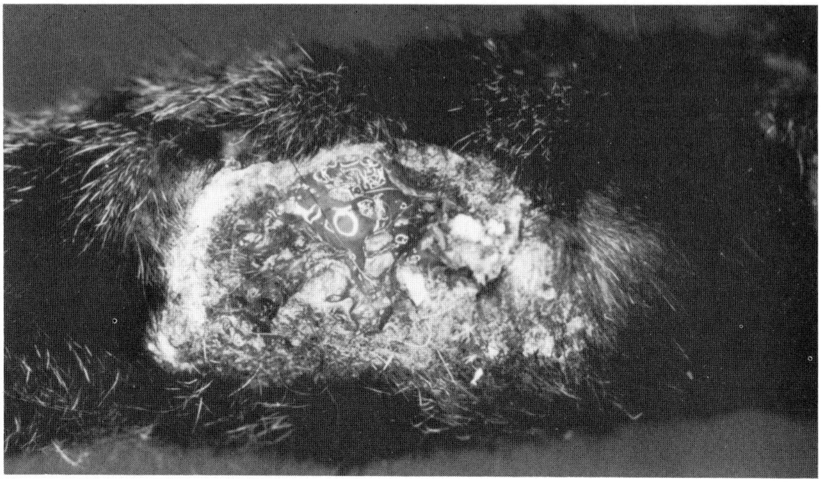

Fig. 5-13. Nodular, ulcerative lesion of feline leprosy.

Feline Leprosy

Feline leprosy is the name given to a granulomatous skin disease of cats associated with the presence of an acid-fast bacilli thought to be *Mycobacterium lepraemurium*, the agent of rat (murine) leprosy.[9,24,25] The mode of transmission is not known, but is hypothesized to be via the bites of infected rats. Lesions are cutaneous nodules, single or multiple, ulcerated or nonulcerated, which seem to have a predilection for the head and limbs (Fig. 5-13). These nodules are usually not painful, and aside from regional lymphadenopathy, systemic signs are generally absent.[9]

Histopathology of the nodules reveals either tuberculoid granulomas with caseation necrosis, or sheets of macrophages with multinucleated giant cells.[26] Acid-fast stains of both formalin-fixed tissues and impression smears of freshly excised nodules usually demonstrate prominent numbers of mycobacteria. *M. lepraemurium* is very difficult to grow in vitro, though some investigators have had success using the Ogawa egg yolk medium.[25] Innoculation does not kill guinea pigs, but usually produces local and lymph node lesions in mice and rats. Diagnosis is based primarily on the presence of acid-fast organisms histologically without either the characteristic animal innoculation pattern of tuberculosis or any growth on tuberculosis or other common media.

Therapy has generally been limited to excisional surgery.[9,24] This is effective in the animal with single or few nodules, but becomes difficult in the cat with multiple lesions. Dapsone, a drug effective in treatment of human leprosy, has been used in Australia in cats with feline leprosy at the daily dosage of 1 mg/kg.[27] This drug may cause hemolytic anemia or neurotoxicity, and is not approved for use in the cat in the United States. Further study of the efficacy, dosage, and toxicities of antimycobacterial drugs in cats is needed before the authors can make specific recommendations.

Cutaneous Atypical Mycobacteriosis

Those mycobacteria which do not cause tuberculosis or leprosy (feline, murine, or human) have been termed the atypical or opportunistic mycobacteria. These organisms may rarely cause cutaneous disease in dogs and cats. Thought to be ubiquitous in the environment, the atypical mycobacteria have been divided into four groups on the basis of physical and laboratory characteristics.[9,28] In Group IV, the "fast-growers," growth will usually be seen within 7 days of media innoculation. Almost all reported cases of cutaneous atypical mycobacteriosis in small animals have been caused by Group IV organisms. The mode of transmission is not completely understood, but the organisms are thought to gain entry through wounds.[9,10] Lesions are usually draining tracts, often associated with subcutaneous nodules (Fig. 5-14). These lesions are painless or only mildly discomforting when palpated. Systemic signs are usually absent.

Histopathology shows pyogranulomatous inflammation, often with areas of caseation necrosis. In contrast to feline leprosy the atypical mycobacteria may be difficult to find with acid-fast stains.[9] Because of this difficulty, impression smears of freshly-excised tissue should also be submitted for acid-fast staining. These organisms may be grown on blood agar and/or Lowenstein-Jensen media. The laboratory should be notified that mycobacteriosis is suspected.

Treatment modalities for cutaneous atypical mycobacteriosis need further research. Surgical excision is occasionally curative, but does not seem to be

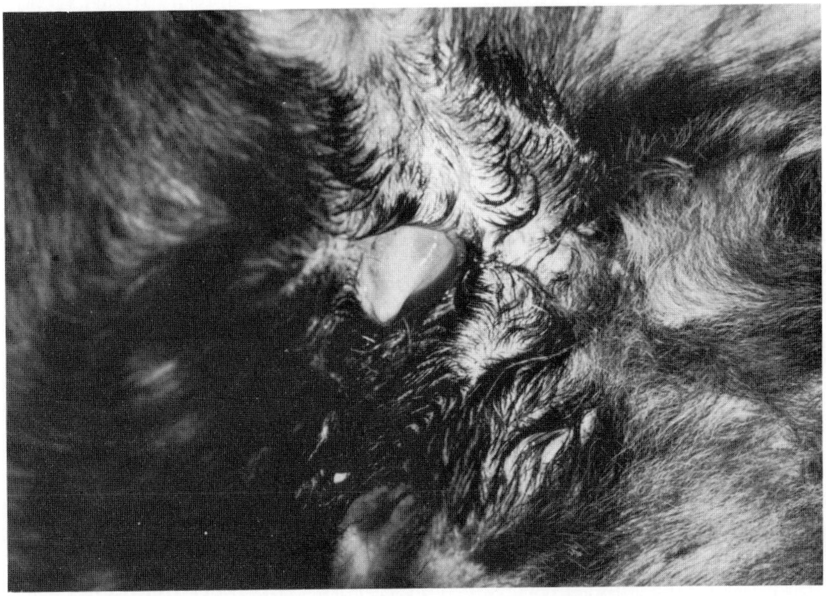

Fig. 5-14. Fistulous tract in cat with atypical mycobacteriosis.

as effective as in feline leprosy. Dehiscence of the incision site and recurrence of the lesions are common. In vitro susceptibility to antimycobacterial drugs is not always reflected by in vivo clinical improvement. In addition, atypical mycobacteriosis may spontaneously regress, rendering an evaluation of therapy difficult.[9,22] The authors' current therapeutic recommendations in otherwise healthy cats with this disease is to keep the affected area clean, and to inform owners of both the difficulty of therapy as well as the possibility of spontaneous remission. If systemic signs (anorexia, fever) develop, the original lesion enlarges, or new lesions occur, antimycobacterial drugs may cautiously be used based on culture and sensitivity tests.

Juvenile Pyoderma

Juvenile pyoderma (juvenile cellulitis, puppy strangles) is a canine disease of unknown etiology frequently classified (and misdiagnosed) as a pyoderma. The condition is most commonly seen in pups less than 4 months of age, though adult dogs have been affected. Certain breeds, such as dachshunds, Brittany and springer spaniels, and Labrador retrievers, have an apparent predilection. Lesions consist of swelling, papules, and pustules, with or without frank exudative pus, in the periorbital, perioral, and periauricular areas.[2,3] A purulent otitis may be seen. The regional lymph nodes are significantly enlarged (Fig. 5-15) and generalized lymphadenopathy may be present. Occasionally these lymph nodes may caseate and fistulate externally. The dogs are usually anorectic, lethargic, and febrile.

Diagnosis is made on clinical signs and negative skin scrapings for demodicosis. Fresh lesions are generally sterile, though staphylococci species may be cultured from older lesions. Although antibiotics conventionally have been used to control secondary infection, the authors (and others) have had the best success using concurrent corticosteroids (prednisone 1 mg/kg, orally, b.i.d.). This dose should be maintained for 1 week, then slowly decreased over

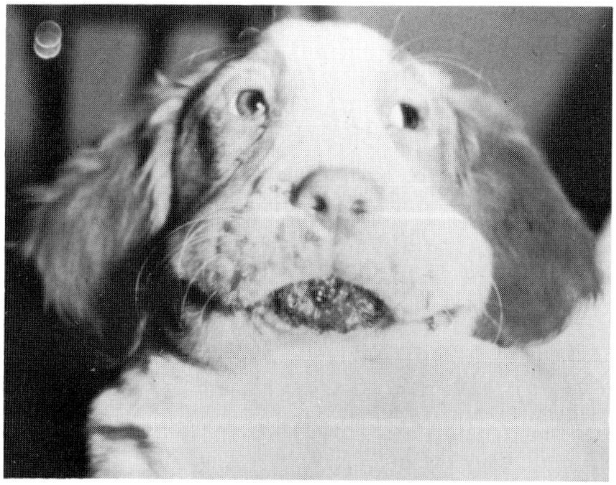

Fig. 5-15. Juvenile pyoderma.

the course of 1 month. If a flare in clinical signs occurs, the dosage given previous to the flare should be reinstituted for 1 week before again attempting to decrease the dosage. Once treated adequately and withdrawn from the prednisone, the dogs do not relapse.

DIAGNOSTIC PROCEDURES

The need for various diagnostic tests depends on the type of pyoderma. The major reason for performing such tests is to confirm the diagnosis and identify the causative bacteria in order to have a rational basis for antibiotic therapy. The two most common tests are microscopic examination of pustule contents and bacterial culture and sensitivity. In most cases of superficial pyoderma, the former is as efficient as the latter in yielding information, and considerably simpler and less costly. Pustules may be opened with a 22-gauge needle or a scalpel blade and the contents collected on a cotton swab and impressions made upon a microscope slide. A rapid stain such as Diff-Quik (Harleco, Gibbstown, NJ) or a Gram's stain may be used. The authors prefer Diff-Quik, as it is both quicker and cleaner than the Gram's stain. In the majority of superficial pyodermas, pustular smears will reveal neutrophils with variable numbers of cocci. These will almost certainly be coagulase-positive *Staphylococcus* species, and the clinician can proceed with empiric choice of antibiotics, as outlined in the therapy section. However, the presence on the smear of many rod-shaped bacteria or fungal organisms warrants a culture of pustule contents. These may be taken as outlined above for the pustular smear, except that 70 percent methyl alcohol is gently dripped on to the intact pustule and allowed to dry, prior to opening. A sterile cotton swab is used to transfer the pustule contents to a culture tube or transport medium. Any superficial pyoderma that has not responded to conventional empiric antibiotic therapy should be cultured. If no pustules can be found, culturing the areas under crusts or epidermal collarettes may be attempted.

Bacterial cultures should always be performed in dogs and cats with deep pyodermas (except acne). This may be done by sterile preparation of the lesion site, followed by either full thickness skin biopsy, sterile cotton applicators introduced into draining tracts, or the sterile collection of purulent material expressed on to the surface.

Biopsy is a neglected diagnostic tool in the investigation of pyodermas. In general, any suspected deep bacterial infection should be biopsied. This is especially useful in cases of demodicosis, mycosis, or mycobacteriosis. Impression smears of any freshly excised tissues also should be made. Superficial pyodermas should be biopsied in cases of persistent pustular eruption unresponsive to conventional systemic and topical therapy.

Often a defect in an animal's immune response may be suspected. Unfortunately, there are currently no readily available, accurate tests to evaluate immune defects in dogs and cats. A complete blood count in an immune competent dog with a moderate to severe pyoderma should show an absolute neutrophilia and a lymphocyte count of 1,000 to 1,500 lymphocytes per cubic milliliter of blood. A broad-based elevation in the beta and gamma range should also be seen on a serum electrophoresis. These tests give only very general information about the immune system and are not function tests.[2]

Both superficial and deep pyodermas will occasionally be secondary to hypothyroidism. While it is beyond the scope of this chapter to review thyroid function, one point is important to remember. Thyroxine (T_4) and triiodothyronine (T_3) serum levels may vary due to illness (euthyroid sick syndrome), time of day, breed, and weather.[3,29,30] The authors recommend the use of the thyroid stimulating hormone (TSH) response test for the diagnosis of hypothyroidism. Protocol and interpretation of this test have been summarized elsewhere.[3] (See Chapter 7.)

THERAPY

Antibiotics

Once the diagnosis of pyoderma is made, the clinician must decide on an antibiotic to initiate therapy. This decision may be empirical or based on culture and sensitivity. Often empirical therapy is necessary while awaiting culture and sensitivity results. Choosing an antibiotic empirically is based on many factors, including route, cost, frequency of administration, and side effects. Perhaps the most important factor is a proven spectrum of activity against the most likely bacterial pathogen. In most pyodermas of small animals, this would be a coagulase-positive *Staphylococcus*. Table 5-2 summarizes drug dosages for various antibiotics effective in small animal pyodermas caused by coagulase-positive staphylococci. Feline abscesses due to bite wounds usually have *Pasturella multocida* as the major pathogen. In those cases ampicillin or amoxicillin are the drugs of choice.

Antibiotics empirically chosen for effectiveness against coagulase-positive staphylococci should be resistant to the beta-lactamases (such as penicillinase) which these bacteria often produce. Because of the long-term therapy usually required in pyoderma treatment, these antibiotics should be in oral form, ideally with a narrow spectrum of activity. Such antibiotics include lincomycin, erythromycin, oxacillin, and dicloxacillin. Lincomycin (Lincocin) is a very effective antibiotic in staphylococcal infections. It requires only twice daily administration, and has few side effects in small animals. Its greatest drawback is its cost. Erythromycin is less expensive, but will frequently cause vomiting. Intact enteric-coated tablets, or some of the newer capsule forms, reduce the gastric side effects. Lincomycin and erythromycin have very similar sensitivity patterns. Bacteria resistant to one of these drugs will probably be resistant to the other. Both of these drugs are less effective empirically once another antibiotic has been tried, consequently they are not recommended as second-line drugs.[31]

The beta-lactamase-resistant synthetic penicillins such as oxacillin and dicloxacillin are excellent agents for staphylococcal pyodermas. Oxacillin has

Table 5-2. Systemic Dosage Levels of Antibiotics Useful in the Management of Pyodermas Caused by Coagulase-Positive *Staphyloccus* sp

Generic Name	Route of Administration	Suggested Dosage Level/kg of Body Weight
Erythromycin	PO[f]	10 to 15 mg, every 8 hr
Lincomycin[a]	PO	22 mg, every 12 hr
Oxacillin[b]	PO	22 mg, every 8 hr
Chloramphenicol	PO	50 mg, every 8 hr
Trimethoprim-sulfadiazine[c]	PO	2.2 mg, (based on trimethoprim fraction) every 12 hr
Cephalexin[d]	PO	22 mg, every 12 hr
Amoxicillin-clavulanic acid[e]	PO	13.75 mg, every 12 hr
Cefadroxil[b]	PO	22 mg, every 12 hr

[a] The Upjohn Co, Kalamazoo, Mich.
[b] Bristol Laboratories, Syracuse, NY
[c] Burroughs Wellcome Co, Research Triangle Park, NC
[d] Eli Lilly and Co, Indianapolis, Ind.
[e] Beecham Laboratories, Bristol, TN
[f] PO = per os

been used frequently by the authors with rare resistance or side effects.[7] Vomiting and inappetance are occasionally noted. Food interferes with absorption, therefore these drugs should be administered 1 hour before or after eating.[32] Initial observations suggest that oxacillin may be more efficacious than dicloxacillin in the treatment of canine pyodermas. The reason for this is not known.[8] This group of antibiotics tends to be moderately expensive.

Broad spectrum antibiotics useful in pyoderma therapy include chloramphenicol, the cephalosporins, trimethoprim-potentiated sulfonamides, and clavulanic acid-potentiated amoxicillin. Chloramphenicol is the only drug of this group requiring three doses daily; the others are administered twice a day. Chloramphenicol has few side effects in the dog, though occasionally vomiting and/or diarrhea is seen. The idiosyncratic aplastic anemias seen in persons have not been reported in the dog. Occasionally a mild reversible anemia may be associated with prolonged administration.[3] Chloramphenicol may cause a more severe anemia as well as anorexia and depression in cats.[13] Because chloramphenicol reversibly causes depression of liver enzymes used to detoxify many drugs, barbituate anesthesia may be prolonged[33] and normal anticonvulsant dosages of primidone may cause extreme depression.[34] Trimethoprim-potentiated sulfonamides (Tribrissen) are also relatively safe drugs. Keratoconjunctivitis and immune hypersensitivity disorders have been reported side effects.[7,35,36] Both chloramphenicol and the trimethoprim-sulfas are relatively inexpensive drugs. Cephalosporins such as cephalexin (Keflex) and cefadroxil (Cefa-Tabs) are very effective antibiotics in staphylococcal pyodermas. They have few side effects, though false-positive Coomb's tests have been noted in human beings.[37] Because of an emerging pattern of cephalosporin resistance, these drugs should be reserved for life-threatening infections, or pyodermas which fail to respond to other antibiotics. They are among the most expensive drugs in pyoderma therapy.

Clavulanic acid-potentiated amoxicillin (Clavamox) is a new concept in antibiotic therapy. It combines a semisynthetic penicillin (amoxicillin) with clavulanic acid, a substance whose structure greatly resembles the beta-lactam ring found in the penicillins. Because of this similarity in structure, clavulanic acid fits into the binding site of the beta-lactamase molecule. This inactivates the enzyme, and allows the amoxicillin to destroy the bacteria. Experimental data on the use of this drug in treating pyodermas is encouraging.[38]

Aminoglycosides such as gentamycin and kanamycin are potent bactericidal antibiotics with a broad range of activity against gram-negative and gram-positive bacteria. Because of the nephrotoxicity and occasional ototoxicity associated with these drugs, as well as their requirement of parenteral administration, they have little place in the therapy of most pyodermas. An exception would be in the treatment of deep pyoderma associated with demodicosis or immunodeficiency where *Pseudomonas* has been isolated and/or sepsis is suspected.

Certain antibiotics are usually not effective against coagulase-positive *Staphylococcus* and are poor empirical choices in pyodermas. These include penicillin, amoxicillin, ampicillin, and the tetracylines.[31] However, should *Staphylococcus* be isolated which is sensitive to one of these drugs, such an antibiotic may then be used. In mixed infections where the bacterial isolates are not all sensitive to one antibiotic the drug effective against *Staphylococcus* should be used. Because the *Staphylococcus* creates an environment favorable to the growth of other bacteria, its elimination is usually sufficient for clinical improvement.[2]

Antibiotic Dosage and Duration of Therapy

Treatment failures in pyodermas are often due to improper dosage or insufficient duration of treatment. Dosage errors are especially common in small or large dogs. All dogs should be accurately weighed to determine dosage. Attempting to save owner expense on a large dog by prescribing less than the recommended dosage of a drug usually results in poor clinical response, development of resistant bacteria, and client dissatisfaction. Over-dosage of small dogs due to the unavailability of pills or capsules of correct dose may result in toxicity. Human pediatric elixirs are useful in such situations.[2]

The duration of antibiotic therapy should be long enough to ensure clinical cure rather than brief remission. This is best done by maintaining the animal on antibiotics for a minimum of 7 to 14 days beyond clinical cure. It should be the veterinarian, rather than the owner, who makes the decision regarding discontinuation of therapy. As stated above, some pyodermas are difficult to cure, even with long-term antibiotic therapy. While a thorough search for underlying causes should always be performed, the clinician should be aware that some cases will need life-long antibiotics. Only in these rare cases should a gradual reduction in frequency of administration of the antibiotic be attempted once clinical remission is achieved. This is done solely for economic purposes. Owners should be aware that recurrence of the disease or the emergence of resistant strains is a possibility. However, in some cases with financial constraints, gradual reduction of drug frequency may be the only alternative to euthanasia.

Topical Therapy

Topical therapy is a valuable adjunct in the treatment of pyodermas. Antibacterial agents in shampoos, gels, and whirlpool baths are especially useful. On the other hand, creams and ointments containing antibiotics have little place in the therapy of pyodermas. This is due to the large surface area usually involved, cost, and animals' tendency to lick such medications off the skin.

Benzoyl peroxide (Oxydex, Pyoben) is an excellent antibacterial agent with an additional follicular flushing effect.[39] It is also useful as a degreaser, debrider, and keratolytic agent.[39] Veterinary formulations are available as 2.5 and 3 percent shampoos and 5 percent gels. The drug is often the only therapy needed for intertrigo, puppy pyoderma, and "acne." The gels are primarily used in long-term management of the latter condition. Erythema, pruritus, and pain are occasionally seen with the use of benzoyl peroxide, especially in cats.[3,39] These reactions have been noted more frequently with the use of generic benzoyl peroxide preparations.[39] Higher concentrations of benzoyl peroxide shampoo at 5 or 10 percent should not be used, as they tend to be more irritating with no advantage over the 2.5 to 3 percent formulas.[39]

Topical antibacterial agents such as povidone-iodine (Betadine) and chlorhexidine (Nolvasan) are excellent for warm water soaks and whirlpool treatments. Six to 8 ounces or more of a solution concentrate are adequate in a 20- to 30-gallon tub. The whirlpools or soaks are administered twice daily as an adjunct to systemic antibiotic therapy. These treatments are especially helpful in cases of deep pyoderma. Povidone-iodine may be irritating to some cats.

Immunotherapy

Various medications have been used in both persons and animals in an attempt to stimulate the immune system in chronic infections. In veterinary dermatology either bacterins or levamisole have most commonly been used. The efficacy of any of these products will vary with each case. Dramatic improvement in one animal may be followed by dismal results in others, and the clinician should advise the owner of the variability of clinical response. These drugs should be used primarily in those cases of chronic superficial or deep pyodermas in which the only alternatives are life-long antibiotics or euthanasia. None of the medications currently used have been shown to be clinically ef-

Table 5-3. Protocol for Staphoid-AB (50–50 with Saline)

Day	Dose (ml)	ID[a]	SC[b]	IM[c]
1	0.25	0.1	0.15	0.00
2	0.50	0.1	0.20	0.20
3	0.75	0.1	0.30	0.35
4	1.00	0.1	0.45	0.45
5	1.25	0.1	0.55	0.60
12	1.50	0.1	0.70	0.70
19	1.75	0.1	0.80	0.85
26	2.00	0.1	0.95	0.95
Booster given every 30 days at same dosage as 26th day				

[a] ID = intradermal
[b] SC = subcutaneous
[c] IM = intramuscular
(Adapted from Baker E: Staphylococcal disease. Vet Clin North Am 4:107, 1974 and Kirk RW: Systemic therapy. p. 454. In Kirk RW (ed): Current Veterinary Therapy VIII. WB Saunders, Philadelphia, 1983.)

fective against the immune suppression thought to cause generalized demodicosis in dogs.

The two most common bacterins used are Staphoid-AB (Jensal Laboratories)[40] and Staphage Lysate (Delmont Laboratories).[21,41,42] The former is a staphylococcal cell wall antigen and toxin mixture. The latter is produced by lysing cultures of *Staphylococcus aureus* with a *Staphylococcus* bacteriophage. After ultrafiltration the lysate contains both antigenic fractions of the bacteria and the active bacteriophage.[41] Both of these drugs must be given parenterally. Suggested dosage schemes are shown in Tables 5-3 and 5-4. While the initial Staphoid A-B protocol takes less time to complete, Staphage Lysate is easier to administer. Side effects are uncommon, but pain, inflammatory reactions and sterile abscesses may be seen at the injection site. The exact mechanism of immune stimulation by bacterins is unclear. It is thought to be due to a favorable effect on cell-mediated sensitivity to staphylococci.[21,41] An improvement in T-cell function has been shown in dogs with *Staphylococcus* pyoderma treated with Staphage Lysate.[21]

Table 5-4. Staph Lysate Schedule for Treatment of Pyodermas

Week	Staph Lysate (ml, SC)[a]
1	0.25
2	0.50
3	0.75
4	1.00[b]

[a] SC = subcutaneous
[b] Can be increased to 2.0 ml weekly if necessary.
(Adapted from Kirk RW: Systemic therapy. p. 454. In Kirk RW (ed): Current Veterinary Therapy VIII. WB Saunders, Philadelphia, 1983.)

Levamisole (Levasole) is an antihelmintic compound with immunotherapeutic properties. Though the exact mechanism of action is not understood, research studies show a restoration of normal function to lymphocytes and phagocytes from immunocompromised hosts. The T-lymphocytes in particular increase in number and improve in function.[43] Any beneficial effect in pyodermas is thought to be due to the stimulation of the cell-mediated branch of the immune system. The drug itself is not toxic to bacteria. Levamisole should be given orally, as parenteral administration has caused severe side effects in small animals. An accurate immune-stimulating dosage is not well defined for dogs and cats. This may be critical, as a ''window effect'' exists, with doses higher or lower than the optimum having no effect, or even causing immune suppression.[21,44] The authors' current dosage is 2.2 mg/kg, given 3 times weekly. Side effects, though uncommon, include vomiting, diarrhea, and neurological signs such as seizures and behavioral changes. Granulocytopenia and allergic skin reactions have been seen in humans.[41,44]

Other drugs which may in the future hold a promise of immune stimulation are thymus fractions such as thymosin,[45] avridine,[46] and bacterins produced from bacteria other than *Staphylococcus*. Further studies are needed before these medications can be recommended.

REFERENCES

1. Weinberg AN, Swartz MN: General consideration of bacterial diseases. p. 1419. Fitzpatrick TB, Eisen AZ, Wolff K, et al (eds): Dermatology in General Medicine. McGraw-Hill, New York, 1979
2. Ihrke PJ: The management of canine pyodermas. p. 505. In Kirk RW (ed): Current Veterinary Therapy VIII. WB Saunders, Philadelphia, 1983
3. Muller GH, Kirk RW, Scott DW: Small Animal Dermatology. WB Saunders, Philadelphia, 1983
4. White SD, Ihrke PJ, Stannard AA, et al: Occurrance of *Staphylococcus aureus* on the clinically normal canine hair coat. Am J Vet Res 44:332, 1983
5. Marples RR: Fundamentals of cutaneous microbiology. p. 482. In Moschella SL, Pillsbury DM, Hurley J (eds): Dermatology. Vol 1. WB Saunders, Philadelphia, 1975
6. Berg JN, Wendell DE, Vogelweid C, et al: Identification of the major coagulase-positive *Staphylococcus* sp. of dogs as *Staphylococcus intermedius*. Am J Vet Res 45:1307, 1984
7. Ihrke PJ: Therapeutic strategies involving antimicrobial treatment of the skin in small animals. J Am Vet Med Assoc 185:1165, 1984
8. Ihrke PJ, Schwartzman RM, McGinley KJ, et al: Microbiology of normal and seborrheic canine skin. Am J Vet Res 39:1487, 1978
9. White SD, Ihrke PJ, Stannard AA, et al: Cutaneous atypical mycobacteriosis in cats. J Am Vet Med Assoc 182:1218, 1983
10. Kunkle GA, Gulbas NK, Fadok V, et al: Rapidly growing mycobacteria as a cause of cutaneous granulomas—report of 5 cases. J Am Anim Hosp Assoc 19:513, 1983
11. Carakostas MC, Miller RI, Woodward MG, et al: Subcutaneous dermatophilosis in a cat. J Am Vet Med Assoc 185:675, 1984

12. Reinke SI, Stannard AA, Ihrke PJ, et al: Histopathologic features of pyotraumatic dermatitis. J Am Vet Med Assoc. In press.
13. Scott DW: Feline dermatology: a monograph; bacterial disorders. J Am Anim Hosp Assoc 16:340, 1980
14. Swartz MN, Weinberg AN: Infections due to gram-positive bacteria. p. 1426. In Fitzpatrick TB, Eisen AZ, Wolf K, et al (eds): Dermatology in General Medicine, McGraw-Hill, New York, 1979
15. Ihrke PJ, Stannard AA, Ardans AA, et al: Pemphigus foliaceus in dogs: A review of 37 cases. J Am Vet Med Assoc 186:59, 1985
16. White SD: Food hypersensitivity in dogs: A review of 27 cases. J Am Vet Med Assoc 188:695, 1986
17. Willemse TA: Report, American Academy of Veterinary Dermatology Annual Meeting, San Antonio, Texas, April 1983
18. Scott DW: Canine pododermatitis. p. 467. In Kirk RW (ed): Current Veterinary Therapy VII. WB Saunders, Philadelphia, 1980
19. Brennan KE, Ihrke PJ: Grass awn migration in dogs and cats: a retrospective study of 182 cases. J Am Vet Med Assoc 182:1201, 1983
20. White SD, Stannard AA: Canine demodicosis. p. 484. In Kirk RW (ed): Current Veterinary Therapy VIII. WB Saunders, Philadelphia, 1983
21. Rosser EJ, Jr: Report, American Academy of Veterinary Dermatology. Annual Meeting, Las Vegas, Nevada, April 1982
22. White SD: Cutaneous Mycobacterioses. p. 529 In Kirk RW (ed): Current Veterinary Therapy IX. WB Saunders, Philadelphia, 1986
23. Parodi A, Fontaine M, Brion A, et al: Mycobacterioses in the domestic carnivora: present day epidemiology of tuberculosis in the dog and the cat. J Small Anim Pract 6:307, 1965
24. Brown LR, Macy CD, Williams SE: A non-tuberculous granuloma in cats. NZ Vet J 10:7, 1962
25. Pattyn SR, Portaels F: *In vitro* cultivation and classification of *Mycobacterium lepraemurium*. Int J Lepr 48:7, 1980
26. McIntosh DW: Feline leprosy: a review of forty-four cases from Western Canada. Can Vet J 23:291, 1982
27. Wilkinson GT: Diseases of cats. p. 19. Vade Mecum No. 3, University of Sydney Post Graduate Foundation in Veterinary Science, Sydney, 1984
28. Runyon EH: Anonymous mycobacteria in pulmonary disease. Med Clin North Am 43:273, 1959
29. Ferguson DC: Canine hypothyroidism. J Am Vet Med Assoc 178:1028, 1981
30. Nachreiner RF: Laboratory diagnosis of endocrine diseases. Proc Am Anim Hosp Assoc 45:55, 1981
31. Ihrke PJ, Halliwell REW, Deubler MJ: Canine pyodermas. p. 513. In Kirk RW (ed): Current Veterinary Therapy VI. WB Saunders, Philadelphia, 1977
32. Marshal AB: Antibiotic therapy of small animal dermatitis. Br Vet Dermatol Newsletter 2:45, 1980
33. Adams HR: Acute adverse effects of antibiotics. J Am Vet Med Assoc 166:331, 1975
34. Campbell CL: Primidone intoxication associated with concurrent use of chloramphenicol. J Am Vet Med Assoc 182:992, 1983
35. Werner LL, Bright JM: Drug-induced immune hypersensitivity disorders in two dogs treated with trimethoprim-sulfadiazine. J Am Anim Hosp Assoc 19:783, 1983
36. Geiger U, Werner LL, Millichamp NJ, et al: Sulfadiazine-induced allergy in six Doberman pinschers. J Am Vet Med Assoc. 186:479, 1985

37. Molthan L, Reidenberg MM, Eichman MF: Positive direct Coomb's test due to cephalothin. N Engl J Med 277:123, 1967
38. Boon RJ, Beale AS, Comber KR, et al: Distribution of amoxicillin and clavulanic acid in infected animals and efficacy against experimental infections. Antimicrob Agent Chemotherapy 22:369, 1982
39. Ihrke PJ: Topical therapy—specific topical pharmacologic agents, dermatologic therapy, part II. Compend Cont Educ Pract Vet 2:156, 1980
40. Baker E: Staphylococcal disease. Vet Clin North Am 4:107, 1974
41. Kirk RW: Systemic Therapy. p. 454. In Kirk RW (ed): Current Veterinary Therapy VIII. WB Saunders, Philadelphia, 1983
42. Anderson RK: Canine pododermatitis. Compend Cont Educ Pract Vet 2:361, 1980
43. Symoens J, Rosenthal M: Levamisole in the modulation of the immune response: the current experimental and clinical state. J Reticuloendothel Soc 21:176, 1977
44. Brunner CJ, Muscoplat CC: Immunomodulary effects of levamisole. J Am Vet Med Assoc 176:1159, 1980
45. Schulof RS, Low TLK, Thurman GB, et al: Thymosins and other hormones of the thymus gland. p. 191. In: The Lymphocyte. Alan R. Liss, New York, 1981
46. Roth JA, Kaeberle ML: Enhancement of lymphocyte blastogenesis and neutrophil function by avridine in dexamethasone-treated and non-treated cattle. Am J Vet Res 46:53, 1985

6 Cutaneous Fungal Diseases

Carol S. Foil

Diseases covered in this chapter are classified according to whether they affect mainly superficial cutaneous structures, deep dermal and subcutaneous tissues, or multiple organ systems. The actinomycetes *Nocardia* and *Actinomyces* are also included. The mycotic diseases all have the potential for causing highly varied clinical syndromes depending on host factors and varying pathogenicity among isolates. A section on pathophysiology is included for each disease so that the practitioner may better predict and understand the clinical spectrum of disease.

A section on antifungal chemotherapy is included at the end of the chapter.

SUPERFICIAL FUNGAL INFECTIONS

Dermatophytosis

The etiology of dermatophytosis in domestic dogs and cats is both simple to cover and complex. Simply, the vast majority of clinical cases in pets are caused by one of three species of fungi: *Microsporum canis, Trichophyton mentagrophytes*, or the geophilic species *Microsporum gypseum*. In cats, 98 percent of cases are caused by *M. canis*. However 20 other species of keratinophilic fungi have been documented in cases of ringworm or in surveys of asymptomatic animals. These include species more commonly pathogenic in man (e.g., *Epidermophyton floccosum*, *Trichophyton rubrum*) or in other animals (e.g., *Trichophyton mentagrophytes* var *erinacei, T. verrucosum, Microsporum gallinae* and *M. nanum*) and geophilic species (e.g., *T. terrestre*).

For each species of dermatophyte that infects human and domestic animals there are unique epidemiologic features. However, the clinical symptoms are quite similar by virtue of a similar pathogenesis for most, once infection has been established.

Pathophysiology

With the exception of *Epidermophyton floccosum*, dermatophyte infections in dogs and cats are infections of the hair shaft and follicle. The lesions that are seen are the result of the loss of infected hairs and of inflammation in and around infected follicles. Inflammation in infected hair follicles and cessation of hair shaft growth quickly brings an end to the dermatophyte infection in those follicles. The classical ring-shaped, spreading lesion of dermatophytosis results as adjacent follicles become infected and follicles in the center of the lesion are cleared of ringworm. As specific humoral and cellular immunity develops, the infection is brought under control rather rapidly in most cases without any intervention. However, there are many variations on this classical pathogenesis. Factors influencing the severity, appearance, and outcome of dermatophyte infections include the species, age and health of the patient, and the pathogenicity of the infecting fungus. Young animals of any species are much more susceptible to severe dermatophyte infections than are adults. Diseases or drugs which interfere with normal host protective mechanisms can be associated with severe dermatophytosis. Also, geophilic and anthropophilic species, once established in the skin of dogs and cats, typically elicit more severe inflammatory reactions than does the relatively host-adapted *Microsporum canis*. Indeed, many cats with widespread hair loss associated with *M. canis* infections of the hair shaft exhibit very little inflammatory skin disease. As inflammation is very detrimental to the fungal infection, these relatively tolerant hosts often develop persistent, if mild, infections.

Clinical Signs

The most consistent clinical sign in dog and cat dermatophytosis is one or more patches of alopecia (Fig. 6-1). There is usually some degree of scaling associated with the hair loss. The other signs and symptoms are highly varied and depend to a great extent on the nature of host-fungus interactions and the amount of inflammation elicited. Table 6-1 outlines some of the clinical syndromes caused by dermatophyte fungi and associated features (Figs. 6-2–6-5).

Dermatophytosis is difficult to diagnose by clinical signs, not only because of the variety of syndromes that can be caused by dermatophytes, but also because there are several other clinical syndromes which mimic the classical ringworm lesion. The most important of these in the dog is the superficial spreading lesion of staphylococcal folliculitis. Some staphylococcal infections of dogs are associated with large erythematous and scaling patches with central

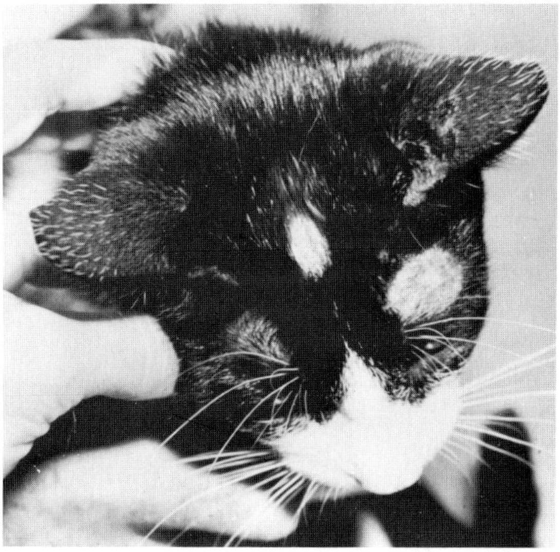

Fig. 6-1. Cat with *Microsporum canis* infection exhibited by circumscribed patches of hair loss on face. Note the patch of crust and scale on the pinna.

healing and hyperpigmentation. This syndrome appears to be commonly misdiagnosed as dermatophytosis. A negative culture for dermatophytes and response to antibiotic therapy will confirm the bacterial cause of such lesions. Other syndromes that can mimic ringworm include demodicosis, seborrheic dermatitis, contact dermatitis and neurodermatitis in cats.

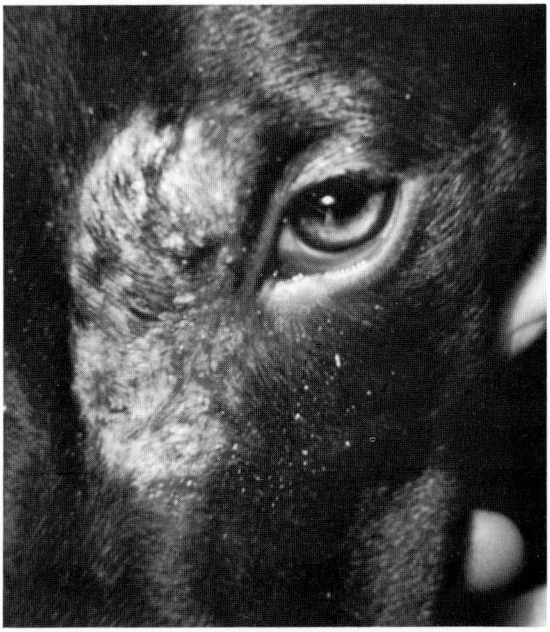

Fig. 6-2. Doberman puppy with localized papular folliculitis caused by *Microsporum canis* infection. This lesion is clinically indistinguishable from localized demodicosis.

Table 6-1. Characteristics of Some Clinical Syndromes Associated With Dermatophytosis in Dogs and Cats

Syndrome	Species Affected	Commonly Associated Fungi	Comments
Classical ringworm	D, C	1	Circular patch of alopecia, scale
Irregular alopecia	C	1, 3	Especially long-haired cats
Miliary dermatitis	C	1	Should always be considered
Folliculitis/furunculosis	D	1, 2, 3	May be localized or generalized
Facial dermatitis	D	3	Mimics pemphigus, DLE
Paronychia/Onychomycosis	D, C	2, 3	Rare
Kerion	D	2, 3	Highly inflammatory, single or multiple
Pseudomycetoma/granuloma	D, C	1, 2, 3	Rare
Asymptomatic carrier	C	1	Especially long-haired cats

1, *M. canis*; 2, *M. gypseum*; 3, *T. Mentagrophytes.*

Diagnosis

Diagnosis is best made by culture. For the practitioner this process has been made much simpler by the availability of the Dermatophyte Test Medium (DTM). There are many possibilities, however, for both false-positive and false-negative findings using the DTM, so that it is important to adhere closely to several principles of use:

1. Clip and clean lesions to be cultured. This greatly reduces contaminant growth on the DTM which may cause false positives. Clip hair to 0.5 cm and pat clean with an alcohol sponge, then dry. Clipping hair will also allow for a larger sample to be cultured.
2. Sample several lesions and include intrafollicular portions of the hair shaft and some scale. Choose hair that is broken, that is near active inflam-

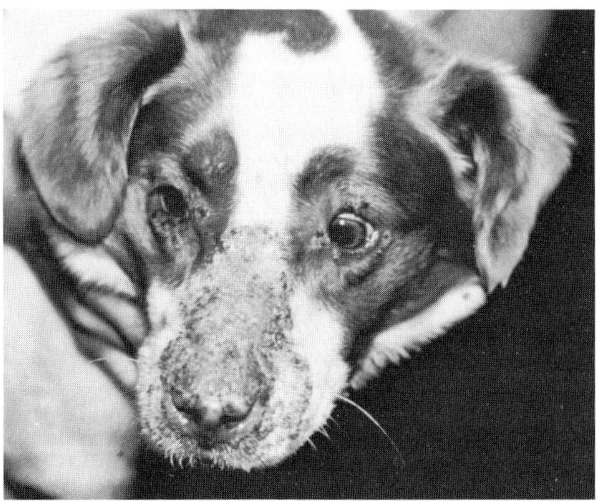

Fig. 6-3. Severe crusting and scaling facial dermatitis due to *Trichophyton mentagrophytes.* Such cases may be mistakenly diagnosed as autoimmune skin diseases. (Courtesy Dr. William Miller, Cornell University, Ithaca, NY.)

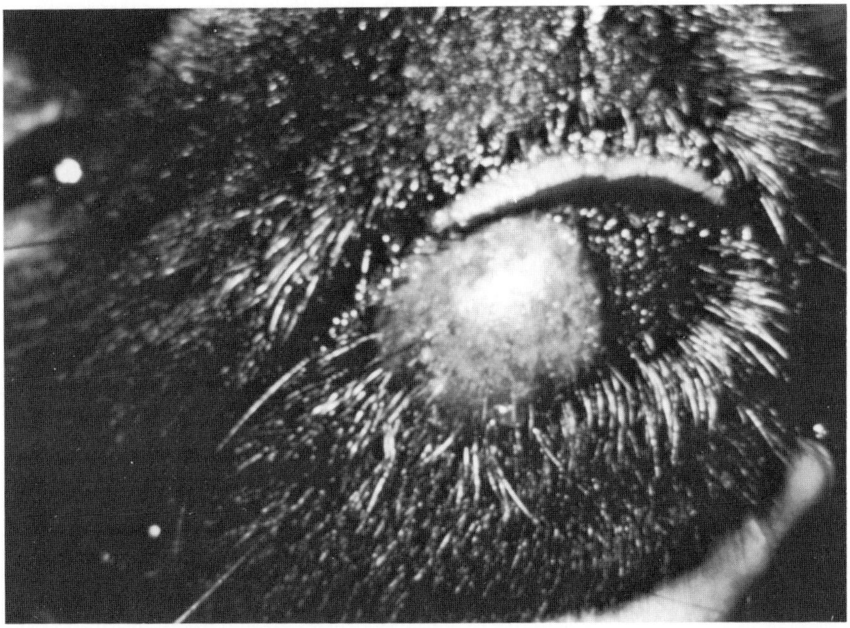

Fig. 6-4. Cutaneous nodule in the lower lip of dog. This lesion is a kerion caused by a dermatophyte. (Courtesy Dr. Peter Ihrke, University of California, Davis.)

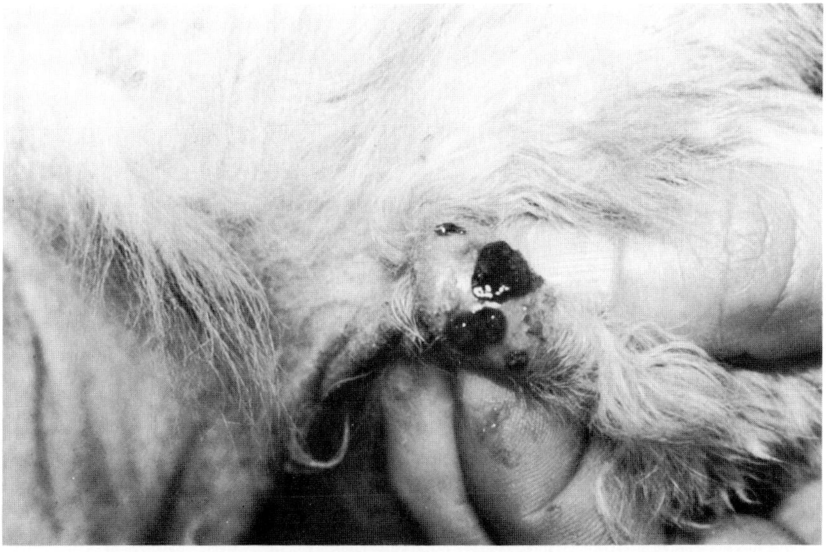

Fig. 6-5. A pseudomycetoma in the axillary fold of a Persian cat with generalized dermatophytosis. This lesion was a manifestation of a *Microsporum canis* infection. (Courtesy Dr. Gail Kunkle, University of Florida, Gainesville, FL.)

matory lesions, and, when possible, use hair which is Wood's lamp positive. Try to avoid putting exudate or antiseptics on the DTM.

3. Leave DTM loosely capped and at room temperature, sheltered from UV light.

4. Inspect DTM samples daily. The color change should occur simultaneously with cottony fungal growth. If it is observed some time after fungal growth has begun, it may be a false-positive.

5. After 7 to 10 days inspect samples of the colony microscopically using lactophenol cotton blue mounting medium. Try to confirm DTM results by identifying the typical macroconidia of the dermatophyte species. Failing this, refer the specimen to a diagnostic laboratory for identification. This information can be important in case management.

6. Discard any specimen which contains blue-, green- or black-pigmented fungi. These are contaminants.

Another diagnostic method is microscopic inspection of hair and scales. 10 percent potassium hydroxide (KOH) is used to clear and mount hair and scale collected from lesions (Figs. 6-6 and 6-7). Even in experienced hands, this technique is diagnostic in only 10 to 50 percent of confirmed cases. It is a time-consuming method and false-positives are possible when saprophytic fungal species are present on an animal's hair coat (Fig. 6-7).

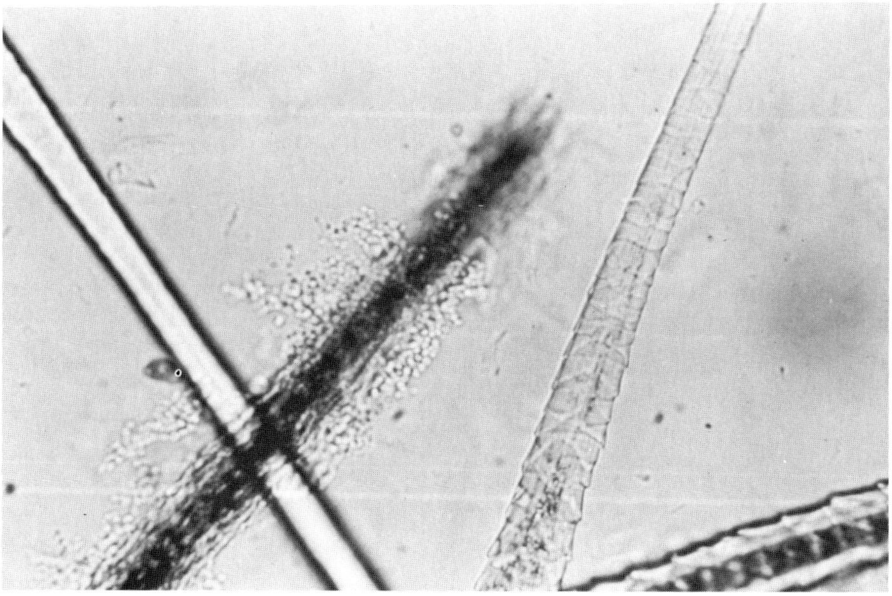

Fig. 6-6. Microscopic preparation of a dermatophyte infected hair after clearing in 10 percent KOH. Note the masses of translucent spores surrounding the broken end of the hair shaft. (Courtesy Dr. Gail Kunkle, University of Florida, Gainesville, FL.)

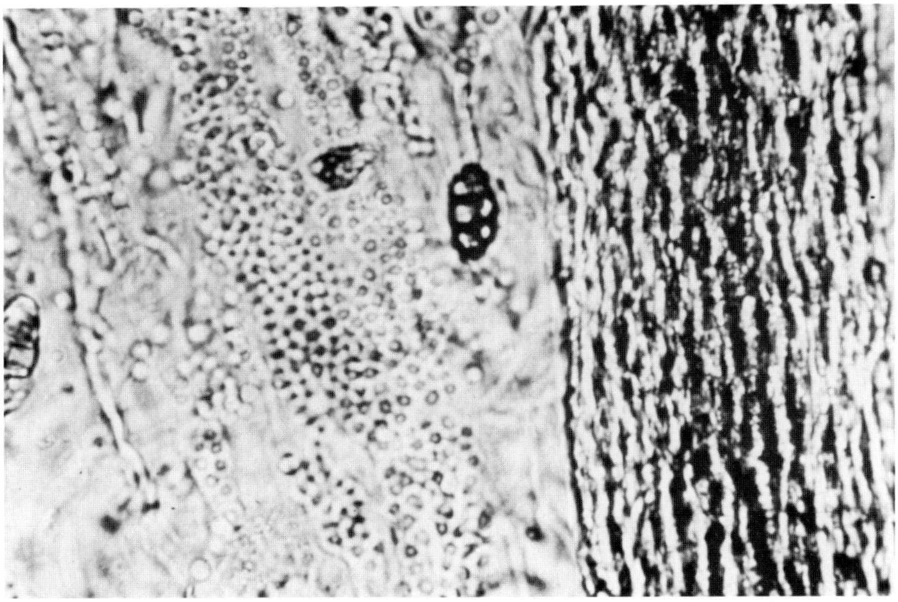

Fig. 6-7. High magnification photomicrograph of a hair shaft on the left with masses of small spherical ectothrix spores. Note the hyphal elements on the periphery. The large multiloculated thick-walled spores are saprophytes. Dermatophytes never form macrospores in tissue.

Wood's light examination may allow a tentative preliminary diagnosis to be made in *Microsporum canis* infections. This is the only common dermatophyte which causes fluorescence and it is positive only 50 percent of the time. False-positives are possible when clinicians are not familiar with the true bright apple-green fluorescence produced in *M. canis* infected hairs. In general, do not rely on this technique unless several hairs can be found on each lesion.

In some situations it is necessary to attempt dermatophyte cultures from asymptomatic cats. This can be useful in trying to eliminate dermatophytosis from a multicat household, in finding the potential source of infection in a human case of dermatophytosis, and in following up therapy, especially in a long-haired cat. The technique preferred by the author is adapted from MacKenzie (Dawson and Noddle, 1968). Clients are asked to purchase a new toothbrush for each animal to be cultured. The toothbrush is used to brush the hair coat, next to the skin, in several sites on the cat's body. The collected hair and scales are then innoculated directly onto DTM by impressing the toothbrush bristles into the medium in several sites. Animals who are not shedding enough spores to be cultured in this way are not likely sources of infection for others.

Table 6-2. Topical Therapy in Dermatophytosis

Product	Brand Name	Administration	Comments
Providone-iodine	Betadine solution	1:4 in water once daily	Irritating, sensitizing
Chlorhexidine	Nolvasan solution	2% solution daily	
	Nolvasan shampoo (Fort Dodge)	Bathe every 5 days	
Lime-sulfur	Lym Dyp (DVM)	2% solution every 5 to 7 days	Odorous, not for white animals
Captan	Orthocide spray (Ortho Chemical)	2% (2 tbs/gal)	
Miconazole	Conofite cream lotion (Pitman-Moore)	Apply b.i.d.	For localized lesions
Clotrimazole	Veltrim (Haver-Lockhart)	Apply b.i.d.	For localized lesions
	Lotrimin (Schering)		

Treatment

In some form, topical therapy is always indicated in dog and cat dermatophytosis. Clipping of affected areas (including the whole body in some cases) and application of topical treatments will remove infected scales, crusts, and hairs and reduce the potential for spread of infection.

There are several antiseptic and fungicidal antibiotic preparations useful in the treatment of dog and cat dermatophytosis. These are described in Table 6-2. Antiseptic preparations include a wide variety of agents which are available as solutions or creams or incorporated into shampoos. Dip solutions and shampoos are useful for the treatment of extensive lesions and are less likely to produce a mycologic cure than are creams or lotions containing antimycotic antibiotics. They are used as adjunctive therapy with systemic treatment. Useful antifungal antibiotics include several imidazole derivatives. Those available in the United States are listed in Table 6-2. In Europe, several other imidazoles are being tested or manufactured for human and veterinary use. Thiabendazole is also available in a lotion in combination with an antibacterial agent and a corticosteroid (Tresaderm, MSD AgVet). This preparation may be used for singular, highly inflammed ringworm lesions on otherwise healthy dogs and cats. Clotrimazole and miconazole preparations are highly effective agents for treatment of localized dermatophytosis. These agents occasionally cause a contact dermatitis.

Systemic therapy is recommended in all nonlocalized dermatophytosis and in any type of infection in long-haired cats or immunocompromised patients. Griseofulvin is the treatment of choice when systemic therapy of dermatophytosis is indicated.

Griseofulvin is a fungistatic antibiotic whose spectrum of action is limited to dermatophytes. Some resistance of ringworm isolates has been documented in *M. canis* and *Trichophyton* sp isolates, but this situation is probably rare in veterinary medicine. Treatment failures are more often due to erratic absorption and underdosing of the drug. Gastrointestinal absorption of griseofulvin is enhanced by administration with a fat-containing meal or by formulations using polyethylene glycol (PEG). Particle size (micronization) also affects oral absorption. Divided dosage regimens also improve absorption of the drug.

There have been widely varying doses published for griseofulvin in veterinary medicine. Microsize griseofulvin is available in tablet formation to veterinarians (Fulvicin-U/F, Schering) or as a pediatric suspension labelled for human use (Grifulvin V, Ortho). Ultramicrosize griseofulvin in PEG tablets are marketed for human use in the United States (GrisPEG, Dorsey). The dose recommended by the author is 50-120 mg/kg for microsize formulations and 10-20 mg/kg for ultramicrosize in PEG. Griseofulvin should be administered in divided doses daily until the patient is rendered symptom-free and culture-negative. This usually requires 4 to 6 weeks of treatment. Relapses are common in long-haired cats. Griseofulvin is teratogenic and causes gastrointestinal disturbances, drug eruptions, hepatotoxicity, and bone marrow suppression. It should not be used except in culture-confirmed dermatologic diseases. When used in cattery situations, breeding must be suspended until mycologic cure has been effected.

Ketoconazole is a broad-spectrum fungistatic synthetic imidazole antibiotic. Its use is limited to severe chronic cases of dermatophytosis caused by griseofulvin-resistant isolates. The recommended dose is 10 mg/kg. Other features of this drug are discussed elsewhere.

Vaccination with killed Trichophyton preparations is widely used in other parts of the world to control epidemic ringworm in cattle. There has been interest in development of an *M. canis* vaccine for use in catteries, but no preparation is currently approved for this use in the United States.

One report of the use of hyperthermia to resolve ringworm lesions has been made in the veterinary literature. As this approach would be applicable only to localized lesions, which are often self-resolving, there will probably be little use of this treatment method in the future.

Management of Dermatophytosis in the Cattery

Once dermatophytosis has been diagnosed in one member of a multi-cat household, or in any human contact of those cats, all of the cats in the household must be suspected as carriers until proven otherwise. Queens who bear litters with affected kittens should be especially suspect as asymptomatic carriers. Especially in long-haired cats, the incidence of asymptomatic carrier states can be quite high. The following provides a guideline for elimination of dermatophytosis from a cattery.

Treatment of Individual Cats. All cats identified as infected must be treated rigorously. This is true whether the animal has lesions or is an asymptomatic carrier. Long-haired cats should be kept clipped off throughout the course of therapy. Therapy should include both topical and systemic treatment and should continue until the animal is culture-negative. As griseofulvin is reliably teratogenic, treatment necessitates cessation of breeding activity. Griseofulvin probably adversely affects semen quality in male cats. Both males and females can be safely and effectively replaced into breeding once treatment has stopped. Any shortcuts in these procedures can lead to persistence of the infection in the colony.

Identification of Carriers and Retesting During Therapy. The Mackenzie toothbrush technique should be used to screen all cats for carrier status and to retest cats who are receiving therapy (see previous section). It should also be used to screen new cats to be introduced into the household. Cats can be placed into affected and unaffected groups on the basis of the culture results, although any negative queen who has had affected litters should be recultured if negative the first time.

Segregation of Affected and Unaffected Cats. Culture-negative cats should be housed in separate quarters and all grooming implements and equipment should be kept separately. Ideally, airflow should be separate or at least there should be no unfiltered airflow from affected to unaffected areas. Handlers should take care to use clean coveralls or to change clothes before moving from affected to unaffected areas. New cats should be completely quarantined until culture results are available.

Cleaning the Environment. Dermatophyte spores are liberated from broken and shedding hairs of infected cats. Spores are extremely long-lived. Therefore, environmental cleanup is necessary. Household bleach or chlorhexidine may be used as disinfectants. Vacuuming and cleaning up corners and other sites where hair has accumulated are very important. Air filters should be changed. Clothing and bedding should be laundered with bleach if possible.

Other Comments. The preceeding protocol is expensive and constitutes a major upheaval in a cattery to be successful, and it requires a highly motivated client. The author does not routinely recommend eradication procedures when dermatophytosis has first been recognized in a cattery. Most cattery owners will eventually come to the conclusion that elimination is the best course when they are provided with the proper information on dermatophytosis.

Cutaneous Candidiasis, Pityrosporum Dermatitis

Both *Candida albicians* and *Malassezia* (*Pityrosporum*) *pachydermatis* have been implicated as rare causes of superficial regional dermatosis in dogs. Both organisms are yeasts which reproduce by unicellular budding. Candida may form pseudohyphae and true hyphae under some conditions, particularly in tissue. *Candida albicans* can be considered part of the normal flora of the lower gastrointestinal tract and the perianal skin in many species, although this has not been studied in the dog. *Malassezia pachydermatis* is part of the normal flora in the ear of dogs.

Pathophysiology

Conditions which may lead to colonization of the skin by these organisms are not well-known for dogs, as few cases have been studied. Some reports of candidal dermatitis following prolonged antibiotic or corticosteroid therapy have been made. One case was shown to have depressed T-cell function by lymphocyte blastogenesis testing. Another case was reported as a superinfection in an undiagnosed case of severe hyperkeratosis. In the only report of a large series of dermatoses associated with *Malassezia*, no predisposing cause was proposed. Experimentally, a self-limiting candidiasis of the skin may be created in dogs by overhydrating the skin under occlusive dressings and exposing the skin to viable cultures. In humans, chronic mucocutaneous candidiasis is almost invariably associated with an immunoincompetent state in the patient or with conditions that lower the pH of moist membranes or chronically moistened skin.

Clinical Signs

Candidiasis has been described as a mucocutaneous disease which also affects intertriginous areas such as the inguinal fold and interdigital webs. The lesions resemble those of contact dermatitis and consist of erythema, surface exudation and, occassionally, superficial pustules and shallow ulcerations (Fig. 6-8). Pruritus and excoriation may be seen. One case has been reported associated with marked production of hyperkeratotic plaques and crusts as may be seen in human candidiasis.

Pityrosporum dermatitis affects abdominal skin of the axilla and inguinal areas and lip folds. Pruritic erythematous plaques occur which may develop pigmented centers. The term "pseudoacanthosis nigricans" was coined to de-

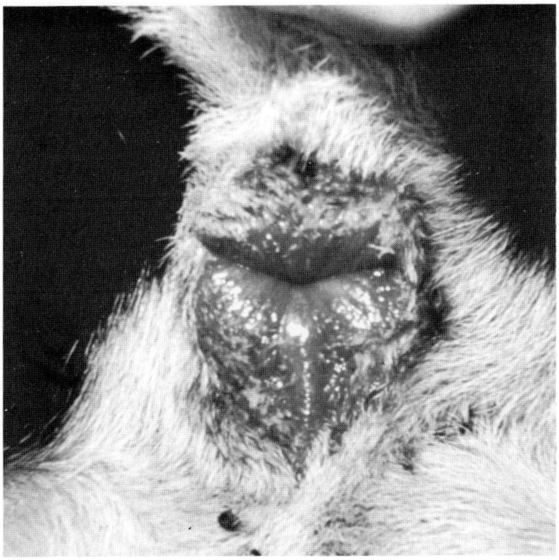

Fig. 6-8. Candidiasis of the perianal mucocutaneous junction in a dog. Note superficial ulceration and exudation. (Courtesy Dr. Valerie Fadok, University of Florida, Gainesville, FL.)

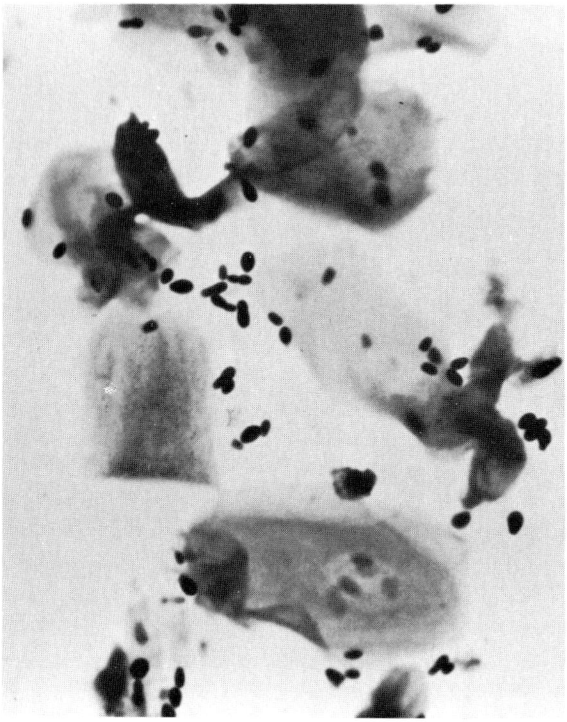

Fig. 6-9. Gram's stain of ear swab containing numerous ovoid and budding gram-positive Malassezia (Pityrosporum) yeasts surrounding epidermal cells.

scribe those lesions. To date, dermatitis associated with this organism has not been described in dogs in the United States.

Diagnosis

Diagnosis may be established by cytology, culture, or biopsy from affected skin. Cytologic preparations are made by scraping surface exudate or hyperkeratotic scale and using a Gram's stain on a smear. Candida is a small (5 to 7 μm), round to oval, gram-positive unicellular organism. Pseudohyphae may be seen. *Malassezia* (*Pityrosporum*) is familiar to most veterinarians. It is slightly larger than Candida (4 to 8 μm) and asymetrical budding is common, so that a characteristic peanut shape is seen on smears (Fig. 6-9). It is amphiphilic, staining both gram-positive and gram-negative. In human skin infections, *M. furfur* characteristically forms short septate hyphae, but this was not reported in the series of cases from dogs.

Scrapings of exudate should be submitted for culture on Sabouraud's dextrose agar (SDA) containing antibiotics. Most microbiology laboratories are well equipped to identify these yeasts.

To make a diagnosis by biopsy, care must be taken not to scrub surface scale and exudate away. If organisms are not found, the likely pathologic diagnosis will be contact dermatitis.

Treatment

Miconazole (or other imidazole-containing) lotions or nystatin-containing creams or lotions may be used topically. Oral ketoconazole would be the drug of choice for systemic therapy. When there is an underlying immunodeficiency, relapses can be expected. Such patients should always have a thorough medical workup.

Actinomycosis and Nocardiosis

Actinomycetes pathogenic to dogs and cats include species of *Nocardia*, *Actinomyces* and, rarely, *Streptomyces*. These are "higher" bacteria, rather than fungi, but are traditionally studied by mycologists because they are filamentous and because they produce pyogranulomatous inflammation and mycetomas.

Actinomycetes grow as fine, straight or branching filaments of less than 1 μm diameter. They may form aerial mycelia on solid media. In tissue as well as in liquid media, they tend to form clumps known as granules.

The species of *Nocardia* affecting dogs and cats include *N. asteroides, N. brasiliensis*, and *N. caviae*. Nocardia are aerobic and partially acid-fast. Filaments may break into coccobacillary gram-positive forms. Spores may be formed in chains. Nocardia are found in soil and fresh water.

Actinomycosis in dogs is usually caused by *Actinomyces viscosus*. Recently, some canine isolates associated with grass awn foreign bodies have been separated from *A. viscosus* into the new species *A. hordeovulnaris*. *Actinomyces* spp are anaerobic or microaerophilic; *A. viscosus* and *A. hordeovulnaris* are more tolerant of aerobic conditions than most. Actinomyces form short, single-branched filaments, coccoid and diphtheroid forms in liquid media and exudate. The tendency to form clumps of organisms in tissue is more pronounced in Actinomyces than in Nocardia. *Actinomyces* spp are normal inhabitants of the oral cavity and other mucosal areas of many species, probably including the dog.

Pathophysiology and Clinical Findings

Actinomycetes becomc pathogenic as a result of invasion after trauma or by local extension of oropharyngeal disease in the case of *Actinomyces* spp. There are no predisposing host factors except for the creation of the portal of entry by trauma. Dissemination may be facilitated by weakened host defenses. This has been suggested to occur in young dogs with disseminated nocardiosis

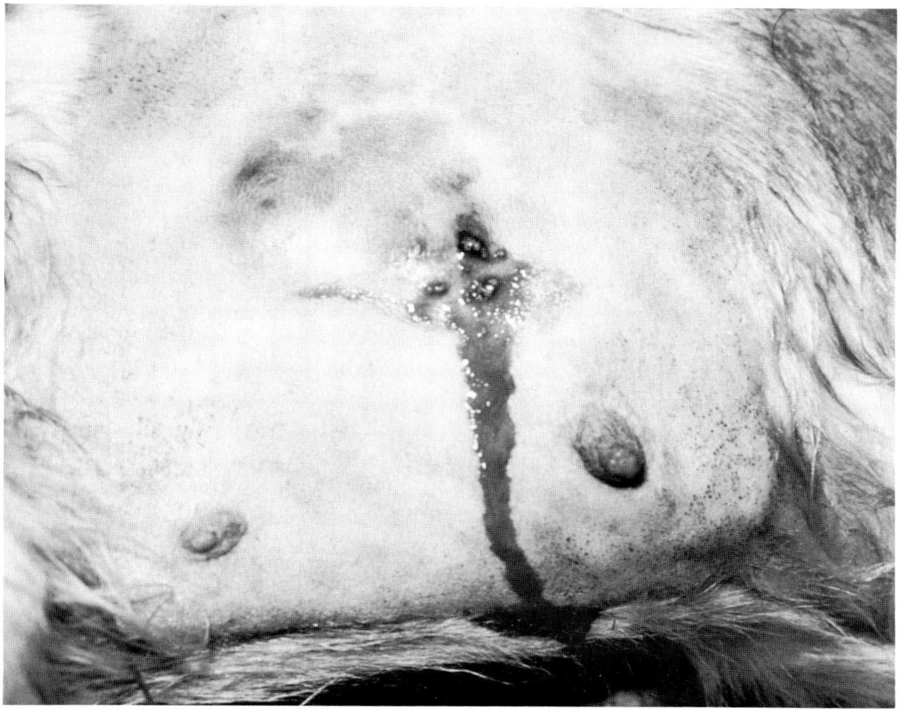

Fig. 6-10. Ruptured chest wall abscess demonstrating exudate with granules on a dog with underlying pleural actinomycosis.

who may also have canine distemper. The more common cause of dissemination is probably penetration of a wound into a body cavity or migration of foreign bodies.

A systemic illness of young dogs resembling canine distemper has been attributed to nocardiosis. Some of these dogs develop cutaneous lesions, osteomyelitis, or septic arthritis.

Cutaneous lesions include dermal and subcutaneous nodules, abscesses, draining fistulous tracts, and deep ulcerations. As with other infectious diseases, young dogs are more often affected, as are active male dogs of large breeds due to the traumatic portal of entry. Skin lesions are more common on the head and extremities.

Other clinical signs vary according to the extent of dissemination of infection. The presence of draining lesions on the chest or abdominal wall may indicate disease in the underlying pleural or peritoneal spaces (Fig. 6-10). Systemic signs, including dyspnea, abdominal effusion, chronic fever, and weight loss often accompany body cavity involvement. Lameness and limb swelling due to osteomyelitis may be seen.

Diagnosis

Diagnosis is made by a combination of cytologic, histologic, and microbiologic means. The ease of diagnosis depends on the accessability of affected tissues and exudate. The development of skin lesions offers the opportunity to diagnose the systemic disease.

Both *Actinomyces* spp and *Nocardia* spp tend to form clumps of organisms in exudate known as granules. The collection of granules is extremely important for diagnostic accuracy. Granules in dogs are often soft and pale when compared to those formed in actinomycosis in other host species.

When exudate or tissue containing granules is obtained by aspiration or at surgery, granules should be isolated and crushed and smeared on glass slides for cytologic examination. The identification by Gram's stain of filamentous gram-positive bacteria ($<1\mu m$ diameter) confirms the presence of an actinomycete. Modified acid-fast stains can then be performed by a microbiology laboratory for guidance in selecting culture techniques. Acid-fast organisms can be assumed to be *Nocardia*. When the acid-fast stain is negative, then cultures for both *Nocardia* and *Actinomyces* will be necessary as *Nocardia* may fail to stain in some circumstances.

Material submitted for culture should consist of exudate containing granules, granules washed in sterile nonbacteriostatic saline, and aseptically-obtained tissue. Submitting small amounts of exudate from surface ulcerations or fistulous tracts or samples obtained with sterile swabs will usually lead to failure to isolate these organisms. When acid-fast stains are negative or not performed, then aerobic, anaerobic, and microaerophilic culture techniques should be employed. Actinomycotic infections are often accompanied by a mixture of other bacteria. Most often the actinomycete will be the primary pathogen, but mixed infections may complicate microbiologic diagnosis.

Pathologic changes include pyogranulomatous inflammation with granule formation. Histologic identification of actinomycetes can be difficult when granules are not present in tissue examined. When organisms are present, the diagnosis is confirmed by tissue Gram's stains and acid-fast stains. Experienced pathologists may be able to differentiate between *Nocardia* and *Actinomyces* in tissue, but in general it is safer to rely on cultural techniques when acid-fast stains are negative. *Actinomyces* spp found in the dog do not form microscopic clubbing at the edge of granules as is typical of *A. bovis* and *A. israelii* infections in other host species.

Treatment

Treatment for actinomycosis and nocardiosis includes surgical and medical modalities. Surgical approaches for both are similar and involve the principles of therapy for body cavity effusions or abscesses caused by any organism. Similarly, prognosis in these diseases is much more favorable when adequate drainage, lavage, and/or debridement is achieved. Cutaneous lesions should be excised, debrided, or lavaged depending on whether nodules, abscesses, or draining tracts are found. As mentioned previously, cutaneous lesions on the abdominal or thoracic skin should alert the clinician to the possibility of disease in the underlying body cavity.

Antibiotic therapy for the two diseases is dissimilar; recommended therapy has been reviewed recently (E. M. Hardie, 1984). Penicillin is the treatment of choice in actinomycosis, although there is some concern that the recently described *A. hordeovulnaris*, which is most often associated with plant awn migration, may be relatively resistant to beta-lactam antibiotics through the production of L-forms. Other choices include erythromycin, lincomycin, clindamycin, rifampin and minocycline. Penicillin must be administered at fairly high doses with 100,000 units/kg being recommended as an original parenteral dose to be followed by oral penicillin V at 50 mg/kg every 8 hours. Duration of therapy should be based on how successfully surgical therapy achieved full debridement or drainage. In incomplete surgical treatment, therapy should be extended for 1 to 3 months or even longer.

Nocardia is relatively more resistent to antibiotic therapy and in vitro testing is recommended in severe or chronic infections. The recommended empirical therapy involves high dose sulfonamides given at 60 to 80 mg/kg every 8 to 12 hours. Sulfadiazine or triple sulfa combinations are recommended for dogs. Trimethoprim–sulfonamide combinations are not always successful, possibly because fixed dose combinations do not allow adequate dosing of the sulfonamide. Therapy should be continued for 2 to 8 months. Long-term sulfonamide therapy probably warrants monitoring of the complete blood count (CBC) for bone marrow suppression.

When the identity of the actinomycete is in question, either before culture results have been reported or when culture methods have failed, combination therapy with penicillin or ampicillin and sulfonamides is indicated. These drugs may be synergistic in either of these infections, so that the only drawbacks to routinely using combination therapy are increased cost and increased chance for adverse reactions.

The prognosis for cutaneous disease caused by either Nocardia or Actinomyces is good, once appropriate therapy is instituted. Prognosis in internal and disseminated disease depends on the organ system affected and the general state of the patient at the time of diagnosis. Aggressively treated empyema associated with Actinomyces most often has a favorable outcome. The prognosis in systemic nocardiosis is poor.

SUBCUTANEOUS MYCOSES

The terminology applied to the miscellaneous mycotic infections caused by less pathogenic, normally free-living fungi is confusing. There are various pathologic and taxonomic terms for overlapping categories of disease. In this chapter the terminology outlined by Chandler, Kaplan and Ajello (1980) will be followed. In dogs and cats, subcutaneous mycoses include mycetomas (eumycotic), subcutaneous phaeohyphomycosis, sporotrichosis, and pythiosis (oömycosis). In addition, there are free-living fungal organisms which may cause systemic disease with cutaneous manifestations. Paecilomycosis and aspergillosis fall into this category and will be discussed with the systemic mycoses. The terms "chromomycosis" and "phycomycosis" are obsolete although still widely used in pathologic diagnoses. Chromoblastomycosis has not been described in dogs and cats.

Eumycotic Mycetomas

Mycetoma is a cutaneous lesion consisting of swelling, fistulous tract formation, and granule production. Eumycotic mycetomas must be distinguished from actinomycotic lesions, and bacterial botryomycosis. Fungal mycetomas may be caused by pigmented (black grain mycetoma) or nonpigmented (white grain mycetoma) fungal organisms. In dogs and cats, black grain mycetoma is caused by *Curvularia geniculata*, a pigmented saprophyte which grows easily on Sabouraud's dextrose agar (SDA). White grain mycetoma caused by *Pseudoallescheria boydii* has been reported in the dog. Both are rare conditons. In addition, a syndrome known as "pseudomycetoma" has been described in cats with *Microsporum canis* infections (Fig. 6-5).

Pathophysiology and Clinical Findings

Mycetomas are localized granulomatous swellings of subcutaneous tissue and sometimes adjacent bone. They are associated with traumatic innoculation of the normally free-living etiologic agents or in the case of dermatophyte pseudomycetomas, with the liberation of fungus-containing hair shafts into the deep dermis or subcutis. Most lesions occur on extremities.

Once established, the agents of mycetoma proliferate in aggregates. These aggregates, as well as host responses to these slowly growing organisms, form the granules. Granule formation is associated with fibrous encapsulation and granulomatous inflammation. The aggregates themselves elicit a pyogenic response which results in abscessation and fistulous tract formation with discharge of granules. The infections are chronic, fibrosing, and locally invasive. Typically, cycles of healing and ulceration lead to firm swelling and scarring. Most such lesions have been treated with a variety of antibiotic agents before the diagnosis is established.

Diagnosis

The diagnosis may be achieved by cytologic examination of the granules and by cultures. Granules may be soft enough to crush and smear, in which case Gram's stain will reveal the mycotic nature (vs. bacterial) of the agent.

If granules are too firm to be crushed, incubation in 10 percent KOH for 2 to 12 hours and examination directly without stain will reveal the pigmented or nonpigmented fungal elements. Culture of granules washed in sterile saline should be attempted for specific identification. The diagnosis may also be easily established by histopathologic examination. When mycetomas are associated with widespread lesions typical of dermatophytosis, DTM cultures should be prepared.

Therapy

Treatment is total surgical excision, possibly including amputation of affected limbs. Relapses are common due to incomplete excision. Antifungal chemotherapy is rarely successful except in the pseudomycetomas associated with dermatophytosis. If antifungal chemotherapy is to be attempted, in vitro sensitivity testing of the isolated agent is recommended as sensitivity patterns of saprophytic fungi are highly variable.

Subcutaneous Phaeohyphomycosis

Phaeohyphomycosis is a granulomatous disease caused by pigmented (dematiaceous) fungi forming hyphal elements in tissue. The disease has been reported more commonly in cats than in dogs. Cases in cats have been associated with the following saprophytic fungi: *Cladosporium bantianum, Exophiala jeanselmei, Drechslera spicifera, Moniliella suaveolens*, and Phialophora verrucosa. In the dog, causative agents have been *Drechslera spicifera* and *Pseudomicrodochium sultonii.*

Pathophysiology and Clinical Findings

Phaeohyphomycosis can be localized or generalized, cutaneous or subcutaneous, or it can be a systemic disease with or without cutaneous lesions. Some cases have been reported as opportunistic infections associated with other infections, systemic disease, or neoplasms. In other cases, no predisposing or immunosuppressing factors have been found.

The inflammatory pattern is pyogranulomatous. In some cases, the presence of pigmented fungi has led to confusion with cutaneous melanomas. In other cases, pigmentation of fungi is only appreciable microscopically. Lesions may be pruritic or necrotizing which leads to ulceration (Fig. 6-11). Distribution of lesions on the body is variable.

Diagnosis

Diagnosis is most often made histopathologically, although in some cases, cytologic examination of lesions has revealed pigmented fungal elements. The causative organisms cannot be identified based on morphology in tissue; cul-

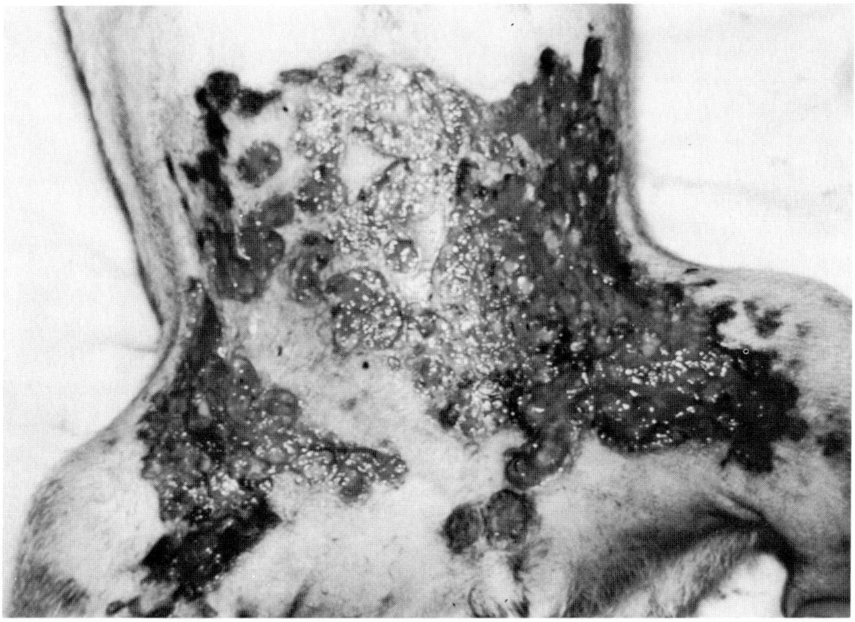

Fig. 6-11. Cutaneous ulceration associated with *Drechslera spicifera* infection in a dog. (Courtesy Dr. Ken Kwochka, The Ohio State University, Columbus, OH.)

tural identification is necessary. Biopsy specimens, aseptically obtained, should be submitted for culture. As these organisms are common laboratory contaminants and saprophytes, any diagnosis must be based on the correlation of histopathologic and cultural data.

Treatment

Treatment should include surgical excision whenever possible. The causative organisms are highly variable in susceptibility to chemotherapeutic agents. In widespread and unresectable disease, in vitro testing of susceptibility of the isolate should be attempted. Agents that have been used with limited success include amphotericin B, flucytosine, and ketoconazole. In some cases, hyperthermia may be used to manage accessible lesions.

Sporotrichosis

Sporotrichium schenkii is a dimorphic fungus found worldwide, occurring naturally in rich organic debris as a saprophytic mycelial fungus. In tissue or at 37°C in culture, the organism grows as a yeast.

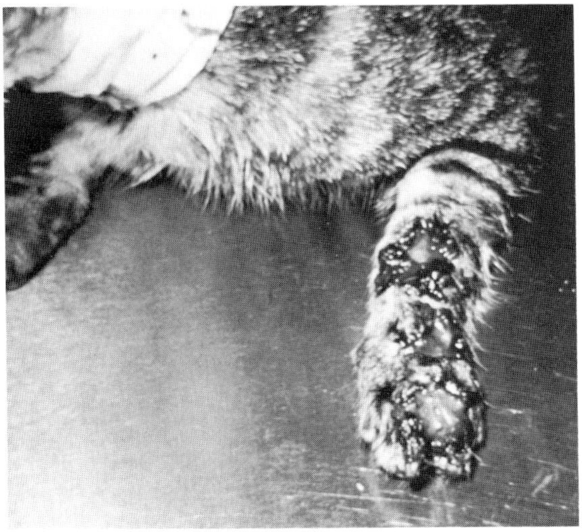

Fig. 6-12. Ulcerative cutaneous lesions on a cat with systemic sporotrichosis. (Courtesy Dr. Nita Gulbas, Phoenix, AZ.)

Pathophysiology

Sporotrichosis is associated with wound contamination. The usual infecting form is the mycelial fungus, but direct exposure to, with or without innoculation of exudate containing yeast, may result in disease; therefore, this disease in dogs and especially in cats is a potential zoonosis.

Once established in the dermis and subcutis, the disease can ascend to the lymphatic system. Rarely, sporotrichosis may become disseminated. This is seen more often in cats than dogs. Cutaneous dissemination may occur by autoinnoculation. It is not clear whether dissemination in cats is limited to immunocompromised individuals as it is in humans and probably in dogs.

Clinical Findings

Cutaneous lesions occur at the site of innoculation. They consist of alopecic nodules and ulcers and most closely resemble lesions of cutaneous blastomycosis (Fig. 6-12). Satellite lesions may develop near the original site. Affected lymph nodes may rupture and drain. The epidermis overlying nodules may become hyperplastic lending a verrucous appearance to some lesions. Lesions are most commonly seen on the head and limbs. The classical lymphocutaneous pattern seen in sporotrichosis of man and the horse is rare in dogs and cats.

Diagnosis

The diagnosis may be difficult to establish either with cytology or by histopathologic examination because the number of organisms is low in many cases. In cases where organisms are abundant, Gram's stains of exudate will

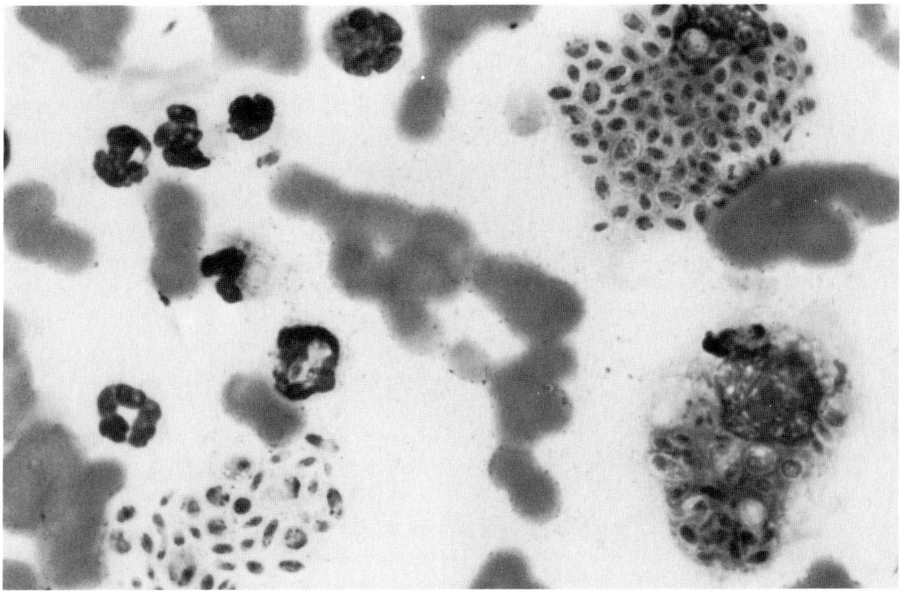

Fig. 6-13. Abundant pyriform nucleated yeasts in macrophages seen on a Wright-Giemsa stain of exudate from the cat in Figure 6-11.

reveal pleomorphic ovoid to pyriform yeasts (2 to 6 μm) within macrophages (Fig. 6-13). Such cases represent a greater zoonotic threat and should be treated with care to avoid exposure of handlers to exudate.

Histopathologically, the inflammatory pattern is granulomatous to necrotizing and pyogranulomatous. When organisms cannot be demonstrated with special stains, hematoxylin-eosin (H & E) stained slides or unstained paraffin-embedded tissues may be used in a commercially available direct fluorescent antibody test. An immunoperoxidase test may also be applied to formalin fixed tissue.

Diagnosis is most often established by culture. Surgically collected biopsy specimens are preferred, but exudate from nonulcerated lesions may be submitted. The organism grows readily on SDA and can be readily identified by microbiology laboratories as a pathogen.

Therapy

In cutancous or lymphocutaneous sporotrichosis, the treatment of choice is sodium iodide. This is usually administered orally to dogs and cats in the form of 20 percent solution. Dogs are given 1 ml of 20 percent iodide solution/5 kg (44 mg/kg) two or three times daily for 6 weeks. The dose for cats is 0.5 ml/5 kg (22 mg/kg) twice daily. Administration should be continued 4 weeks beyond apparent clinical remission. Potassium iodide may be substituted but is less palatable. These drugs may be mixed with milk or cream to increase palatability.

Side effects will sometimes limit the dosage regimen, especially in cats. Side effects include anorexia, nausea, salivation, lacrimation, sneezing, and dry scaly skin. In such cases, the dosage may be reduced by half.

Hyperthermia may be a useful adjunctive therapy in localized lesions. This can be applied by means of local hot compresses several times daily. Alternatively a hyperthermia unit may be used; unfortunately this requires anesthesia.

In disseminated sporotrichosis, treatment with ketoconazole is recommended. The recommended dose is 10 mg/kg. Not all isolates are susceptible, in which case treatment with amphotericin B and flucytosine, as in cryptococcosis, should be substituted.

Pythiosis

Synonyms for subcutaneous pythiosis include subcutaneous phycomycosis and oömycosis. The causative organisms are unidentified members of the genus *Pythium* (*Hyphomyces destruens*). These organisms are dimorphic flagellate protozoa, not true fungi. In culture and in tissue the growth form is mycelial. The infective agent is an aquatic flagellated zoospore. The organisms are parasites of aquatic plants in tropical and subtropical areas worldwide. The habitat is stagnant water with high organic content. Zoospore production may be seasonal, as cases are more common in summer and early fall.

Pathophysiology and Clinical Signs

Cutaneous infections are relatively common in horses in endemic areas. The disease has also been reported in cattle. Pythiosis has two forms in dogs, gastrointestinal and subcutaneous. Both diseases are uncommon and are not usually coexistent. Disseminated disease has rarely been reported.

Infection is established after exposure to the aquatic zoospore either orally or percutaneously. It is likely that some minor antecedent trauma or excoriation is necessary for cutaneous invasion. The primary lesion is a dermal nodule which may ulcerate. Once established, the infection progresses rapidly, expanding locally in the subcutis and forming satellite lesions (Fig. 6-14). The inflammatory response is pyogranulomatous and occasionally necrotizing as the organism tends to exhibit angiocentric invasion. Pruritus is often marked and self-mutilation may be prominent. When infection occurs on distal extremities, lesions may resemble acral lick granulomas.

The cutaneous disease has been most often reported in large dogs. Lesions most commonly occur on the limbs, the face, and the dorsal lumbar area.

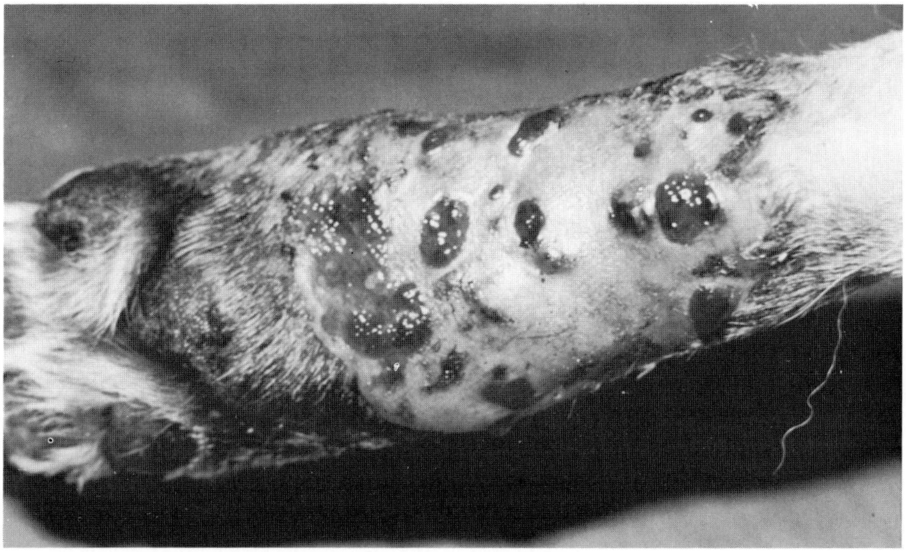

Fig. 6-14. Multiple ulcerated cutaneous nodules developing within a split-thickness skin graft in a dog with relapsing cutaneous pythiosis.

Diagnosis

The diagnosis may be established by cultural, cytologic, and histopathologic examination of biopsy material. Aspiration cytology is seldom rewarding. Digestion of affected tissue in 10 percent KOH for 2 to 12 hours will allow microscopic visualization of the nonpigmented hyphal forms. These are short robust hyphae with parallel walls, occasional right-angled branching, and rare septations.

The histopathologic pattern consists of multiple microscopic pyogranulmatous foci surrounded by fibrosis. Organisms are more prominent in the necrotizing centers of granulomatous foci. Special stains (Grocott's methenamine silver [GMS] is preferred) are often needed as the organism is difficult to visualize on H&E slides.

Necrotizing centers are often visible grossly as yellow foci and these should be sterilely dissected and placed whole on solid culture media. The organism will grow on blood agars and SDA, but growth is most rapid on vegetable extract agar. In culture, *Pythium* resembles the early growth of some zygomycetes. Special techniques are necessary to induce zoospore formation in vitro, which allows cultural identification.

Therapy

To date only surgical therapy has been successful in pythiosis. As the disease is aggressively invasive locally, wide surgical margins are required.

Preliminary data from clinical observations and limited in vitro testing suggest that *Pythium* is not susceptible to antifungal agents. As cell membrane composition of this protozoal agent is dissimilar to that of true fungi, this is not an unexpected finding. Similarly, limited experience with other modalities used in equine pythiosis, such as potassium iodide or autogenous vaccine, have been disappointing. Current research efforts center on the use of an agricultural agent, metalaxyl, which is useful when crops are attacked by pathogenic *Pythium*.

CUTANEOUS MANIFESTATIONS OF SYSTEMIC MYCOSIS

The dog appears to be a natural host for the systemic mycoses histoplasmosis, blastomycosis, and coccidiodomycosis; these diseases are rare in the cat. Cryptococcosis occurs in the dog and cat, and it may be either a systemic or localized cutaneous or nasal mycosis. Opportunistic systemic infections with normally saprophytic fungi are uncommon in dogs and cats. *Aspergillus* and *Paeciliomyces* have been best described as pathogens in small animals.

Any of the systemically disseminated mycoses may have cutaneous lesions. Skin lesions are most often thought to derive from hematogenous spread, but there is abundunt evidence for local infection after percutaneous exposure for most of these diseases. The systemic mycoses that are most commonly accompained by cutaneous lesions are blastomycosis and cryptococcosis.

Blastomycosis

Blastomyces dermatitidis is a dimorphic fungus which exists in nature as a mycelial saprophyte. The infectious form consists of conidiospores which are released into the air from the colony and may be inhaled. The tissue form is a large (8 to 12 μm), thick-walled yeast which reproduces with broad-based buds.

Pathophysiology

Dogs are extremely susceptible to blastomyces infection. Infection is acquired by inhalation of spores from the fungus in its saprophytic stage. Classically, thoracic infection develops as a disseminated granulomatous interstitial pneumonitis. Occasionally granulomatous pleuritis and/or thoracic granulomatous lymphadenopathy develop. The majority of infected dogs develop disseminated blastomycosis; no predisposition or immunosuppression is necessary. Dissemination is hematogenous and may affect any organ system. However, cutaneous, musculoskeletal, ocular, and nervous system tissues are most often infected. Affected dogs are primarily young (2 to 4 years), male (72 percent), and of large breeds.

Until recently, knowledge of the habitat and growth requirements of *Blastomyces dermatitidis* in nature is limited. A recent report has described the natural habitat to be associated with beaver lodges (Klein, Vergeront, Weeks et al, 1986). The geographic distribution of the disease or limited to North and Central America and Africa. The disease is limited in the United States to the east and generally includes the Mississippi-Ohio River drainage system, Appalachia, and the St. Lawrence River system. States with the highest incidence are Arkansas, Illinois, Indiana, Iowa, Kentucky, Louisiana, Mississippi, North Carolina, Ohio, Tennessee, and Wisconsin.

The disease is not contagious but cutaneous lesions at the site of direct innoculation of infective materials have been reported in veterinarians and pathologists. Cutaneous infection has not been reported to disseminate.

Clinical Signs

General signs of systemic illness in blastomycosis include fever and weight loss. Other signs are variable and depend on the organ system most severely affected. Respiratory signs are most common, followed by ophthalmic disease, lameness, and cutaneous lesions.

Skin lesions are ulcerative and granulomatous (Fig. 6-15). In general, lesions present as poorly circumscribed swellings with ragged necrotic ulcera-

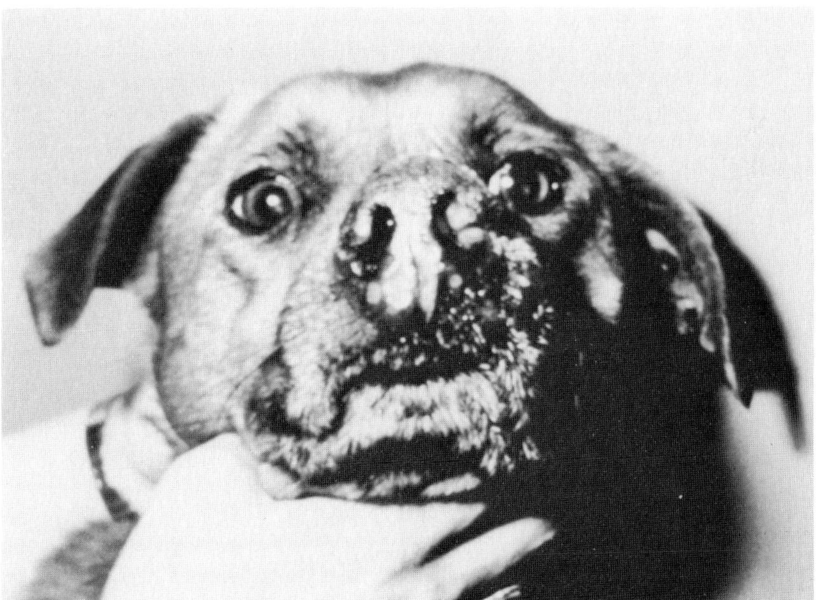

Fig. 6-15. Nasal and cutaneous ulcerative granuloma in a dog with blastomycosis. (Courtesy Dr. Marilyn Stiff, North Carolina.)

tions. Digits and limbs are most commonly affected. Peripheral lymphadenopathy is present in the majority of cases. Lymph nodes may abscess and drain. Exudate is usually blood-tinged and is not copious. Lesions are usually not pruritic. The practitioner should suspect blastomycosis in any dog which presents with one or more ulcerating nodules or localized cellulitis that does not respond to antibiotic therapy. If the dog has been within an endemic area in its lifetime, specific diagnostic tests should be undertaken. Not every patient with skin lesions will have overt signs of systemic disease at the time of presentation.

Diagnosis

A battery of diagnostic tests are available to rule-in blastomycosis. Cutaneous lesions are most readily investigated cytologically. Dry smears should be prepared from aspirations of nodules or lymph nodes or by impressions made from ulcers. Wright's stain or Gram's stain may demonstrate the characteristic organisms (Fig. 6-16). Cutaneous lesions have variable numbers of organisms, however, so the infection cannot be ruled out cytologically if negative.

Chest radiographs should be taken in all suspect cases. Radiographic lesions may be marked even in dogs without respiratory signs. Radiographic findings include diffuse nodular interstitial densities (snow-storm) (Fig. 6-17),

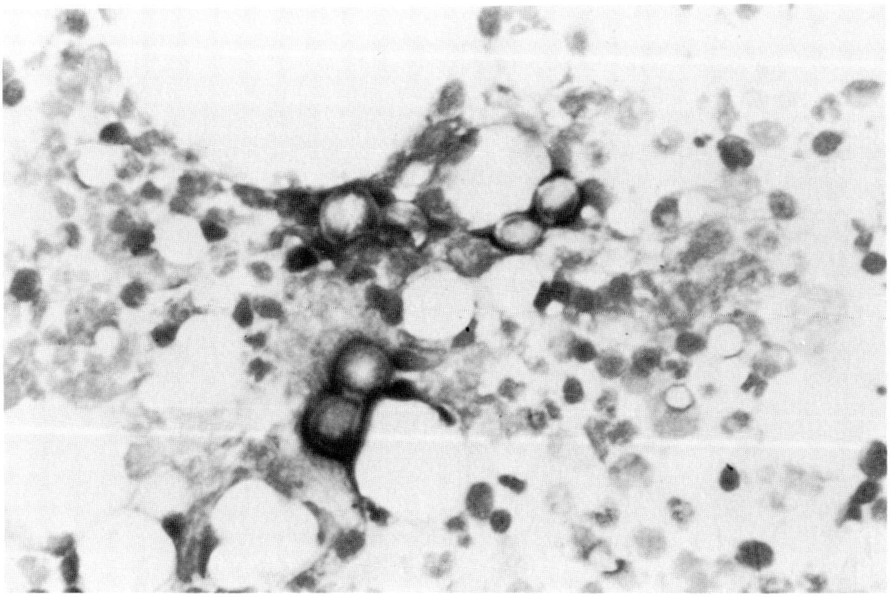

Fig. 6-16. Wright's stain of a lymph node aspiration from a dog with blastomycosis. Note three pairs of thick-walled yeasts demonstrating broad-based budding.

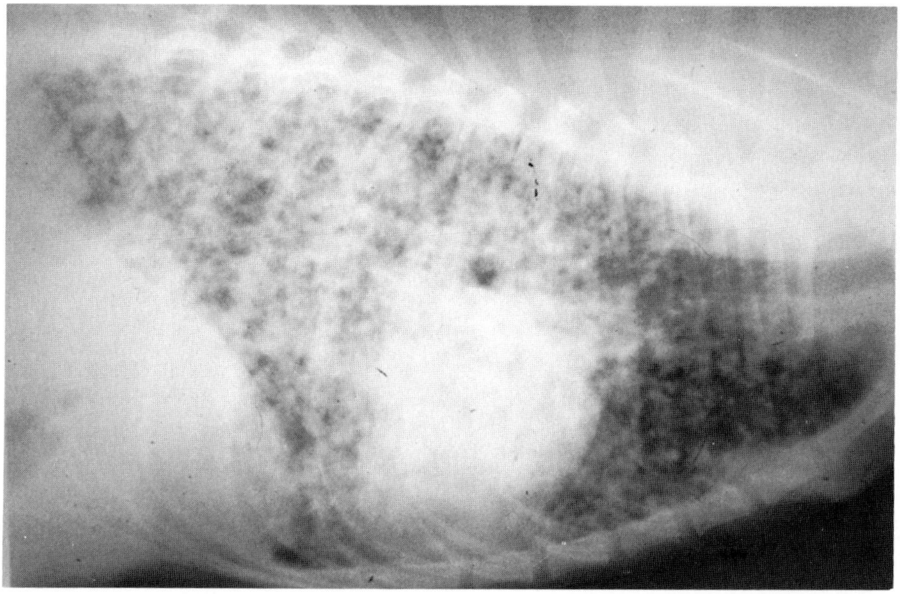

Fig. 6-17. Lateral chest radiograph of a dog with blastomycosis demonstrating nodular and diffuse interstitial pneumonioa. (Courtesy Dr. John Watters, Louisiana State University, Baton Rouge, LA.)

bronchointerstitial lung density, pleural effusion, and/or thoracic lymphadenopathy.

The serologic test of choice in the dog is the agar-gel immunodiffusion (AGID). This test is widely available commercially and does not have to be modified for use with dog serum. It has excellent specificity and fair sensitivity. False-negative results are most often a problem in end-stage disease.

Culture is most successful when surgically obtained tissues are submitted en bloc. Excisional or incisional biopsies of nonulcerated cutaneous nodules or lymph nodes may be submitted for culture. (These tissues may be examined cytologically as well by means of 12-hour maceration in 10 percent KOH; Fig. 6-18.) Cultural identification requires some expertise and also represents a hazard to laboratory personnel so cultures should be submitted to state reference laboratories.

Therapy

Therapeutic approaches to this disease have been markedly changed by the introduction of ketoconazole to treatment regimens. By using a combination of amphotericin B and long-term ketoconazole administration, toxicity and relapse rates have been reduced. The success rate has been reported to be as high as 75 percent.

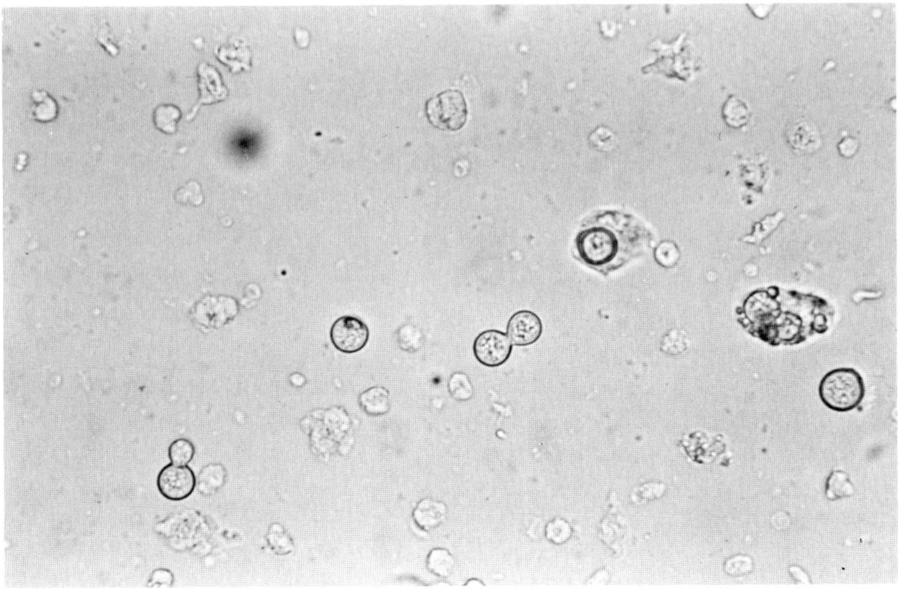

Fig. 6-18. KOH digest preparation of exudate from a dog with blastomycosis. Note budding pairs and double-walled appearance of some yeasts. (Courtesy Dr. Richard Miller, Louisiana State University, Baton Rouge, LA.)

The current protocol most widely used calls for amphotericin B at 0.5 mg/kg given three times weekly to a total dose of 4 to 6 mg/kg and ketoconazole 10 to 30 mg/kg daily for 3 to 6 months. Higher doses of ketoconazole and longer treatment regimens should be used in cases of central nervous system (CNS), bone, eye, or cutaneous involvement. See the section on antifungal chemotherapy for specific details of administration and toxicity.

Cryptococcosis

Cryptococcus neoformans is an encapsulated saprophytic yeast which reproduces by narrow-based budding. The size of the yeast varies, from 4 to 20 μm. The mucopolysaccharide capsule is also of variable thickness, but may equal twice the diameter of the cell.

Pathophysiology

The route of infection is by inhalation of organisms. The infection may be established in the upper respiratory tract where nasal granulomatous disease is produced. In the lower respiratory tract, local or disseminated granulomas result. Dissemination occurs in some patients and the CNS is most often affected. CNS involvement may occur by direct extension of nasal granuloma or by hematogenous spread. Dissemination occurs most readily in man in states of immunosuppression, and this is postulated to be the case in dogs and cats where the use of glucocorticoids or the presence of neoplastic disease or feline leukemia virus (FeLV) infection have all been associated with cryptococcosis. On the other hand, nasal cryptococcosis has been reported in both dogs and cats with no detected immunosuppressive disease. Infection by percutaneous innoculation is possible. It is not known whether skin lesions on animals with nasal granulomas are derived from hematogenous spread or by self-innoculation. Skin lesions on or near the planum nasale probably occur by direct extension of mucosal lesions.

In all organ systems, affected lesions consist of granulomas or pyogranulomas. On gross examination of lesions and exudate, a mucoid quality is often observed. On histologic sections, yeast cells are often abundant but are usually collapsed and the identifying capsule is not readily apparent without special stains. Older lesions may have few organisms.

Cryptococcus neoformans exists as a saprophyte worldwide in nitrogen-rich debris. It has been isolated most often in association with pigeon droppings. Cryptococcosis occurs as a sporadic opportunistic infection in a wide range of mammalian species. It is the most common systemic mycotic infection of cats. The strains or serotypes that have been studied have exhibited varying degrees of virulence in laboratory and domestic animals.

Clinical Signs

Signs of the disease vary with the organ system affected. Nasal granuloma and granulomas of the facial skin are by far the most common presentations (Fig. 6-19). Nasal granulomas usually begin as unilateral obstructions with mucoid nasal discharge. The disease may progress to involve both nasal passages. Presentation for respiratory distress is uncommon, more often lower airway disease is accompanied by vague constitutional signs such as weight loss and fever. The CNS is next most often affected. Animals may present with signs of meningoencephalitis or may have localized CNS lesions. Ocular, musculoskeletal, hepatic, and urinary tract involvement has been noted.

Cutaneous lesions consist of well-circumscribed dermal or subcutaneous nodules. These may be pruritic. Nodules may ulcerate and discharge scant to copious quantities of mucoid exudate. Skin lesions are most commonly described on the face and ears, but may be multiple and widespread. As previously noted, cutaneous lesions may or may not accompany disseminated disease.

Diagnosis

The diagnosis is most readily achieved by cytologic methods. The organism may be demonstrated in exudate from nasal passages, from cutaneous lesions, in CSF, and in urine. However, preparation of dry smears often leads to col-

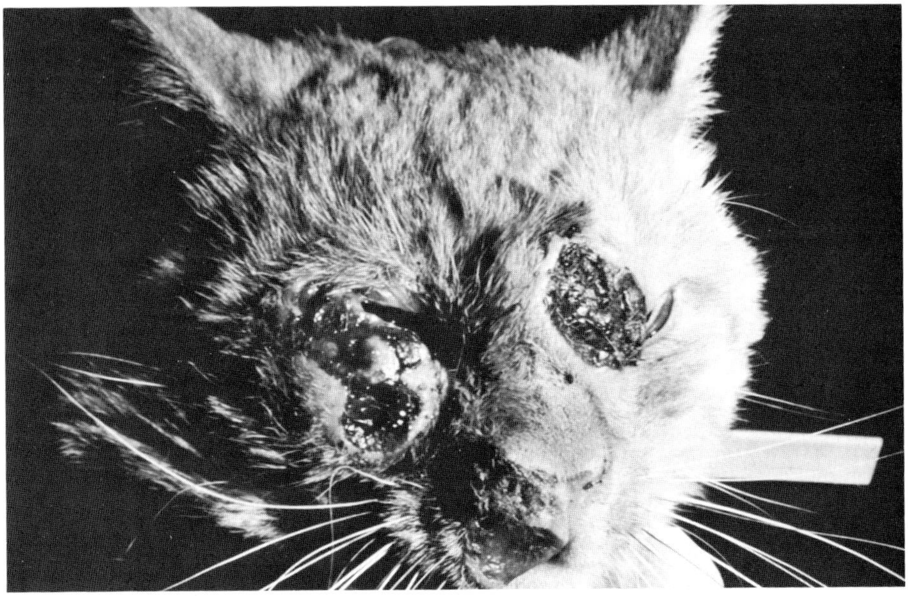

Fig. 6-19. Disfiguring nasal and facial granulomas in cat with cryptococcosis. (Courtesy Dr. Nita Gulbas, Phoenix, AZ.)

lapse of the thin-walled yeast cells and the characteristic capsule does not stain readily. For dry smears Gram's stain is preferred. Wet mounts of tissue or exudate are most satisfactory. Exudate may be diluted and macerated in 10 percent KOH which will allow the organism to be seen under low light. New methylene blue may be used alone or added to KOH to stain the capsule and the organism (Fig. 6-20). Alternatively, India ink may provide negative staining as the capsule appears light against a dark background. In the author's experience, this type of preparation requires more experience to interpret.

Detection of serum antibody levels is not very useful in diagnosis. The indirect fluorescent antibody test has been used but it not very sensitive or specific. The most useful diagnostic test when organisms cannot be isolated is the latex agglutination test for capsular antigen. The test can be used to detect Cryptococcus antigen in serum, CSF, and urine and is reported to be very specific and highly sensitive, especially for CSF samples.

Diagnosis may be attempted by culture of tissue or exudate, but this is generally used to confirm cytologic findings. As there are saprophytic yeasts which resemble *C. neoformans* morphologically, biochemical tests are necessary to confirm identification of isolates from exudate, nasal tissue, or open cutaneous lesions.

Histopathologic examination using special fungal stains and capsular stains provide a diagnosis along with cultural attempts when cytologic examination has been negative. In dense, cellular tissue and where the strain has a poorly-

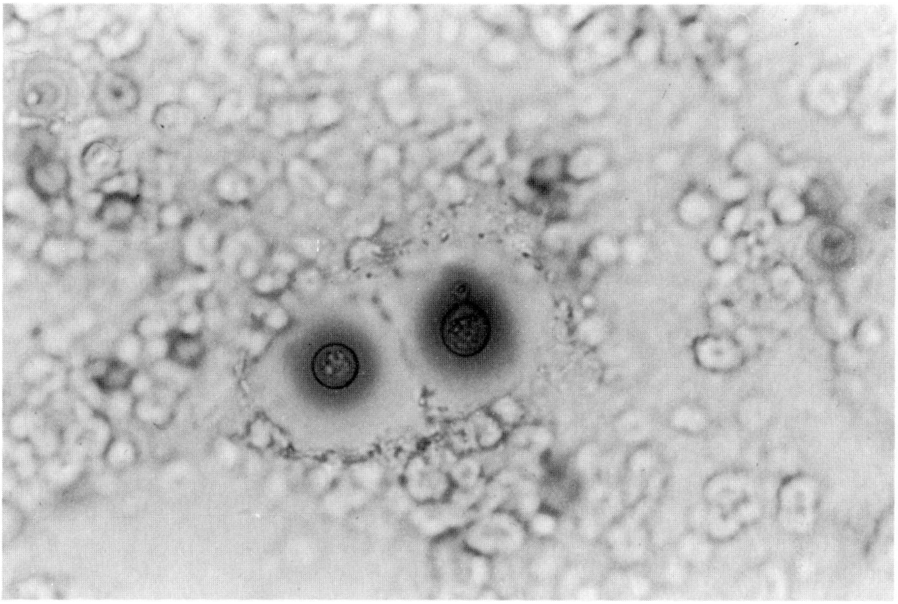

Fig. 6-20. New methylene blue stain of exudate containing two *Cryptococcus neoformans* yeasts. Note capsular staining and small narrow-based bud.

formed capsule, direct immunofluorescence testing may be necessary for identification.

Treatment

When surgical removal of granulomas is possible, this is the treatment of choice. More often, chemotherapy is required. At present, the treatment of choice for cryptococcosis in dogs and cats is not well defined. In CNS or life-threatening systemic disease a combination of amphotericin B and flucytosine is recommended. In nasal granuloma and primary cutaneous cryptococcus, ketoconazole alone has been effective. However, in human cases, isolates have shown highly variable susceptibilities to ketoconazole. The use of flucytosine alone is associated with a high rate of emergence of resistance and is not recommended.

Amphotericin B should be administered at 0.25–0.5 mg/kg twice weekly for a total dose of 4 to 6 mg along with flucytosine at 200 mg/kg given in 3 to 4 divided dosages daily. Once remission is achieved, maintenance therapy can consist of ketoconazole 10 mg/kg daily or 20 mg/kg every other day in cats. Refer to the section on antifungal chemotherapy for specifics about administration and side effects.

Histoplasmosis, Coccidiodomycosis

Histoplasmosis and coccidiodomycosis are caused by the dimorphic fungi *Histoplasma capsulatum* and *Coccidioides immitis*. Each disease has a very specific geographic distribution based on the ecologic requirements of the free-living mycelial phase of the fungus.

In tissue, *H. capsulatum* forms small (2 to 4 μm), uniformly ovoid yeasts that reproduce by narrow-based budding. The disease is unique among the systemic mycoses in that the organism reproduces intracellularly. Widespread dissemination in the reticuloendothelial system is seen in fatal cases.

Histoplasmosis has a widespread distribution worldwide in major temperate and tropical river valleys. In the United States, the disease is most common in the Mississippi-Ohio River Valley. The organism is found in nitrogen-rich soils especially associated with bird or bat droppings.

Coccidioides immitis in tissue forms large (20 to 100 μm) spherules which reproduce by internal budding forming endospores (2 to 3 μm). Dissemination of endospores occurs hematogenously and locally after which each matures in tissue to form new spherules.

Coccidioides immitis is found in nature in desert areas of North and South America. In the southwestern United States the disease is prevalent in southern California, Arizona, and Texas. The saprophytic phase is associated with rodent burrows and spores are most likely to be formed in large numbers following a rainy period.

The route of infection in both diseases is by inhalation of spores from the free-living saprophyte when habitat is disturbed. The primary infection is pulmonary, but in most cases is subclinical and self-limiting. Factors that contribute to dissemination are unclear, although there is some evidence of breed-associated susceptibility for coccodioidomycosis in a way that mimics racial susceptibility among humans.

In both diseases, cutaneous lesions are uncommon and when they do occur, it usually represents extension from underlying pathologic processes such as lymphadenopathy or osteomyelitis. As such, draining tracts appear in limbs overlying fungal osteomyelitis. Lameness would be a common concomitant finding. Although subcutaneous granulomatous panniculitis has been reported in disseminated histoplasmosis, these lesions are rare. Patients are seldom presented to veterinarians for cutaneous lesions.

In neither disease are organisms readily identified in exudate draining from skin lesions. Identification of underlying pathology and appropriate diagnostic tests are therefore dictated by the presenting signs which accompany cutaneous lesions.

Aspergillosis and Paecilomycosis

Various species of the free-living saprophytes *Aspergillus* and *Paecilomyces* show pathogenic potential for vertebrates. In dogs and cats there are sporadic reports of disseminated aspergillosis and paecilomycosis; some of these patients have had cutaneous manifestations of the disease. Little is known of the epidemiology or pathogenesis of the disease in dogs and cats but there is evidence in most cases of either prior debilitating disease or the use of immunosuppressive drugs similar to what is observed when the disease occurs in humans. The more common form of aspergillosis of dogs—aspergilloma of the nasal cavity—has not been reported to be associated with disseminated disease.

Widespread cutaneous lesions are seen rarely in disseminated aspergillosis or paecilomycosis. They are derived from hematogenous spread and infected vascular thrombosis. The lesions are necrotizing and ulcerative and may contribute greatly to the general morbidity of the disease state. Cutaneous lesions may facilitate diagnosis in the systemic disease. Ulcerated lesions should be biopsied en bloc and submitted for histopathologic and cultural evaluation. Cytologic preparations would rarely be rewarding. Only by comparison of histopathologic morphology and culture results can a confident diagnosis be rendered when the etiologic agent is such a common free-living form as are the species of *Aspergillus* and *Paecilomyces*. It is difficult to recommend a therapeutic regimen in these diseases as the prognosis is grave. Amphotericin B would be the antifungal agent of choice.

ANTIFUNGAL AGENTS FOR CHEMOTHERAPY

The ideal antifungal agent should have a broad spectrum of antifungal activity, high efficacy, low toxicity, broad tissue distribution, and oral dosage form. Until the recent introduction of ketoconazole, the systemic antifungals available to the clinician were very far from this ideal. Most of the other agents to be discussed in this section have a low therapeutic index.

Ketoconazole has disadvantages as well. It lacks efficacy and does not penetrate well into bone and the CNS. Many of the traditional antifungal agents must be relied on in treating many of the mycoses that affect the skin. Unfortunately, the development of new agents for antifungal chemotherapy has been hampered by the relative rarity and great diversity of the mycotic infections. Several new imidazoles and triazoles are being tested and used in Europe, but will not likely be made available for veterinary use.

Iodides

Sodium and potassium iodide were the only systemic antifungal agents available until the 1940s. The mechanism of action is unknown. The iodides are well absorbed by oral routes, are widely distributed, and are excreted in the urine.

The spectrum of activity is wide but efficacy is not high. Curent indications for use include lymphocutaneous sporotrichosis and certain subcutaneous mycoses. The available formulation is a saturated (20 percent) oral solution. Dogs are given 1 ml/5 kg on a once to three times basis for 6 weeks. The dose for cats is 0.5 ml/5 kg once or twice a day.

Adverse reactions are fairly common and include anorexia, nausea, salivation, lacrimation, sneezing, and dry scaly skin.

Flucytosine

Flucytosine (Ancobon, Roche Lab) is a fluorinated pyrimidine antimetabolite. Fungi that possess the enzyme cytosine deaminase convert the drug to 5-fluorouracil which is the active compound. It inhibits nucleotide synthesis and activity.

Flucytosine is available as an oral agent and is well absorbed by this route. Good CSF levels are reported for this drug. Excretion is impaired in states of reduced renal function.

The indications for flucytosine include only candidiasis, cryptococcosis, sporotrichosis, and infections with Cladosporium. Emergence of resistance during therapy is a problem and combination therapy with amphotericin B is recommended. The drug is particularly useful in cryptococcosis of the CNS.

The dose for dogs and cats is 100 to 200 mg/kg divided into three or four doses daily. As 250 and 500 mg capsules are available, the drug may have to be recompounded for cats.

Toxicity includes bone marrow suppression. Serum levels should be monitored when renal impairment is present. Toxic levels are 100 μg/ml in humans. Flucytosine may cause neurologic impairment in cats.

Amphotericin B

Amphotericin B (Fungizone, Squibb) is a polyene macrolide antibiotic. It is not water soluble and is unstable in liquid suspensions, which makes in vitro testing with the drug difficult.

Amphotericin B (AMP-B) binds to cell membrane ergosterol and disrupts membrane function. It has some affinity for membrane cholesterol which is one basis for its toxicity.

The drug is supplied in a lyophilized form with deoxycholate and buffer. It is suspended in buffered 5 percent dextrose solutions prior to administration. It is for intravenous use only. Pharmacokinetics are poorly known. Distribution to the CNS is poor.

The spectrum of activity against fungi is broad but effectiveness is variable. AMP-B is the drug of choice in all life-threatening systemic mycoses. Many saprophytic fungi are susceptible. *Aspergillus* species are most often resistant. As noted previously, *Pythium* is not susceptible to AMP-B.

Most dosage regimens have been developed empirically. Most call for doses of 0.5 mg/kg given two or three times weekly to a final total dose. The drug is diluted in dextrose 5 percent by weight (D5W) either as a slow drip in 250 ml or as a slow bolus in 50 to 100 ml.

Acute adverse reactions include vomiting, shivering, fever, and collapse. Renal toxicity occurs in virtually every patient treated with AMP-B. The blood urea nitrogen (BUN) must be monitored during therapy and treatment must be suspended when BUN rises over 50 mg/dl. Preexisting renal disease is not a contraindication to use AMP-B as decreased glomerular filtration rate (GFR) does not limit metabolism. Phlebitis and anemia are additional adverse reactions.

There are two techniques for trying to reduce renal toxicity in AMP-B therapy. The drug may be given with mannitol (12.5 g) added to 250 ml of prepared solution. Also, sodium-loading by means of administration of 0.9 percent NaCL (5 ml/kg) prior to dosing has been helpful, especially in debilitated, anorexic patients.

Ketoconazole

Ketoconazole (Nizoral, Janssen Pharm.) is a fungistatic benzimidazole derivative with broad-spectrum antifungal activity. Ketoconazole (KCZ) inhibits cell membrane synthesis by interfering with ergosterol production. It is labelled for human use for candidiasis, coccidioidomycosis, histoplasmosis, chromomycosis (sic), and paracoccidioidomycosis. It receives wide usage in cases of chronic trichophytosis as well.

In veterinary medicine, successful treatment has been reported with ketoconazole in trichophytosis, coccidioidomycosis, blastomycosis, cryptococcosis, histoplasmosis, and nasal aspergillosis.

The drug is absorbed with variable efficacy after oral administration to dogs. It is metabolized in the liver. Lowest concentrations are found in the CSF, bladder, bone, and skin after oral administration.

Ketoconazole is provided as 200 mg tablets. The recommended dose is 5 to 30 mg/kg given in one or two daily doses. Dogs and cats should be treated after an acid-containing meal as stomach acidity is necessary for absorption.

The major side effect in animals is anorexia. This may be alleviated in some cases by administering divided dosages. Other side effects are rare and may include hepatotoxicity and inhibition of steroid hormone synthesis. Icterus has been seen as a reversible side effect in cats.

SUGGESTED READINGS

Ackerman N, Grain Jr. E, Castleman W: Canine nocardiosis. J Am Anim Hosp Assoc 18:147, 1987

Barsanti, JA. Sporotrichosis in Greene CE (Ed.) Clinical Microbiology and Infectious Disease of the Dog and Cat. W.B. Saunders, Philadelphia, 1984

Buchanan AM, Scott JL: Actinomyces hordeovulnaris, a canine pathogen that produces

L-phase variants spontaneously with calcium deposition. Am J Vet Res 45(12):2552, 1984

Chandler FW, Kaplan W, Ajello L. Color Atlas and Text of the Histopathology of Mycotic Diseases. Year Book Med Pub Inc, Chicago, 1980

Chester DK. Superficial fungal infection of the skin. Comp Cont Enduc 1:910, 1979

Coyle V, Isaacs JP, O'Boyle DA. Canine mycetoma: a case report and review of the literature. J Small Anim Pract 25:261, 1984

Davenport AA, Carter GR, Schirmer RG: Canine actinomycosis due to *Actinomyces viscosus*; report of six cases. Vet Med/Small Anim Clin November: 1442, 1974

Dawson CO, Noddle BM. Treatment of *Microsporum canis* ringworm in a cat colony. J Small Anim Pract 9:613, 1968

Dufait R: Pityrosporon canis as the cause of canine chronic dermatitis. Vet Med/Small Anim Clin July:1055, 1983

Fadok VA: Dermatologic manifestations of the subcutaneous and deep mycoses. Comp Cont Educ 2:506, 1980

Fadok VA: Dermatophytosis. Dermatol Rep. 2:1, 1983

Foil CS: Antifungal agents in dermatology. In Kirk RW (Ed). Current Veterinary Therapy IX Small Animal Practice. W.B. Saunders, Phil. p 560, 1986.

Foil CSO, Short BG, Fadok VA, Kunkle GA: A report of subcutaneous pythiosis in five dogs and a review of the etiologic agent Pythium sp. J Am Anim Hosp Assoc 20:959, 1984

Georg LK, Brown JM, Baker HJ, et al: Actinomyces viscosus as an agent of actinomycosis in the dog. Am J Vet Res 33:1457, 1972

Hardie EM: Actimomycosis and Nocardiosis. In Green CE. Clinical Microbiology and Infectious Diseases of the Dog and Cat. W. B. Saunders, Philadelphia, 1984

Klein BS, Vergeront JM, Weeks RJ *et al*: Isolation of *Blastomyces dermatitidis* in soil associated with a large outbreak in Wisconsin. N Eng J Med 314:529, 1956

Kwochka KW, Calderwood Mays MB, Ajello L, Padhye A: Canine phaeohyphomycosis caused by *Drechslera spicifera*: A case report and literature review. J Amer Anim Hosp Assoc 20:625, 1984

Levine HB. Ketoconazole in the Management of Fungal Disease. ADIS Press, New York, 1980

Miller GH, Kirk RW, Scott DW. Fungal Diseases in Small Animal Dermatology 3rd Ed. W.B. Saunders, 1983

Moriello KA: Ketoconazole. Clinical pharmacology and therapeutic recommendations. J Amer Vet Med Associ 188:303, 1986

Pichler ME, Gross TL, Kroll WR: Cutaneous and mucocutaneous candidiasis in a dog. Comp Cont Educ 7:225, 1985

Scott DW: Feline Dermatology 1900–1978: A monograph. J Am Anim Hosp Assoc 16:303, 1980

7 Endocrine Dermatoses

David K. Chester

HYPOTHYROIDISM

Etiology

The inability to utilize circulating thyroid hormones, or the lowering of serum or plasma active thyroid hormone levels that is severe enough to cause disease is defined as hypothyroidism.

Causes of hypothyroidism are numerous (Table 7-1). Primary hypothyroidism accounts for approximately 95 percent of the disease in dogs; with idiopathic thyroid atrophy and chronic lymphocytic (autoimmune) thyroiditis most common.[1–8] Lymphocytic thyroiditis has been reported to be familial in laboratory dogs.[9,10] Clinical signs are similar regardless of the cause. Secondary and tertiary hypothyroidism are rare and treatment is the same as for primary disease.

Thyroid Physiology

Thyroid physiology is complex, involving absorption and utilization of iodine as well as control, secretion, and metabolism of thyroid hormones.[4] Dietary iodine is reduced to iodide and rapidly absorbed from the gastrointestinal tract. Iodide ions are then actively "trapped" by thyroid follicular epithelial cells, oxidized and incorporated into tyrosine moieties of thyroglobulin within the follicular lumen. The resulting mono- and diiodotyrosines undergo oxidative condensation to form the active hormones triiodothyronine (T_3) and tetraiodothyronine (T_4) and the inactive hormone 3,3′,5′ triiodothyronine (reverse T_3).[11]

Thyroid hormone production and release is regulated by at least four in-

Table 7-1. Some Potential Causes of Hypothyroidism

Primary
Aplasia or hypoplasia (congenital)
Autoimmune lymphocytic thyroiditis
Idiopathic follicular atrophy
Tumors
Defects in hormone or thyroglobulin synthesis
Iodine deficiency
Surgical or radiation removal of the thyroid
Use of antithyroid drugs
Thiocyanates (raw soybeans, cabbage)
Perchlorates
Thiouracil, propylthiouracil
Secondary
Tumors of the pituitary
Negative feedback from other diseases, i.e., hyperadrenocorticism
Pituitary damage from trauma or disease
Congenital pituitary malformation, i.e., cysts
Tertiary
Lack of TRH production
Lack of peripheral utilization of thyroid hormones

(Chester DK: The Thyroid Gland and Thyroid Diseases. p. 90. In Drazner FH (ed): Small Animal Endocrinology. Churchill Livingstone, New York, 1987.)

dependent systems: (1) the hypothalamus, which produces thyrotropin-releasing hormone (TRH), a peptide hormone that stimulates synthesis and release of thyroid-stimulating hormone (TSH), (2) the pituitary adenohypophysis, which produces TSH, which stimulates iodine trapping, hormone synthesis, and hormone release from the thyroid, (3) the thyroid gland itself, which responds to blood levels of iodine, TSH and perhaps other materials to trap iodine, form thyroid hormones and release them into circulation, and (4) the blood levels of free thyroid hormones, which regulate TRH and TSH production but are internally regulated by many chemicals or events that alter their binding to proteins.

The metabolic effects of thyroid hormones relate directly or indirectly to increasing oxidative thermogenesis and metabolic activity of most tissues. T_3 is reported to be the most active thyroid hormone at the cellular level.[3,11] Normally, T_4 is readily converted to T_3 in the peripheral circulation allowing T_4 to be used alone in treatment protocols.

Hypothyroidism is a relatively common disorder. One epidemiologic study of 1.1 million dogs seen at 15 veterinary schools revealed hypothyroidism in 1 out of every 343 patients.[12] Golden retrievers, Doberman pinchers, dachshunds, Shetland sheepdogs, Irish setters, Pomeranians, miniature schnauzers, cocker spaniels, and Airedales were breeds in which the prevalence of the disease was significantly higher than the general population. German shepherd and mixed breed dogs had a significantly lower prevalence. Hypothyroidism as a clinical entity has not been well documented in the cat.[13] Cats with clinical signs similar to those seen in dogs are known to respond to thyroid supplementation.

Diagnosis

The clinical presentation of a hypothyroid dog can vary. The disease must be diagnosed by combining the animal's history, clinical signs, laboratory data, and response to therapy. Considered separately, these sources of information are rarely sufficient to confirm a diagnosis of hypothyroidism.

History

The history of the animal is often helpful. Hypothyroidism is most likely to occur in dogs 4 years of age or older; however, it is not unusual to find the disease in 1- to 2-year-old dogs of the predisposed breeds. Signs of hypothyroidism develop insidiously; therefore, the owner may have ignored signs such as decreased activity, dull attitude, or loss of stamina, which a thorough history reveals. Daily caloric intake should be determined. Hypothyroid dogs, while rarely grossly overweight, will maintain normal or increased body weight on a caloric intake that is well below what would be expected for maintenance. Intolerance to cold is another sign obtained in the history. It is suggested by the dog not wanting to go out in the cold or staying in warm places in the house.

Clinical Signs

Clinical signs of hypothyroidism affect several body systems (Tables 7-2 and 7-3). Because degrees of thyroid hormone deficiency vary, different patients manifest different patterns and severities of clinical signs. Owners often seek medical attention when signs are associated with the integumentary system; therefore, this system is often overemphasized. It has been observed that up to 40 percent of hypothyroid dogs do not have clinical involvement of their integument. (Chester DK, unpublished data)

Loss of hair is one of the more common signs associated with the integument.[14] Lack of thyroid hormones causes hairs to stay in the telogen phase longer.[13] These hairs become dull and epilate easily, producing alopecia in frictional areas such as the tail, abdomen, or under the collar. Undercoat (secondary, lanuga) hairs are often lost first while guard (primary) hairs remain, resulting in a sparse hair coat. Hair fails to grow in areas where it has been clipped or shaved.

The skin is often dry and scaly, a result of epidermal atrophy, abnormal keratinization, and sebaceous gland atrophy.[15] Secondary Staphylococcal infections occur frequently because normal skin defenses are impaired.[13] Follicular plugging with comedone formation and folliculitis are commonly seen.

Table 7-2. A Summary of Some of the Changes Reported in the Integumentary and Cardiovascular Systems with Canine Hypothyroidism

Integumentary Changes
Hair Coat
Thin, dull, not growing, epilates easily
Loss of undercoat (lanuga hair)
Alopecia in areas of friction
Skin
Thickened (myxedema), puffy
Hyperpigmentation
Seborrheic
Changed bacterial flora (secondary infection present)
Follicles plugged—comedones
Inelastic
Cool to the touch
Poor wound healing, easy bruising
Cardiovascular Changes
Heart
Slowed rate, weak apex beat and pulse
ECG changes—low voltage, inverted T waves
Blood–Vascular Changes
Mild nonregenerative, normocytic normochromic anemia
Hyperlipidemia–Hypercholesterolemia
Hypertension–Hypotension
Thrombosis

(Chester DK: The Thyroid Gland and Thyroid Diseases. p. 93. In Drazner FH (ed): Small Animal Endocrinology. Churchill Livingstone, New York, 1987.)

Accumulation of hyaluronic acid in the interstitial ground substance causes dermal thickening.[13] Clinically this is most often observed around the face and eyes, and is the cause for the "tragic expression" of many hypothyroid dogs. Hyperpigmentation is an inconsistent finding seen most often in areas of alopecia. Uncomplicated hypothyroidism is characteristically nonpruritic; however, when secondary seborrhea or infections are present, pruritus may be the presenting complaint.

The clinical signs associated with the other body systems will not be discussed in detail in this review. However, it is important that these systems be evaluated, since they may give the clinical evidence needed to confirm the diagnosis.

Laboratory Diagnosis

Technology available for laboratory testing of thyroid function in animals has greatly improved in the last 10 to 15 years. However, a single laboratory test that will reliably confirm a diagnosis of hypothyroidism still does not exist. Available tests measure only one aspect of thyroid function at a given time and clinicians have expected too much from these function tests. To properly use thyroid function tests, the clinician must understand what specific tests measure, what laboratory difficulties are encountered, what clinical conditions alter

Table 7-3. A Summary of Some of the Changes Reported in the Gastrointestinal, Neurological, Musculoskeletal, Reproductive and Ophthalmologic Systems with Canine Hypothyroidism

Gastrointestinal Signs
Constipation—diarrhea
Decreased appetite—normal to increased body weight
Neurologic or Musculoskeletal Signs
Lethargy, confusion, decreased mental awareness
Behavioral change—aggressive, very good
Swollen joints—lameness
Reluctance or inability to walk
Head tilt
Facial paralysis
Myopathy
Decreased body temperature—lack of shivering
Voice change
Reproductive Signs
Reduced spermatogenesis and libido in the male
Reduced length and number of estrus cycles
Reduced fertility in the female
Abortion or weak puppies if conception occurs
Galactorrhea
Testicular atrophy
Ophthalmologic Signs
Retinal and pre-retinal hemorrhage
Retinal edema
Swelling of the optic disc
Retinal detachment
Chronic uveitis
Lipid effusion into the aqueous humor
Corneal lipidosis

(Chester DK: The Thyroid Gland and Thyroid Diseases. p. 93. In Drazner FH (ed): Small Animal Endocrinology. Churchill Livingstone, New York, 1987.)

test results, what information will be gained by further testing, and whether tests are cost-effective. Results of laboratory testing must be carefully correlated with clinical signs, history, and response to therapy before a final diagnosis of hypothyroidism is made. A systematic approach to the laboratory diagnosis of hypothyroidism is suggested in Table 7-4.

Routine data-base testing with a complete blood count (CBC) and biochemical panel helps identify or exclude other diseases more than it permits diagnosis of hypothyroidism. The only hematologic abnormality seen frequently is mild reduction of the hematocrit. Serum cholesterol and glucose levels are the only biochemical tests that are likely to be altered. Cholesterol levels exceed the normal range in about 60 percent of the cases, sometimes reaching high values. Serum glucose levels are usually normal or decreased. This finding may help to differentiate hypothyroidism from hyperadrenocorticism, which frequently has an elevated glucose level.

The most reliable single screening test for diagnosis of hypothyroidism that is currently available is the total serum thyroxine level as determined by

Table 7-4. An Outline of a Suggested Approach to the Diagnosis of a Potential Hypothyroid Dog

Dog is presented with one or more historical or clinical signs suggestive of hypothyroidism.
- Minimum data: CBC, biochemical panel and baseline T_4.
  - Results all normal:
    - Normal dog, no treatment
    - Other disease, specific diagnostic tests
    - If signs continued or get worse, retest or perform TSH stimulation within one month
  - Questionable results and/or several clinical or historical signs of hypothyroidism present:
    - Perform TSH stimulation test.
  - Elevated cholesterol, anemia and low T_4 without history of medication or other disease to account for it:
    - Hypothyroid; start treatment
- TSH stimulation.
  - Normal response with normal or low prevalues
    - Euthyroid—look for other disease
  - Questionable response:
    - Further testing such as:
      - Thyroid biopsy
      - Thyroid scan
      - RIU or others if available
  - No response or poor response:
    - Hypothyroid; begin therapy

(Chester DK: The Thyroid Gland and Thyroid Diseases. p. 104. In Drazner FH (ed): Small Animal Endocrinology. Churchill Livingstone, New York, 1987.)

radioimmunoassay (RIA T_4,T_4).[3,4] However, there are several factors that the clinician must consider to accurately interpret T_4 results. (1) Many laboratories use kits that have been developed for measuring T_4 in human serum or plasma where values below 157.6 nmol/l (2 μg/dl) are considered unimportant and some of these kits cannot be altered to measure T_4 values below 78.8 nmol/l (1 μg/dl) as is needed for canine or feline specimens. A reliable laboratory that has validated their procedure to measure the low T_4 values in canine and feline blood specimens must be chosen. Sending specimens to a reference laboratory is made easier by the fact that T_4 values are not altered significantly during storage at room temperature for as long as one week.[16] (2) Certain drugs will alter T_4 results. Some of those known to lower T_4 values are glucocorticoids,[17,18] phenylhydantoin, phenobarbital, phenylbutazone and o,p′ DDD.[13] Estrogens have been found to elevate T_4 values in some animals. (3) T_4 values are often lowered in animals that are fasted or affected with diseases[5,11,13] such as generalized demodicosis, systemic fungal infections, malignancy, and immunologic skin diseases. It is likely that other conditions that have not yet been identified also cause lowered T_4 values. (4) There also appear to be minor changes in T_4 values as a result of the animal's age, the time of day the sample is taken,[19] and the environmental temperature where the animal is housed.

Single random T_4 values within the normal range (118 to 275 nmol/L, 1.50 to 3.48 μg/dl) are observed in hypothyroid animals, and single random low T_4 values are observed in apparently normal animals.[5,13] When values are obtained that do not correlate with the historical or physical findings, testing should be repeated later or other tests (e.g., TSH stimulation, TSH measurement) should be performed.

Total serum or plasma T_3 (RIA T_3, T_3) concentration is measured by radioimmunoassay in many commercial laboratories. Reported normal values of 3.94 to 15.76 nmol/L (50 to 200 ng/dl) in the dog[3,13] and 3.15 to 8.67 nmol/L (40 to 110 ng/dl) in the cat[13] vary with the laboratory. The value of the T_3 measurement for diagnosis of hypothyroidism is controversial. The same diseases, drugs, and physiological conditions that alter T_4 values also alter T_3 values, and in most cases they alter them more rapidly. When both test values fall below the normal range with no known contributing factors, a diagnosis of hypothyroidism is supported. Results must be considered equivocal when either test is normal while the other is abnormal. Resting low T_3 or T_4 values alone are unreliable for diagnosis when clinical, historical, or other clinicopathologic evidence of hypothyroidism is lacking.

Response of the thyroid gland to stimulation by exogenous TSH has become accepted as the most reliable method of evaluating thyroid function in the dog and cat.[19–22] Measurement of T_4 values before and after TSH administration is most often used to evaluate this response. Cost of the TSH and laboratory services, confusion regarding optimum sampling times and proper interpretation of results, and occasional inability to obtain TSH have prevented routine use of this test in many practices. The test is most valuable for differentiating between low resting T_4 values produced by abnormally functioning thyroid glands and low resting T_4 values caused by drug therapy and/or physiologic or disease conditions.

Two protocols, based on whether the route of administration of TSH was intravenous or subcutaneous, are commonly used for the TSH response test. A prestimulation T_4 serum sample is collected in the morning. Five to ten units of bovine TSH is administered by either route. A poststimulation T_4 sample is obtained 4 hours after intravenous or 8 hours after subcutaneous administration of TSH. The measurement of T_3 serum concentrations pre- and post-TSH has questionable diagnostic value.

Normal T_4 values before TSH with a two-to fourfold increase 4 hours (IV route) or 8 hours (SC route) after TSH is given is considered a normal response. When the T_4 value is low for the pre-TSH sample and fails to increase following stimulation, hypothyroidism is confirmed. When extrathyroidal factors such as drugs or systemic disease (euthyroid sick syndrome) are present, the basal T_4 level may be low while the response to TSH is normal. Interpreting test results becomes difficult when the presample is normal but a poor response is obtained (low thyroid reserve), or when the presample is borderline and only a partial response is obtained (possible secondary hypothyroidism.) Authorities do not agree on how to interpret these results. Usually further testing procedures will be required in these animals. Fortunately the number of animals that produce these types of results is small.

Thyroid gland biopsy and measurement of thyroidal radioiodine uptake (RIU) are other tests that can be used to study thyroid gland function. Because of technical difficulties and expense, these tests are used infrequently by most clinicians. Measurement of free thyroxine or TSH would be helpful, but care should be taken to ensure that the test has been validated for use in dogs and cats. A test for measuring canine TSH has been recently reported and is commercially available in some laboratories.[23] RIA tests using human TSH have been shown to be inaccurate for measuring dog TSH.[5,24]

Findings that are suggestive of hypothyroidism may be revealed by skin biopsy. Epidermal changes associated with hypothyroidism include thinning or thickening, hyperkeratosis, follicular keratosis, dilation and plugging of the hair follicles, and epidermal melanosis. Mucin accumulation in the dermis and subcutis, atrophic sebaceous glands, increased numbers of telogen hair shafts, swollen and separated collagen bundles, and hypertrophy of arrector pili muscles may also be observed.[13,15] None of these changes are sufficiently specific to confirm a diagnosis of hypothyroidism by themselves.

Diagnosis of hypothyroidism is through a combination of historical and physical findings, laboratory results, and correct interpretation of response to therapy. Reliance on any of the parts as the single diagnostic method will often result in misdiagnosis and improper therapy. Apparent response to thyroid therapy is no more proof that hypothyroidism exists than is a single abnormal laboratory test. Classic clinical signs of hypothyroidism are also inadequate proof that the disease exists since many diseases produce similar clinical signs. Diagnosis of this disease is challenging, but the results can be rewarding if proper procedures are followed.

Treatment

The treatment of hypothyroidism is aimed at replacing the insufficient hormones in quantities sufficient to correct the clinical signs. Dogs with severe deficiencies will therefore require larger doses of replacement hormone than those with a mild deficiency. This author prefers administration of replacement therapy twice daily while others have found treatment once daily to be satisfactory.[5,25–27] Controlled studies proving one method superior to the other have not been reported.

Sodium levothyroxine (L-thyroxine, T_4) is the synthetic hormone product most commonly used for treatment of hypothyroidism. Most circulating T_3 in dogs and cats comes from peripheral conversion of T_4; therefore, T_4 is the only drug necessary for treatment of most animals.[27] Following oral administration, peak blood levels of T_4 occur in 4 to 6 hours with minor individual variations. Canine dosage recommendations vary from 20 μg/kg (0.1 mg/11 lb) given once daily to 20 μg/kg b.i.d.[27] Others suggest dosages based on body surface areas.[5,25] Favorable response is usually manifested by improved activity and mental status within 2 weeks. Regardless of the initial dosage, treatment should be monitored using clinical signs and/or laboratory tests, and the dose should be increased or decreased as needed. Dosage recommendations for the feline vary from 0.05 to 0.3 mg daily.[27] Although it is difficult to produce hyperthyroidism in dogs by overdosing with thyroid hormones, care should be taken to prevent overdose in cats.

Liothyronine (sodium L-triiodothyronine or T_3) is the other synthetic product used in treatment for hypothyroid dogs and cats. Compared with T_4, advantages of this product are greater biological potency, faster action, and better absorption from the gastrointestinal tract. Disadvantages include shorter half-life, greater cost, and difficulty in therapeutic monitoring. Most clinicians use this drug only as a supplement to T_4 therapy when there is laboratory evidence that T_4 is not being converted to T_3. When used as the only treatment, a dose of 4.4 μg/kg given every 8 hours is recommended.[27]

Crude hormone products are prepared from thyroid tissue of animals from slaughter houses and include desiccated thyroid (thyroid USP) and thyroglobulin (thyroglobulin USP). Disadvantages of these crude products are inconsistant biologic value[28] and loss of potency during storage. Recommended dosage for desiccated thyroid is 15 to 20 mg/kg/day.[27] The author prefers synthetic products.

Laboratory monitoring of therapeutic response using postmedication measurement of T_4 and T_3 levels is recommended. Samples are drawn 4 to 6 hours following drug administration to determine maximum levels, and/or at 12 or 24 hours (i.e., just prior to the next treatment) to determine minimum posttreatment blood levels. Both T_4 and T_3 values should be in the normal range regardless of the sampling times chosen. Adjustments in therapy must be made if the values are abnormal. When products containing T_3 are used for therapy, postmedication laboratory monitoring will not be valuable because the T_4 value will be low.

Therapeutic Complications

Complications are rarely associated with thyroid therapy in dogs. Thyrotoxicosis due to excessive thyroid supplementation is rare in dogs, but can be produced easily in cats. Clinical signs observed with thyrotoxicosis are polyuria, polydipsia, nervousness, weight loss, panting, tachycardia, and increased pulse pressure.[27] Since cardiac signs are the most serious, a lower starting dosage should be used in hypothyroid animals with cardiac disease.[27]

Thyroid hormones increase demand for corticosteroids by stimulating increased metabolism. When the conditions coexist, adrenal insufficiency should be treated before hypothyroidism is corrected to prevent precipitating an adrenal crisis.

Diabetics should also be monitored very closely when thyroid therapy is initiated, because insulin requirements may be markedly increased in some animals.[27]

Improper dosage, owner's inability or unwillingness to give medication, poor gastrointestinal absorption, and incorrect diagnosis are possible causes for therapeutic failure. Changing to a different type of medication, crushing the tablets before administration, or treating a malabsorption disorder may help when poor absorption is the problem. Therapeutic monitoring, client education, and further testing to determine the presence of other diseases are all helpful in eliminating other causes of therapeutic failure.

HYPERADRENOCORTICISM

Etiology

Hyperadrenocorticism (canine Cushing's syndrome) is the disease produced by an excessive circulating level of cortisol. Causes of the disease are grouped into three main categories: (1) pituitary-dependent hyperadrenocorticism (PDH), (2) functional adrenal neoplasia, and (3) iatrogenic hyperadrenocorticism.

Excessive secretion of adrenocorticotropic hormone (ACTH) by the pituitary gland causes PDH. Secreting pituitary tumors can cause such high ACTH levels. Alternately, pituitary or hypothalamic failure to respond to high cortisol levels by reducing ACTH production causes the same high ACTH levels. PDH represents approximately 85 to 90 percent of spontaneous hyperadrenocorticism in dogs.[29] The remaining cases of spontaneous hyperadrenocorticism are represented primarily by cortisol-secreting adrenal tumors. These tumors produce cortisol, which lowers circulating ACTH levels, but production of cortisol is not reduced by the low ACTH levels.[30]

Iatrogenic hyperadrenocorticism occurs when corticosteroids are given in quantities large enough to cause changes in the body. Clinical manifestations are indistinguishable from those seen with spontaneous hyperadrenocorticism. A single treatment or therapy for weeks, months, or years with corticosteroids may produce the disease.[31] The condition is difficult to produce in cats, but signs are similar to those seen in dogs.[32,33] The iatrogenic disease is common in dogs and may account for as much clinical hyperadrenocorticism as the spontaneous disease.[32]

Physiologic Effects of Corticosteroids

Corticosteroids have many physiologic effects that produce substantial clinical and laboratory signs when these compounds are present in excess.[34] Increased gluconeogenesis and inhibition of peripheral glucose utilization cause high blood glucose levels and are accompanied by increased hepatic glycogen storage. Increased peripheral catabolism of proteins, inhibition of fibroblast formation and collagen deposition, and reduced transport of amino acids across extrahepatic cell membranes cause retarded tissue repair and growth, increased conversion of amino acids to glucose, and increased liver formation of proteins. Increased fat catabolism causes shifting body fat stores, increased circulating fatty acids, hyperlipemia, and hypercholesterolemia.

Glucocorticosteroids increase free water clearance and promote water excretion resulting in polyuria and polydipsia. They increase renal excretion of calcium, reduce calcium absorption from the bowel, cause tissue catabolism of bone matrix, which interferes with bone ossification, and decrease conversion of vitamin D to the active form by the kidney. These effects combine to cause calcification abnormalities of bone and soft tissues.[34]

The glucocorticosteroids have marked antiinflammatory and immunosuppressive activity.[34] They suppress fibroblastic activity and granuloma formation and stabilize lysosomal and cellular membranes. Phagocytosis, chemotactic responses, antigen processing, and complement formation and action are all inhibited.

Effects on the hemopoietic system include reduction of circulating eosinophil numbers by suppressing their production, reduction in lymphocyte numbers by causing their lysis and suppression of their production, and increasing neutrophil numbers by stimulating production and mobilizing sequestered cells and those in the bone marrow pool.[34]

The gastrointestinal system is affected because glucocorticoids increase production of hydrochloric acid and pepsin by the stomach which can result in gastric ulcers. High levels may cause acute pancreatitis. Another common effect is increased appetite.

Diagnosis

History and Clinical Signs

Diagnosis of hyperadrenocorticism is made by combining patient history with clinical signs and laboratory data. Spontaneous disease is most often seen in dogs older than 6 years and is seldom seen in dogs less than 4 years old. A significant sex predisposition has not been reported. Boston terriers, poodles, dachshunds, and boxers are consistently reported breeds in which the disease has high prevalence.[29,35–40] However, many breeds may be affected, and the diagnosis should not be excluded because of breed. Signs of the disease are slowly progressive. The patient's history is valuable in diagnosing iatrogenic hyperadrenocorticism, especially if the dog has received corticosteroids prior to development of clinical signs.

Clinical signs of the disease are often dramatic and diagnostic even though some animals show only mild signs that can be confused with other endocrine diseases.[38] Polyuria and polydipsia are early signs that are seen in 85 percent or more of the dogs.[35] This sign may precede skin changes by as much as 6 months to 1 year. Polyphagia is reported to occur in 67 to 100 percent of dogs.[38] A poor appetite is seldom seen except in late stages of the disease.

Skin or hair coat changes are seen in 55 to 90 percent of the cases. A generalized thinning of the hair coat in a symmetrical pattern is caused by poor hair growth. The head and extremities are less often affected. Short coated breeds tend to lose less hair then dogs with long coats. The hair is often dry, brittle, and can be epilated easily. Color changes toward lighter colors can be marked when present. The disease results in skin that is very thin, fine textured, inelastic, easily bruised, and dehydrated in appearance. Subcutaneous vessels of the ventral abdomen are often strikingly visible through nonpigmented skin. Excessive scale formation and keratin plugging of the hair follicles (comedones) are other skin changes that are seen. Cutaneous mineralization (calcinosis cutis) is seen in up to 40 percent of the dogs,[38] most often in later stages of disease. The skin heals slowly following trauma or injury and decubitus ulcers may result. Secondary bacterial infections of the skin and other body systems are seen in some cases.

Accelerated catabolism of protein frequently produces generalized muscle wasting.[36] Muscles of the shoulders, thighs, pelvis, and temporal area are most often involved. Weakness and atrophy of abdominal muscles results in a "pot belly" appearance. Enlargement of the liver contributes to this appearance. Myotonia is seen in a small number of cases.[36] Lethargy, exercise intolerance, or both are seen in about 75 percent of hyperadrenocortical dogs as a sequela to muscle wasting.

Osteoporosis or osteomalacia occurs in about one third of the animals with this disease. Lameness and/or pathologic fractures may be seen as a result. Frequent panting is seen in approximately half of the cases. This sign is often interpreted as intolerance to heat, but may be seen in animals that are not exposed to high temperatures.

In some female dogs with PDH, stimulation of adrenal androgens produces prolonged anestrus and clitoral enlargement. In males, decreased hypothalamic gonadal releasing hormone release may produce testicular atrophy. Neurologic signs are seen in some dogs with encroaching pituitary tumors. Depending on the nerve tracts affected, these signs vary in type and severity and may include impairment of pupillary reflexes, vision, or locomotion.

Diabetes mellitus and hyperadrenocorticism as concurrent diseases are not unusual since prolonged elevation of blood glucose by excessive glucocorticoids can produce pancreatic islet cell exhaustion. One study found 30 of 137 dogs with hyperadrenocorticism also had diabetes mellitus.[41]

Laboratory Diagnosis

Pretreatment laboratory confirmation of the diagnosis of hyperadrenocorticism is very important because the treatment can be life-threatening. Database testing with a CBC and biochemical panel is very helpful. The most consistent change in the CBC is a total eosinophil count of less than 100/μl. Response to internal or external parasites may offset this change. The next most frequent change is a total lymphocyte count of less than 1,000/μl. Less consistently, the neutrophil count will be seen to elevate to within a range of 6,000 to 65,000/μl.[38]

Blood biochemical changes frequently seen are elevations in cholesterol, glucose, alkaline phosphatase, and glutamic pyruvic transaminase (SGPT). Serum or plasma levels of T_3 and T_4 are frequently lowered, causing problems in differentiating this disease from hypothyroidism if the clinical signs and other laboratory changes are not carefully observed.

The measurement of plasma cortisol before and after either ACTH stimulation or dexamethasone suppression is the most reliable way to confirm the diagnosis of hyperadrenocorticism. Cortisol is measured by several methods,

Table 7-5. Plasma Cortisol Findings Expected

	Before Maneuver		After Maneuver	
Condition	Resting Value	ACTH Stimulation	Low Dose Dex—Supp[b]	High Dose Dex—Supp[c]
Normal	Normal	Two- to fourfold elevation	Suppressed	Suppressed
Dog under stress	Normal or elevated	Normal response	Suppressed	Suppressed
Pituitary-dependent hyperadrenal	Normal or elevated	Fivefold or more increase or above 15 μg/dl RIA[a]	Should not suppress	Suppressed
Adrenal tumor	Usually elevated	May or may not show an increase	Should not suppress	Should not suppress
Iatrogenic hyperadrenal	Normal or depressed	Little or no response	Not needed	Not needed

[a] The normal and abnormal values vary among reference laboratories. The clinician must verify these before interpreting results.
[b] Low dose dexamethasone suppression test.
[c] High dose dexamethasone suppression test.

but the most common is by RIA. There is variation in normal values between laboratories even when the same methods are used. Normal values for the specific reference laboratory used must be considered when interpreting test results. It is important to centrifuge blood samples soon after they are obtained and to freeze the serum or plasma for storage and shipment in order to prevent spurious lowering of the values.[16,42,43]

There is agreement among clinicians[29,44] that the diagnostic value of a single resting cortisol determination is so questionable that response tests should always be conducted to confirm hyperadrenocorticism. Of these tests, the easiest to perform is the ACTH response test because it can be conducted on an inpatient or outpatient basis in less than 3 hours. A blood specimen for resting cortisol determination is obtained between 8 and 10 AM. Synthetic ACTH (0.25 mg IV) or ACTH gel (1 unit per lb. IM) is then administered. A blood specimen for cortisol determination is then obtained one hour after synthetic ACTH or 2 hours after gel administration.[45] Expected responses are summarized in Table 7-5. This test is considered approximately 85 percent reliable in confirming the diagnosis of hyperadrenocorticism.[29,34,42,46,47] It is, however, unreliable in the diagnosis of hyperadrenocorticism caused by adrenal tumors.[30,39,48]

The low dose dexamethasone suppression test is advocated by some as the test of choice for diagnosis of spontaneous hyperadrenocorticism.[29,32,46,47,49] It has been shown to be over 90 percent reliable in confirming this diagnosis. A blood specimen for baseline cortisol determination is drawn in the morning, and then 0.01 mg/kg of dexamethasone is administered intravenously. The second sample is drawn at 4 hours following the dexamethasone injection and a third sample is drawn after 8 hours. The second cortisol value should be less than 50 percent of the baseline value and not more than 1.4 μg/dl. The cortisol value should remain suppressed at the 8 hour sampling time. This is an important sample since some affected dogs will suppress at the earlier time but will not remain suppressed. Neither this test nor the ACTH stimulation test will accurately differentiate between PDH and adrenal tumors. To differentiate between these conditions, it is necessary to combine either or both of these screening tests with the high dose dexamethasone suppression test (Table 7-5).[29,37,46,47,49,50]

The procedure for a high dose dexamethasone suppression test is exactly the same as for the low dose test, except for the dexamethasone dosage that is used. For high dose response testing, the dosage is 0.1 mg/kg IV or 1.0 mg/kg IM. Normal animals and those with PDH will have postsuppression cortisol values below the least amount that the test can measure. Dogs with hypercortisolemia caused by adrenal tumors should have postsuppression cortisol values only slightly depressed from the baseline value and greater than 1.4 μg/dl.[46]

This amount of testing is both time-consuming and expensive; therefore, workers[51–53] have tried to shorten the process by combining the ACTH and high dose dexamethasone suppression tests into a 1-day procedure requiring 6 hours or less. The author no longer uses the method because results obtained using this approach have been difficult to interpret. Clinicians planning to treat all spontaneous hyperadrenocorticism with o,p′-DDD (Mitotane) need only confirm the diagnosis.

Treatment

The two general methods of treating hyperadrenocorticism are surgical and medical. Surgery should be attempted only by competent and experienced surgeons. Surgical removal of adrenal tumors is the treatment of choice for that disease. Bilateral adrenalectomy corrects the signs of PDH, but the procedure requires performing surgery on an animal with a compromised immune system and poor wound healing. However, these dogs must be treated for hypoadrenocorticism for the rest of their lives. Hypophysectomy can successfully correct the symptoms of PDH by removing the source of ACTH, but this requires a surgeon with considerable experience. Furthermore, surgery would require the animal to receive lifelong treatment for hypoadrenocorticism, hypothyroidism, and diabetes insipidus.

Chemotherapy with o,p′-DDD (Mitotane) is a satisfactory treatment for pituitary-dependent spontaneous hyperadrenocorticism and has become the most common therapy for this disease.[54] Dogs with functional adrenal tumors may also be treated by this same protocol even though surgery is the treatment of choice. Therapy is begun by giving o,p′-DDD at a rate of 50 mg/kg/d for 7 to 10 days. Low dose (0.01 mg/kg) prednisone or prednisolone is often recommended starting within the first 3 days of o,p′-DDD therapy to minimize side effects of the drug. It is necessary to monitor the therapeutic response to the loading dose of o,p′-DDD. Normal water consumption (60 ml/kg or less) may return in as few as 2 days or may take up to 2 weeks. Return of normal eosinophil and/or lymphocyte levels is a less reliable guide for terminating initial therapy, but is helpful in dogs with normal water consumption when therapy is begun. Monitoring cortisol levels before and following ACTH stimulation is the most accurate way to determine therapeutic response. The time required to get test results returned from the laboratory often precludes reliance on this test alone in clinical practice. A commonly used protocol is to perform the ACTH response test 1 to 4 days after discontinuing the loading dose of o,p′-DDD. The oral glucocorticoid may be given for an additional 3 or 4 days. If signs of hypocortisolism (weakness, vomiting, anorexia) occur when the glucocorticoid is discontinued, the glucocorticoid should be reinstituted immediately. Successful o,p′-DDD therapy results in normal (1.4 to 4.0 μg/dl) resting (i.e., baseline) cortisol values and little or no increase in cortisol levels following ACTH administration.[29,54,55] If the post-ACTH cortisol levels are higher than 4.0 μg/dl, the o,p′-DDD loading protocol is continued until the post-ACTH cortisol levels fall within the normal baseline range.

The maintenance protocol involves the weekly administration of 50 mg/kg or biweekly dosage of 25 mg/kg to maintain control of the disease. Therapeutic response is usually monitored by clinical and/or laboratory evaluation (ACTH response test) every 3 to 6 months and adjustments made in the treatment schedule based on the results obtained. Occasionally, the symptoms are completely relieved with the initial therapy and no maintenance therapy is required.

Therapy for iatrogenic hyperadrenocorticism requires reduction of excessive exogenous glucocorticoid administration while continuing maintenance therapy for secondary hypoadrenocorticism. Return of adequate adrenal function may take months to years depending on the duration of the excessive corticosteroid therapy. Prednisone, prednisolone, or hydrocortisone are the corticosteroids of choice for maintenance therapy. Treatment is initiated by starting the animal on an equivalent of half the steroid level it was receiving when signs developed. Maintenance therapy is gradually reduced every 2 weeks until the dog is free of signs of hypoadrenocorticism without corticosteroid supplementation. The initial reductions are made only on alternate days until the dog is receiving medication every other day. Reductions are then continued in the alternate day dose. The author prefers not to use ACTH injections for this disease since it is so short in its action and antibodies to it can be developed. Laboratory evaluation may be used as a guide to therapy. Cortisol levels in response to ACTH stimulation should return to normal when the adrenal glands have recovered normal function.

Treatment Complications

Administration of o,p′-DDD is not without hazard. Careful attention should be given to initiating therapy only in dogs that have hyperadrenocorticism and to monitoring for adverse effects in those that need therapy. Overdose can lead to complete destruction of the adrenal cortex and a hypoadrenal crisis.[56] Anorexia, nausea, vomiting, and diarrhea are signs that may signal overdose. When these signs occur, the dose should be reduced or the drug discontinued. In some cases vomiting is caused by gastric irritation and dividing the daily dose into two treatments or giving the medication with food may provide relief. Weakness, depression, disorientation, head pressing, and ataxia are other toxic effects of the medication that can be overcome by dividing the daily dose into 2 treatments. When any of these symptoms persist, however, corticosteroids should be given at the lowest dose that corrects the clinical signs.

SEX HORMONE ABNORMALITIES

Etiology

The area of endocrine dermatology that is least understood and most poorly documented is sex hormone dermatoses. Excesses or deficiencies of estrogens, testosterone, and/or progesterone have been hypothesized but seldom proven.

Hyperestrogenism is thought to be the cause of two dermatoses: hyperestrogenism in intact female dogs (ovarian imbalance type I)[57] and feminization of male dogs with a functional Sertoli cell tumor,[58–64] interstitial cell tumor[60,65] or seminoma[60,66] of the testicle. Similar syndromes are produced in dogs by estrogen supplementation.[67–70] An estrogen requirement for normal skin and hair coat has not been established. Animals with low serum estrogen levels do not develop skin disease. However, it has been speculated that hypoestrogenism causes estrogen-responsive dermatoses (ovarian imbalance type II) of spayed females.[71]

Skin disease caused by androgen excess is rare.[72] A testosterone-responsive dermatosis of male dogs is thought to be due to hypoandrogenism. Male feminizing syndrome without testicular tumor is another rare disease of male dogs for which hypotestosteronism is the suspected etiology, but abnormal serum levels of estrogen or testosterone were not found.[73] Detailed clinical reports proving androgen abnormalities to be the causes of these diseases were not found.

Skin disease as a result of an excess or deficiency of progesterone has not been documented except for the influence that progesterone has on growth hormone production. This is discussed later in this chapter.

Physiologic Effects on the Skin

Estrogen's physiologic effects on skin vary with the dose, route of administration, and type of estrogen used.[68,74,75] Estrogens increase skin pigmentation in guinea pigs and hyperpigmentation is also a feature of canine hyperestrogen syndromes.[71] Estrogens produce atrophy of sebaceous glands in dogs.[76,77] Estrogens also produce alopecia when administered either orally, subcutaneously, intramuscularly, or topically.[68] Subcutis thickness was reduced in dogs given stilbesterol for 400 days.[68] Bone marrow suppression is another serious effect of estrogens that has been reported with both spontaneous and experimentally induced disease.[78–85]

Androgens cause increased epidermal mitotic activity, cell turnover time, and skin thickness in humans. They increase cutaneous pigmentation especially in genital skin of men. Androgens increase the size and production of sebaceous glands in several species. In humans, the rate of hair growth is increased by androgens, and thickening of the dermis due to an increase in collagen content is a result of increased androgens.[71]

Progesterone compounds bind to cytosol receptors for dihydrotestosterone and inhibit 5-αreductase, the enzyme that converts testosterone to dihydrotestosterone. Physiologic effects of this binding give progestational compounds an androgenic, synandrogenic, or antiandrogenic effect depending on the compound, dose, and product used.[71]

Diagnosis of Sex Hormone Skin Disease

Diagnosis of sex hormone-related skin disease is based on the patient's history, clinical findings, and only rarely on distinctive laboratory findings.

Feminization Associated with Sertoli Cell Tumor

Feminization of male dogs is most often seen with Sertoli cell tumors. Only one-third of dogs with scrotal Sertoli cell tumors have signs of feminization[61] while dogs with Sertoli cell tumors in abdominal testicles show a comparative sevenfold higher incidence of feminization.[63] Feminization has been seen on rare occasions in dogs with other types of tumors of the testicle.[60,61,65,66,82] The disease is seen most frequently in older dogs. The average age of affected dogs is 9 years, but the disease has been reported in dogs as young as 3 years.[58,61,64,81] Owners may complain that their male dog has developed behavioral abnormalities including sexual attractiveness to male dogs, lack of libido, and an irritable or aggressive temperament.

Clinical signs include: alopecia with dry, brittle, and poor-growing hair that epilates easily; hyper- or hypopigmented skin especially of the genital area, medial thighs, and ventral abdomen; gynecomastia; pendulous prepuce; one enlarged or retained testicle and the other small and soft; and enlarged prostate gland. Alopecia is usually seen in a symmetrical pattern that starts in the flank or genital area and spreads to the lower abdomen or total trunk. The skin may be thin and soft, but becomes thick and seborrheic as the disease progresses.

Histologic skin changes are suggestive of an endocrine alopecia. Changes include acanthosis, hyperkeratosis, and hyperpigmentation of the basal cell layer. Dermal thinning with atrophic hair follicles and normal to atrophic sweat and sebaceous glands is reported.[71,76,77]

Complete blood count changes are seldom diagnostic. A few dogs will have anemia and thrombocytopenia as a result of bone marrow suppression.[82] When this occurs there will usually be clinical signs as intestinal hemorrhage or petechial hemorrhages in the skin or mucous membranes which suggest bleeding abnormalities.

Normal estradiol values for male dogs are approximately 15 to 60 pg/ml.[71] Unfortunately, measurement of estrogen levels is not very helpful in the diagnosis of this disease since most laboratories measure only one of the several estrogens produced; therefore test results are not reliable. However, elevated estrogen levels in an intact male is consistent with a testicular tumor. The test's cost also discourages its use.

Male Feminizing Syndrome

Male feminizing syndrome is a rare disease of middle-aged dogs. Clinical signs include symmetrical alopecia, severe seborrheic skin disease including ceruminous otitis, hyperpigmentation especially in the inguinal and flank areas, gynecomastia with attraction of male dogs and decreased libido, and normal testicles. Clinical disease is similar to hyperestrogenism in either males or females from other causes. Laboratory evaluation of testosterone and estradiol has failed to reveal differences from normal dogs.[73] Skin biopsy reveals changes consistent with an endocrine dermatosis.

Female Hyperestrogenism (Ovarian Imbalance Type I)

Clinical features of female hyperestrogenism (ovarian imbalance type I) are similar to male hyperestrogenism except for estrus cycle abnormalities. Irregular cycles, anestrus, prolonged estrus, and severe pseudopregnancy are frequently part of the history. Middle-aged intact bitches are most often affected. There is no breed predisposition. Hair is easily epilated, and symmetrical alopecia beginning in the perineal and genital areas and spreading to most of the body except the head is characteristic of this disorder. Skin is often seborrheic and may be pruritic as a result of secondary infection. Hyperpigmentation around the vulva and in the flank area with enlargement of the nipples and vulva is often seen.

Histologic examination of skin is nondiagnostic, revealing changes consistent with endocrine skin disease. Those changes include hyperkeratosis, follicular keratosis, follicular dilation or atrophy, and sebaceous gland atrophy. Inflammatory change such as perivascular dermatitis is seen in some cases. Functional ovarian tumors,[57] cystic ovaries, or normal ovarian and uterine tissue may be seen on microscopic examination of the genital tract. Laboratory test abnormalities are not routinely reported and estrogen measurements in our laboratory have not been diagnostic. Normal estradiol levels for female dogs are approximately 10 to 80 pg/ml.[71]

Testosterone-Responsive Dermatosis (Hypoandrogenism)

A rare symmetrical alopecia of older male dogs is testosterone-responsive dermatosis (hypoandrogenism). Intact male dogs with normal or diseased testicles and castrated male dogs may develop the disease. Alopecia usually begins in the perineal or genital area and spreads to other parts of the trunk and legs. Pigmentary changes and pruritus are rarely seen. The skin is thin and hypotonic, and inflammatory changes are rare. Histopathology of the skin reveals the same changes as are seen with other endocrine dermatoses. There is no laboratory confirmation of this disease other than that required to exclude more common endocrine dermatoses such as hypothyroidism and hyperadrenocorticism.

Estrogen-Responsive Dermatosis (Ovarian Imbalance Type II)

Estrogen-responsive dermatosis (ovarian imbalance type II, hypoestrogenism) is a rare symmetrical alopecia of neutered female dogs. Alopecia begins in genital and perineal areas and spreads to the trunk and upper legs. Hair is easily epilated. Grossly, skin is usually uninvolved, and infantile nipples and vulva are usually seen. Urinary incontinence is seen in some animals. Skin biopsy and other laboratory data are nondiagnostic. Final diagnosis is based on history, clinical signs, and exclusion of hypothyroidism, hyperadrenocorticism, or other metabolic and endocrine alopecias.

Hyperandrogenism

Hyperandrogenism is another rare and poorly documented endocrine alopecia. It is seen in intact male dogs and in dogs of either sex when androgenic hormones are administered in excess. Middle-aged or older dogs are more likely to be affected. This author has seen this condition in one spayed female dog that had hyperadrenocorticism as the source of both glucocorticoids and androgens. Characteristically, aggressive male sexual behavior is part of the history. The alopecia is usually diffuse over the trunk and is associated with severe seborrhea. Pruritus and secondary infection may be seen later in the course of the disease. Histopathology of the integument is typical of an endocrine alopecia except that the sebaceous glands are often dilated. Laboratory findings are not diagnostic. Final diagnosis is based on history, clinical findings, and exclusion of common causes of seborrheic dermatitis.

Treatment

Testicular tumors should be treated by total castration because dogs with tumors of one testicle frequently have tumors in the opposite testicle.[63] Testosterone supplementation is usually not necessary following castration because recovery of normal skin and hair coat is usually seen within 3 months. Recovery followed by relapse is an indication of tumor metastasis and should be treated accordingly.

The treatment of choice for other male feminizing syndromes is castration. Treatment with methyl testosterone (1 mg/kg, up to a maximum total dose of 30 mg) given orally every other day is effective in treating male feminizing syndrome without testicular tumor and testosterone-responsive dermatosis of male dogs.[71] Maintenance doses given once or twice per week may be needed in some dogs. Response is usually seen within 3 months. Repositol testosterone given intramuscularly at the rate of 2.2 mg/kg every 6 months is also effective.[71]

Ovariohysterectomy is the treatment of choice for ovarian imbalance type I. Diethylstilbestrol (0.1 to 1 mg) given orally every other day is recommended for estrogen-responsive dermatosis. Since bone marrow suppression is a danger in animals on prolonged estrogen therapy, select the lowest effective dose and never treat longer than 3 weeks without a 1 week or longer nontreatment period.

Symptomatic antiseborrheic therapy should be used in those dogs with scaling and crusting. This includes shampoos with coal tar, sulfur, benzoyl peroxide, or salicylic acid as their base. Antibiotics should be used when secondary infection is present. In all cases, response should be expected within 3 months. The diagnosis should be reevaluated if a response is not observed.

GROWTH HORMONE ABNORMALITIES

Etiology

Skin and hair coat abnormalities can be seen with increases or decreases in growth hormone (GH) levels. Causes of increased GH levels (acromegaly) include functional pituitary tumors[86] and spontaneous or iatrogenic high levels of progestogens.[87–91] GH deficiency is seen as a genetic recessive hereditary disease in German shepherds which results in dwarfism.[92–94] An adult onset GH deficiency (pseudo-Cushing's) of unknown etiology has also been identified.[95,96] Suppressed GH response to zylazine has been reported in association with hyperadrenocorticism.[97]

Physiologic Effects of Growth Hormone

Growth hormone influences tissue growth indirectly by stimulating activity of insulin-like growth factors I and II (IGF I and IGF II, somatomedins).[98,99] The dependency of epidermal, fibroblast, and nerve growth factors on GH is unknown.[98] The combined effects of these factors and thyroid hormones is chondrogenesis, protein synthesis, increased mitosis, and growth. In addition to this indirect action, GH has a direct insulin antagonism, which causes lipolysis, insulin resistance, and hyperglycemia.[98,99]

There are relationships between GH and corticosteroid, thyroid, estrogen, and progesterone hormones in the normal growth process. Glucocorticoids inhibit the metabolic actions of GH.[100] Estrogens enhance GH response to some stimuli, but, in high doses, may block some of the peripheral metabolic actions of GH.[100] Spontaneous and iatrogenic increases in progestogens can cause increased levels of GH.[87–91,99] The mechanism by which progestogens cause this increase in GH is not understood.

Diagnosis of Growth Hormone Excess (Acromegaly)

Acromegaly is an endocrine disorder characterized by overgrowth of soft tissue and/or bony structures due to GH overproduction in adult animals. In dogs, spontaneous acromegaly can occur during diestrus (progesterone phase).[88–90] The use of progesterone compounds for estrus control or treatment of skin disease has produced acromegalic symptoms in some dogs and cats.[86–89,99,101] History suggesting recent completion of the estrus cycle, pseudocyesis, or use of progestogens requires including acromegaly in the differential diagnosis when the proper clinical signs are present.

The clinical signs seen with either form of this disorder are visible increase in soft tissue mass resulting in inspiratory stridor; prominent skin folds and an enlarged abdomen; enlargement of the interdigital spaces; and polyuria/polydipsia.[87,89,90,91] The excessive skin folds are more prominent around the head, neck, and distal extremities. The skin may become palpably thickened and feel puffy. The hair coat may become coarse,[91] excessively thickened, or long and curly.[87,90] Excessive toenail growth is reported.[87]

Microscopic changes in acromegalic dog skin exhibit variable degrees of orthokeratotic hyperkeratosis, hypergranulosis, and epidermal hyperplasia. Increased amount of dermal collagen and number of fibroblasts results in a thickened dermis, which appears inordinately dense, compact, and cellular. Mucinous degeneration (myxedema) may also be seen.[91]

Laboratory abnormalities include increased blood glucose levels,[86,89] increased serum alkaline phosphatase levels,[89] lowered packed cell volume,[89] and high T_4 values;[89] however, all of these have been found normal in some acromegalic dogs.[86,89,90] These changes are not diagnostic. Suggestive historic findings, proper clinical signs, and measurement of GH levels are necessary for diagnosis. Canine GH assays are species specific. Therefore, they are not commercially available. Normal serum GH values approximate 1 to 2 ng/ml.[102] Persistent GH values of 10 ng/ml or higher which can not be suppressed by intravenous glucose load (1 g/kg) are diagnostic of acromegaly.[87–89,99] IGF I is also elevated in acromegalic dogs. Twenty acromegalic dogs had levels of 679 $\pm$ 116 ng/ml while 13 normal German shepherds had levels of 280 $\pm$ 23 ng/ml.[99] This compound does not have species specificity and therefore may be easier to have assayed.

Diagnosis of Growth Hormone Deficiency Disease

Growth hormone deficiency in the immature animal results in short stature and severe skin and hair coat changes.[98,100,103–108] The same skin and hair coat changes occur in mature animals with GH deficiency regardless of the cause.[95,96,109,110] The first change is failure of development or loss of primary or guard hairs. This leaves a soft woolly undercoat of lanugo hair. All hair is easily epilated and with time the entire coat is lost over the trunk, resulting in a bilaterally symmetrical alopecia. Hair is usually retained on the head, face and distal extremities. The alopecic skin has normal pigmentation at first, but with time it becomes pigmented to varying degrees. The skin is thin, hypotonic, scaly, and has excessive folds or wrinkles. Follicular plugging (comedones) is often seen.

These changes suggest GH deficiency but are also similar to changes seen with the more common endocrine diseases hypothyroidism and hyperadrenocorticism; therefore, it is necessary to use the patient's history laboratory data, and response to therapy to confirm the diagnosis. Pituitary dwarfism is most often seen in the German shepherd breed.[92–94,98,100,103,105,107,108,111,112] Adult onset growth hormone deficiency has most often been reported in poodles, Pomeranians, chow chows, and keeshonds.[95,96] One Samoyed[96] and one Lhasa apso[95] with the disease have been reported. GH deficiency is usually seen in young adult dogs (less than 5 years at onset) compared to other endocrine diseases, which are seldom seen in dogs less than 4 years of age.

Laboratory tests for adrenal, thyroid, and sex hormone abnormalities are normal in adult onset GH deficiency[95,96] but may be abnormal in dwarfism[100,103,106] due to loss of pituitary function. Microscopic examination of the skin reveals changes consistent with other endocrine diseases. Special elastin stains reveal moderate to marked decreases in dermal elastin as compared to normal skin.[100] Hyperadrenocorticism is another endocrine disease that produces this histologic change.

Basal GH levels will be low, but they do not reliably separate normal and GH deficient dogs. It is necessary to confirm the diagnosis by measuring GH levels 15, 30, 45, 60, and 90 minutes following administration of clonidine (10 μg/kg, slowly IV) or xylazine (Rompum) (100 to 300 ng/kg, IV.).[102] GH deficient dogs show clearly subnormal responses to this stimulation compared to normal animals.[95,103,109]

Treatment

Successful treatment of adult onset GH deficiency with bovine and porcine GH (5 IU per injection given every other day for 10 treatments) has been reported.[96] Two IU of porcine GH given subcutaneously every other day for 100 days followed by 2 IU every fourth day for 6 months was partially successful in a pituitary dwarf.[98] Synthetic (genetically engineered) GH is produced in Israel and the United States. This form of GH is being used on an experimental basis for treatment of GH deficiency dermatosis in dogs. Response to therapy is usually seen within 4 to 6 weeks after initiation of therapy.[96] There is potential for hypersensitivity reactions and either transient or permanent diabetes mellitus with GH administration in dogs.[110] The author recommends a dose of no more than 0.1 IU/kg/SC every other day for 12 treatments. The need for treatment should be carefully considered since dogs with adult onset GH deficiency do very well without treatment except for their baldness.

Iatrogenic growth hormone excess is treated by discontinuing the progesterone therapy. Spontaneous growth hormone excess is treated by ovariohysterectomy.

FELINE ENDOCRINE ALOPECIA

Feline endocrine alopecia (FEA) is a rare symmetrical alopecia of unknown etiology seen exclusively in neutered male (90 percent) or female cats. Sex hormone deficiency or imbalance is hypothesized but not proven to be the cause. It has been shown that thyroid hormone levels are normal in FEA.[113,114] Affected cats range in age from 2 to 12 years with an average age of 6 years.[115,116]

FEA is characterized by bilaterally symmetrical alopecia, which begins in the genital and perineal regions. Diffuse hair loss progresses to total baldness in affected areas. Partial alopecia of the lateral thorax, flanks, and front limbs may occur but total alopecia seldom develops in these locations. It is this author's opinion that no skin involvement or pruritus are seen with FEA and cats with those signs are misdiagnosed as having FEA. With the exception of alopecia, cats with FEA are normal. The diagnosis of FEA is based on the history and clinical signs. All laboratory tests should be normal.

Recommended therapy consists of combination estrogen–androgen injections, estrogen or androgen used alone, or progestational compounds. Repositol testosterone (12.5 mg/cat) in combination with repositol stilbestrol (0.625 mg/cat) given intramuscularly has given excellent results.[116] A second dose is given in 6 weeks if new hair has not grown in that period of time. Intramuscular injections of repositol progesterone (2.2 to 20 mg/kg) or medroxyprogesterone acetate (50 to 175 mg/cat) are also reported to be effective. Repeat injections are given in 6 weeks if new hair growth has not occurred.[115,116] Megestrol acetate (2.5 to 5 mg/cat) may be given orally, every other day, until regrowth of hair is evident. A maintenance dose of 2.5 to 5 mg/cat, once or twice weekly is usually required.[115,117] Although all of these treatments are reportedly effective, the author recommends no therapy for true FEA. The author has seen six cats with FEA that were given no therapy recover within the 6 week period usually needed for recovery with treatment. It is the author's opinion that many cats would spontaneously recover if no treatment were given. FEA causes no harm to the cat other than the alopecia, which some owners are willing to tolerate. Therapy with hormones has potential serious complications, therefore, the owner has the option of no treatment before using hormonal therapy. A relapse rate of 55 percent is reported with all forms of therapy.[116]

REFERENCES

1. Anderson RK: Canine hypothyroidism. Compend Cont Ed Pract Vet I:103, 1979
2. Belshaw BE: Diagnosis and treatment of hypothyroidism in dogs. Proc Kal Kan Vet Sympos 6:85, 1982
3. Belshaw BE: Thyroid diseases. p. 1592. In Ettinger SJ (ed): Textbook of Veterinary Internal Medicine. 2nd ed. Vol. 2 WB Saunders, Philadelphia, 1983
4. Capen CC, Belshaw BE, Martin SL: Thyroid gland. p. 1378. In Ettinger SJ (ed) Textbook of Veterinary Internal Medicine. Vol. 2 WB Saunders, Philadelphia, 1975
5. Chastain CB: Canine hypothyroidism. J Am Vet Med Assoc 181:349, 1982
6. Gosselin SJ, Capen CC, Martin SL: Histologic and ultrastructural evaluation of thyroid lesions associated with hypothyroidism in dogs. Vet Pathol 18:299, 1981
7. Gosselin SJ, Capen CC, Martin SL et al: Autoimmune lymphocytic thyroiditis in dogs. Vet Immunol Immunopath 3:185, 1982
8. Gosselin SJ, Capen CC, Martin SL et al: Biochemical and immunological investigations on hypothyroidism in dogs. Can J Comp Med 44:158, 1980
9. Musser E, Graham WR: Familial occurrence of thyroiditis in purebred beagles. Lab Anim Care 18:58, 1968
10. Tucker WE Jr: Thyroiditis in a group of laboratory dogs. A study of 167 beagles. Am J Clin Path 38:70, 1962
11. Ferguson DC: Thyroid function tests in the dog. Recent concepts. Vet Clin North Am 14:783, 1984
12. Milne KL, Hayes HM Jr: Epidemiologic features of canine hypothyroidism. Cornell Vet 71:3, 1981
13. Muller GH, Kirk RW, Scott DW: Cutaneous endocrinology. p. 492. In Small Animal Dermatology. (3rd ed.) WB Saunders, Philadelphia, 1983
14. Nesbitt GH, Izzo J, Peterson L, et al: Canine hypothyroidism: A study of 108 cases. J Am Vet Med Assoc 177:1117, 1980
15. Martin SL, Capen CC: Hypothyroidism and the skin. Vet Clin North Am 9:29, 1979
16. Reimers TJ, McCann JP, Cowan RG, et al: Effects of storage, hemolysis, and freezing and thawing on concentrations of thyroxine, cortisol, and insulin in blood samples. Proc Soc Exp Biol Med 170:509, 1982
17. Kemppainen RJ, Thompson FN, Lorenz MD, et al: Effects of prednisone on thyroid and gonadal endocrine function in dogs. J Endocrinol 96:293, 1983
18. Woltz HH, Thompson FN, Kemppainen RJ, et al: Effect of prednisone on canine thyroid gland and plasma T_4 and T_3. J Am Vet Med Assoc 184:817, 1984
19. Oliver JW, Waldrop V: Sampling protocol for thyrotropin stimulation test in the dog. J Am Vet Med Assoc 182:486, 1983
20. Hoenig M, Ferguson DC: Assessment of thyroid functional reserve in the cat by thyrotropin-stimulation test. Am J Vet Res 44:1229, 1983
21. Lorenz MD, Stiff M: Serum thyroxine content before and after thyrotropin stimulation in dogs with suspected hypothyroidism. J Am Vet Med Assoc 177:78, 1980
22. Reimers TJ, Concannon PW, Cowan RG: Changes in serum thyroxine and cortisol

in dogs after simultaneous injections of TSH and ACTH. J Am Anim Hosp Assoc 18:923, 1982
23. Quinlan WJ, Michaelson S: Homologous radioimmunoassay for canine thyrotropin: Response of normal and x-irradiated dogs to propylthiouracil. Endocrinol 108:937, 1981
24. Larsson M: Evaluation of human TSH radioimmunoassay as a diagnostic test for canine primary hypothyroidism. Acta Vet Scand 22:589, 1981
25. Evinger JV, Nelson RW: The clinical pharmacology of thyroid hormones in the dog. J Am Vet Med Assoc 185:314, 1984
26. Rosychuk R: Management of hypothyroidism. p. 869. In Kirk RW (ed) Current Veterinary Therapy VIII. WB Saunders, Philadelphia, 1983
27. Rosychuk RAW: Thyroid hormones and antithyroid drugs. Vet Clin North Am 12:111, 1982
28. Levy G, Knox F: The biological activity of orally administered desiccated thyroid. Am J Pharm 133:255, 1961
29. Peterson ME: Hyperadrenocorticism. Vet Clin North Am 14:731, 1984
30. Feldman EC: Effect of functional adrenocortical tumors on plasma cortisol and corticotropin concentrations in dogs. J Am Vet Med Assoc 178:823, 1981
31. Scott DW, Greene CE: Iatrogenic secondary adrenocortical insufficiency in dogs. J Am Anim Hosp Assoc 10:555, 1974
32. Muller GH, Kirk RW, Scott DW: Clinical aspects of endocrine skin disease hyperadrenocorticism. p. 511. In Small Animal Dermatology 3rd ed. WB Saunders, Philadelphia, 1983
33. Scott DW, Manning TO, Reimers TJ: Iatrogenic Cushing's syndrome in the cat. Feline Prac 12:30, 1982
34. Feldman EC: The adrenal cortex. p. 1650. In Ettinger SJ (ed): Textbook of Veterinary Internal Medicine. 2nd ed. Vol. 2 WB Saunders, Philadelphia, 1983
35. Ling GV, Stabenfeldt GH, Comer KM, et al: Canine hyperadrenocorticism: Pre treatment clinical and laboratory evaluation of 117 cases. J Am Vet Med Assoc 174:1211, 1979
36. Lorenz MD: Canine hyperadrenocorticism: Diagnosis and treatment. Compend Cont Ed Proc Vet I:315, 1979
37. Lorenz MD: Diagnosis and medical management of canine Cushing's syndrome: A study of 57 consecutive cases. J Am Anim Hosp Assoc 18:707, 1982
38. Scott DW: Hyperadrenocorticism (hyperadrenocorticoidism, hyperadrenocorticalism, Cushing's disease, Cushing's syndrome). Vet Clin North Am 9:3, 1979
39. Stolp R, Meijer JC: Differential diagnosis and laboratory evaluation of hyperadrenocorticism in dogs. Proc Kal Kan Vet Sympos 6:9, 1982
40. Willeberg P, Priester WA: Epidemiological aspects of clinical hyperadrenocorticism in dogs (canine Cushing's syndrome). J Am Anim Hosp Assoc 18:717, 1982
41. Peterson ME, Nesbitt GH, Schaer M: Diagnosis and management of concurrent diabetes mellitus and hyperadrenocorticism in thirty dogs. J Am Vet Med Assoc 178:66, 1981
42. Feldman EC, Tyrrell JB, Bohannon NV: The synthetic ACTH stimulation test and measurement of endogenous plasma ACTH levels: Useful diagnostic indicators for adrenal disease in dogs. J Am Anim Hosp Assoc 14:524, 1978
43. Olson PN, Bowen RA, Hustad PW, et al: Effects of storage on concentration of hydrocortisone (cortisol) in canine serum and plasma. Am J Vet Res 42:1618, 1981
44. Halliwell REW, Schwartzman RM, Hopkins L, et al: The value of plasma corticosteroid assays in the diagnosis of Cushing's disease in the dog. J Small Anim Pract 12:453, 1971

45. Feldman EC, Stabenfeldt GH, Farver TB, et al: Comparison of aqueous porcine ACTH with synthetic ACTH in adrenal stimulation tests of the female dog. Am J Vet Res 43:522, 1982
46. Feldman EC: Comparison of ACTH response and dexamethasone suppression as screening tests in canine hyperadrenocorticism. J Am Vet Med Assoc 182:506, 1983
47. Peterson ME: Use of o,p'-DDD in treatment of canine hyperadrenocorticism. Proc Kal Kan Vet Sympos 6:91, 1982
48. Peterson ME, Gilbertson SR, Drucker WD: Plasma Cortisol response to exogenous ACTH in 22 dogs with hyperadrenocorticism caused by adrenocortical neoplasia. J Am Vet Med Assoc 180:542, 1982
49. Meijer JC, de Bruijne JJ, Rijnberk A, et al: Biochemical characterization of pituitary-dependent hyperadrenocorticism in the dog. J Endocr 77:111, 1978
50. Meijer JC, Lubberink AAME, Rijnberk A, et al: Adrenocortical function tests in dogs with hyperfunctioning adrenocortical tumours. J Endocr 80:315, 1979
51. Eiler H, Oliver J: Combined dexamethasone suppression and cosyntropin (synthetic ACTH) stimulation test in the dog: New approach to testing of adrenal gland function. Am J Vet Res 41:1243, 1980
52. Eiler H, Oliver JW, Legendre AM: Stages of hyperadrenocorticism: Response of hyperadrenocorticoid dogs to the combined dexamethasone suppression/ACTH stimulation test. J Am Vet Med Assoc 185:289, 1984
53. Kemppainen RJ, Thompson FN, Lorenz MD: Effects of dexamethasone infusion on the plasma cortisol response to cosyntropin (synthetic ACTH) injection in normal dogs. Res Vet Sc 32:181, 1982
54. Peterson ME: O,p'-DDD (mitotane) treatment of canine pituitary-dependent hyperadrenocorticism. J Am Vet Med Assoc 182:527, 1983
55. Kirk GR, Boyer S, Hutcheson DP: Effects of o,p'-DDD on plasma cortisol levels and histology of the adrenal gland in the normal dog. J Am Anim Hosp Assoc 10:179, 1974
56. Willard MD, Schall WD, Nachreiner RF, et al: hypoadrenocorticism following therapy with o,p'-DDD for hyperadrenocorticism in four dogs. J Am Vet Med Assoc 180:638, 1982
57. McCandlish IAP, Munro CD, Breeze RG, et al: Hormone producing ovarian tumours in the dog. Vet Rec 105:9, 1979
58. Brodey RS, Martin JE: Sertoli cell neoplasms in the dog (The clinicopathological and endocrinological findings in thirty-seven dogs). J Am Vet Med Assoc 133:249, 1958
59. Capen CC, Martin SL: Ultrastructural evaluation and pathophysiology of testicular sertoli cell neoplasms from dogs with a syndrome of hyperestrogenism. Proc Electron Micro Soc Am 31:384, 1973
60. Comhaire F, Mattheeuws D, Vermeulen, A: Testosterone and oestradiol in dogs with testicular tumours. Acta Endocrinol 77:408, 1974
61. Lipowitz AJ, Schwartz A, Wilson GP, et al: Testicular neoplasms and concomitant clinical changes in the dog. J Am Vet Med Assoc 163:1364, 1973
62. Pulley LT: Sertoli cell tumor. Vet Clin North Am 9:145, 1979
63. Reif JS, Brody RS: The relationship between cryptorchidism and canine testicular neoplasia. J Am Vet Med Assoc 155:2005, 1969
64. Weaver AD: Survey with follow-up of 67 dogs with testicular sertoli cell tumors. Vet Rec 113:105, 1983
65. Kahan H: An atypical case of interstitial cell tumor of the testicle in a dog. J Am Vet Med Assoc 126:471, 1955

66. Barsanti JA, Duncan JR, Nachreiner RF: Alopecia associated with a seminoma. J Am Anim Hosp Assoc 15:33, 1979
67. Barsanti JA, Medleau L, Latimer K: Diethylstibestrol-induced alopecia in a dog. J Am Vet Med Assoc 182:63, 1983
68. Dow C: Oestrogen-induced atrophy of the skin of dogs. J Path Bact 80:434, 1960
69. Eigenmann JE, Doortman J, Koeman JP: Estrogen-induced flank alopecia in the female dog: Evidence for local rather than systemic hyperestrogenism. J Am Anim Hosp Assoc 20:621, 1984
70. Jabara AG: Some tissue changes in the dog following stilboestrol administration. Aust J Exp Biol 40:293, 1962
71. Muller GH, Kirk RW, Scott DW: Sex hormones. p. 505. In Small Animal Dermatology 3rd ed. WB Saunders, Philadelphia, 1983
72. Schwartzman RM: The androgenic dog. Gaines Vet Sympos 13:14, 1964
73. Mattheeuws D, Comhaire F: Oestradiol and testosterone in male dogs with alopecia and feminization without testicular neoplasia. Br Vet J 131:65, 1975
74. Schwartz E, Thornaben JA, Boxill GC: Effects of chronic oral administration of long-acting estrogen, quinestrol, to dogs. Toxicol Appl Pharmacol 14:487, 1969
75. Williams WL, Gardner WU, DeVita J: Local inhibition of hair growth in dogs by percutaneous application of estrone. Endocrinol 38:368, 1946
76. Conroy JD: Dermatopathologic signs of internal disease: Metabolic and toxic diseases. Vet Clin North Am 9:137, 1979
77. Scott DW: Histological findings in endocrine skin disorders of the dog. J Am Anim Hosp Assoc 18:173, 1982
78. Castrodale D, Bierbaum O, Helwig EB, et al: Comparative studies of the effects of estradiol and stilbestrol upon the blood, liver, and bone marrow. Endocrinol 29:363, 1941
79. Legendre, AM: Estrogen-induced bone marrow hypoplasia in a dog. J Am Anim Hosp Assoc 12:525, 1976
80. Lowenstine LJ, Ling GV, Schalm OW: Exogenous estrogen toxicity in the dog. Calif Vet 26:14, 1972
81. Maddux JM, Shaw SE: Possible beneficial effect of lithium therapy in a case of estrogen-induced bone marrow hypoplasia in a dog: A case report. J Am Anim Hosp Assoc 19:242, 1983
82. Morgan RV: Blood dyscrasias associated with testicular tumors in the dog. J Am Anim Hosp Assoc 18:970, 1982
83. Pyle RL, Hill BL, Johnson JR: Estrogen toxicity in a dog. Canine Pract 3:39, 1976
84. Schalm OW: Exogenous estrogen toxicity in the dog. Canine Pract 5:57, 1978
85. Sherding RG, Wilson GP, Kociba GJ: Bone marrow hypoplasia in eight dogs with sertoli cell tumor. J Am Vet Med Assoc 178:497, 1981
86. Eigenmann JE, Wortman JA, Haskins ME: Elevated growth hormone levels and diabetes mellitus in a cat with acromegalic features. J Am Anim Hosp Assoc 20:747, 1984
87. Concannon P, Altszuler N, Hampshire J, et al: Growth hormone, prolatin, and cortisol in dogs developing mammary nodules and an acromegaly-like appearance during treatment with medroxyprogesterone acetate. Endocrinol 106:1173, 1980
88. Eigenmann JE: Naturally occurring and iatrogenic acromegaly in the dog. Proc Kal Kan Vet Sympos 6:81, 1982
89. Eigenmann JE, Venker-van Haagen AJ: Progestagen-induced and spontaneous canine acromegaly due to reversible growth hormone overproduction: Clinical picture and pathogenesis. J Am Anim Hosp Assoc 17:813, 1981

90. Rijnberk A, Eigenmann JE, Belshaw BE, et al: Acromegaly associated with transient overproduction of growth hormone in a dog. J Am Vet Med Assoc 177:534, 1980
91. Scott DW, Concannon PW: Gross and microscopic changes in the skin of dogs with progestagen-induced acromegaly and elevated growth hormone levels. J Am Anim Hosp Assoc 19:523, 1983
92. Andresen E, Willeberg P: Pituitary dwarfism in German Shepherd dog: Additional evidence of simple, autosomal recessive inheritance. Nord Vet Med 28:481, 1976
93. Andresen E, Willeberg P, Rassmussen PG: Pituitary dwarfism in German Shepherd dogs: Genetic investigations. Nord Vet Med 26:692, 1974
94. Nicholas F: Pituitary dwarfism in German Shepherd dogs: A genetic analysis of some Australian data. J Small Anim Pract 19:167, 1978
95. Eigenmann JE, Patterson DF: Growth hormone deficiency in the mature dog. J Am Anim Hosp Assoc 20:741, 1984
96. Parker WM, Scott DW: Growth hormone responsive alopecia in the mature dog: A discussion of 13 cases. J Am Anim Hosp Assoc 16:824, 1980
97. Peterson ME, Altszuler N: Suppression of growth hormone secretion in spontaneous canine hyperadrenocorticism and its reversal after treatment. Am J Vet Res 42:1881, 1981
98. Eigenmann JE: Diagnosis and treatment of pituitary dwarfism in dogs. Proc Kal Kan Vet Sympos 6:107, 1982
99. Eigenmann JE: Acromegaly in the dog. Vet Clin No Am 14:827, 1984
100. Scott DW, Kirk RW, Hampshire J, et al: Clinicopathological findings in a German Shepherd with pituitary dwarfism. J Am Anim Hosp Assoc 14:183, 1978
101. Muller GH, Kirk RW, Scott DW: Canine acromegaly. p 527, In Small Animal Dermatology 3rd ed, WB Saunders, Philadelphia, 1983
102. Hampshire J, Altszuler N: Conidine or zylazine as provocative tests for growth hormone secretion in the dog. Am J Vet Res 42:1073, 1981
103. Eigenmann JE: Diagnosis and treatment of dwarfism in a German Shepherd dog. J Am Anim Hosp Assoc 17:798, 1981
104. Jensen, EC: Hypopituitarism associated with cystic Rathke's cleft in a dog. J Am Vet Med Assoc 135:572, 1959
105. Muller GH: Pituitary dwarfism. Vet Clin Am 9:41, 1979
106. Muller GH, Jones SR: Pituitary dwarfism and alopecia in a German Shepherd with a cystic Rathke's cleft. J Am Anim Hosp 9:567, 1973
107. Muller GH, Kirk RW, Scott DW: Pituitary dwarfism. P 525, In Small Animal Dermatology 3rd ed, WB Saunders, Philadelphia, 1983
108. Roberg JW: Dwarfism in the German Shepherd. Canine Pract 6:42, 1979
109. Eigenmann JE, Lubberink AAME, Koemann JP: Panhypopituitarism caused by a suprascellar tumor in a dog. J Am Anim Hosp Assoc 19:377, 1983
110. Muller GH, Kirk RW, Scott DW: Growth-hormone responsive dermatosis in the mature dog. p 529, In Small Animal Dermatology 3rd ed, WB Saunders, Philadelphia, 1983
111. Cassel SE: Ovarian imbalance in a German shepherd dwarf VM/5AC 74:162, 1979
112. Willeberg P, Kastrup KW, Andresen E: Pituitary dwarfism in German Shepherd dogs: Studies on somatomedin activity. Nord Vet Med 27:448, 1975
113. Doering GG, Jensen H: Feline Endocrine Alopecia. p 102 In Clinical Dermatology of Small Animals, CV Mosby Co. St. Louis, 1973
114. Scott DW: Thyroid function in feline endocrine alopecia. J Am Anim Hosp Assoc 11:798, 1975

115. Muller GH, Kirk RW, Scott DW: Feline endocrine alopecia. p. 531, In Small Animal Dermatology 3rd ed, WB Saunders, Philadelphia, 1983
116. Scott DW: Feline dermatology: 1900–1978: A monograph. Hormonal and metabolic disorders. J Am Anim Hosp Assoc 16:390, 1980
117. McDougal, BJ: The use of megesterol acetate for treatment of feline endocrine alopecia. Texas Vet Med Assoc 37:12, 1979

8 Nutritional Dermatoses

Candace A. Sousa

Due to the development of guidelines and standards for proper canine and feline nutrition, nutritonal dermatoses are uncommon. The availability of commercial canned, dry, and semimoist foods enable pet owners to meet their pet's nutritonal requirements.[1,2]

Cutaneous manifestations of malnutrition may belie other problems, and internal changes in various body systems also may occur. The integumentary system manifests signs of poor nutrition primarily because continuous growth occurs throughout life and because it is the most visible organ of the body.

The effect of nutrition may be direct or indirect. The direct impact may be a result of a frank dietary deficiency, insufficient intake, an inability to digest or absorb the proper nutrients, nutrient binding, failure to metabolize, excess urinary or fecal loss, abnormally high requirements, or an improper nutrient balance. Food processing and storage also have many effects on the availability or utilization of various nutrients.

Indirectly, poor nutrition may alter the skin's environment allowing pathogenic bacteria (i.e., *Staphylococcus* sp, coagulase positive) to proliferate. Parasites such as fleas and lice may find conditions conducive to optimal growth. Nutritional imbalances that affect other organs may also induce integumentary alterations. For example, a dietary iodine deficiency could result in hypothyroidism that, in some cases, results in alopecia, lichenification, hyperpigmentation, and secondary infections. The development of allergy to certain foods with resultant pruritus and self-induced lesions is another indirect effect.

Vitamin and mineral deficiencies are presented here as solitary deficiencies, but this is seldom the case. Generally, deficiencies of several nutrients are concurrent.

PROTEIN DEFICIENCY

Most commercial dog foods are usually adequate in protein content. Consequently, protein deficiency is rare. Protein should supply at least 25 percent on a dry-matter basis of the caloric intake for the dog and 33 percent for the cat.[1,2]

Hair is composed of 95 percent protein and contains a high percentage of sulfur-containing amino acids. Protein deficiency may result in patchy alopecia as the hair coat becomes thin, rough, dry, dull, and brittle. There is also loss of pigmentation and vitality of the hair. Edema of the feet and legs, hyperkeratosis, and epidermal hyperpigmentation are often noted. Erythematous and edematous lesions have been reported on the head, back, chest, axilla, and inguinal areas. Vesiculation, watery discharge, scales, and crusts may also develop in these areas.[3,4]

Protein deficiency is reported most often in growing puppies and kittens whose protein needs are higher. It may result from an inadequate intake in quality or quantity, excessive growth or catabolic states, or excessive loss via the kidney. Rapidly growing dogs may have energy needs in excess of that which can be supplied by fat and carbohydrate in the diet and thus utilize protein for energy, with subsequent depletion of the protein available for tissue growth.[4]

Treatment involves correction of the protein deficiency or imbalance. To insure adequate protein quality, an animal source product should be one of the first two ingredients listed in a canned ration and one of the first four in a dry ration.[3]

FATTY ACID DEFICIENCY

Fats perform a multiplicity of functions in the diet. Fats are an excellent energy source, act as a carrier for fat-soluble vitamins, provide substances known as essential or unsaturated fatty acids, and confer palatability to food. Essential fatty acids are used by the body to synthesize prostaglandins and parts of the cell membrane.[5,6] Polyunsaturated linoleic acid is essential in the diet of all animals. Arachidonic and linolenic acids are also required but except for arachidonic acid in the cat, they can be synthesized from linoleic acid.[7] Both are found naturally only in fats of animal origin.

The symptoms of fatty acid deficiency are usually seen only in animals fed dry food or special human food diets. Deficiency may also occur in association with intestinal malabsorption, pancreatic disease, and chronic hepatic disease. Animals must be fed a diet deficient in fatty acids for several months before skin problems become evident.[8] It has been reported that they develop a fine, flaky desquamation and a generalized dry, lusterless hair coat followed by hair loss, pruritus, and resultant areas of acute moist dermatitis (''hot spots''.) The skin and hair coat are reported to develop a greasy seborrhea due to increased activity of the sebaceous glands.[3] Moist dermatitis and exudation may occur from the ear canals and interdigital spaces.[8,9] A generalized erythema with marked alopecia and cyclic desquamation has been reported with chronic fat deficiency. Changes in temperment have been noted with the dog at first becoming excitable, then tremulous.

Histologically, the epidermis becomes acanthotic with thickening of the stratum granulosum. Both hyperkeratosis and parakeratosis occur. The dermis thickens due to edema and an infiltrate of white blood cells. All of these changes increase the susceptibility of the skin to secondary infections.[10] Impetigo-like lesions develop on the abdomen, back, and pinnae.[4] Fatty acid deficiency causes changes in the lipid film of the skin surface, which leads to changes in the bacterial flora.

The fat content of most dry foods is low. Unsaturated fatty acids contain double bonds and therefore oxidation (rancidity) may occur if sufficient antioxidants are not present when the food is stored for longer than 6 months or subjected to high temperatures. Rancidity also interfers with the availability of other nutrients and destroys vitamins D, E, and biotin. Antioxidants, such as vitamin E, must be present in amounts high enough to prevent fats from becoming rancid and losing their value as a source of essential fatty acids.[3]

Dogs should be fed a canned food diet containing a minimum of 3 percent fat or a dry diet with 7 to 8 percent (5 percent per kilogram dry weight.)[2] Cats usually need 35 to 40 percent of their calories provided by fat (90 percent per kilogram dry weight).[1] In the dog, treatment of suspected deficiency should consist of changing to a well-balanced diet containing a high fat content supplemented with 10 ml (2 tsp) of vegetable oil per cup of dry dog food. Soybean, safflower, and corn oil contain a high percentage of unsaturated fatty acids. Greater supplementation is not recommended as it will decrease consumption of the diet to the extent that other nutritional deficiencies may occur. Response to treatment is usually seen within 2 to 3 weeks. Cats should be fed animal fats to meet their requirement for polyunsaturated fatty acids.

VITAMIN IMBALANCES

Vitamin A (Retinol) Deficiency

Vitamin A, a fat-soluble vitamin, is found only in fish oils and in animal tissues such as liver and kidney. Plants contain carotinoids, such as beta-carotene, which function as pigments which the dog can convert to retinol in the intestinal tract. However, the cat cannot convert carotinoids to retinol.[11] Deficiency is usually not a problem if the cat consumes vitamin A-rich organ meats. Retinol deficiency seen in cats is primarily due to the destruction of the vitamin in food preparation or from prolonged storage.

The maintenance of skin and epithelial cells is an important function of vitamin A.[12] Vitamin A also aids in the synthesis of mucopolysaccharides and cortisone. It appears to influence the stability of mitochondria and lysosomal membranes. A deficiency results in epithelial cell atrophy and excess keratinization.[13,14] Hyperkeratosis, particularly of the follicle, is prominant. When it occurs in the ducts of skin glands it occludes the lumens thus blocking secretion. Papular eruptions with a firm central core are formed. These may be localized or generalized. Varying degrees of alopecia develop and there is an increased susceptibility to bacterial infections of the skin. In cats, vitamin A deficiency produces focal atrophy of the skin, "eczema," and a scaly mouth.[15,16]

The National Research Council (NRC) recommends 5,000 IU vitamin A per kilogram of dry diet for dogs and 10,000 IU vitamin A per kilogram of dry diet for cats.[1,2] Treatment of a deficiency with a single injection of aqueous vitamin A, 6,000 IU/kg, is usually sufficient to reverse the signs of deficiency.[3] The injectable dose equals the liver's storage capacity, thus repeated dosages need not be employed for at least two months. Oral vitamin A given at a dose of 400 IU/kg per day for 10 days is also effective.

Because vitamin A stores well in the system, toxicity may be of more concern than is deficiency. An excess of retinol produces exfoliation of the epithelium, pruritus, skin rash, and alopecia. There may also be anorexia, exopthalmos, vomiting, pain, hepatomegaly, and painful, swollen joints. Dogs may be irritable and drowsy. Degenerative and proliferative bone changes occur in cats. A good history is essential to differentiate vitamin A toxicity from deficiency.

Vitamin A-Responsive Dermatosis

Several authors have reported on a seborrheic dermatitis in the dog that responded to treatment with oral vitamin A.[17,18] The dogs had generalized scaling and multiple severe, thickened focal, crusty dermatitic lesions that were worse on the ventral abdomen and thorax (Fig. 8-1). All of the animals were fed commercial brands of kibble or canned dog food that met the NRC requirements for the dog. Routine laboratory results were within normal limits. In one dog with this diagnosis, the serum vitamin A level was within normal limits.[18]

Histopathologic changes consisted of severe follicular hyperkeratosis and mild surface hyperkeratosis. The epidermis was acanthotic with some rete ridge formation. A few dyskeratotic cells were seen. In the superificial dermis there was a mild to moderate mononuclear cell infiltrate consisting of lymphocytes, mast cells, neutrophils and plasma cells. Sebaceous and apocrine glands varied from normal to hypertrophic.

In three cases, treatment with oral vitamin A at 10,000 IU daily resulted in improvement over a 5 to 8 week period.[17] In the fourth case, 50,000 IU b.i.d. was needed to maintain normalcy.[18] The effect of vitamin A in these cases was probably not due to replacement of an absolute deficiency, but by either meeting needs brought about by a localized deficiency or by overriding partial metabolic impairment of utilization.

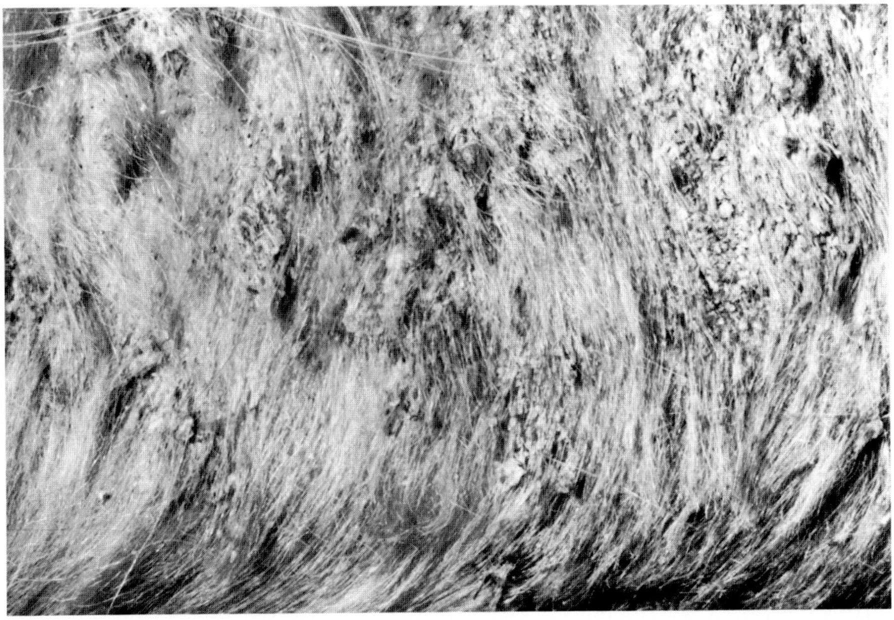

Fig. 8-1. Vitamin A-responsive dermatosis. Thick scales and crusts adhere to the hair and skin of a 6-year-old male cocker spaniel.

Vitamin B Complex

Deficiency of single B vitamins occurs very rarely. The clinical manifestations resulting from deficiencies of single or multiple B vitamins are quite similar (dry hair coat, seborrhea, anorexia, weight loss). All B vitamins are synthesized by the intestinal bacteria of herbivores. They are water soluble and only small amounts are stored by the body. Any condition that causes excessive water loss from the body (polyuria, diarrhea) can lead to a deficiency, but toxicities do not occur as excesses are easily excreted in the urine. All deficiencies can be effectively treated with Brewer's yeast or B-complex injections or both.

Thiamine (Vitamin B_1) Deficiency

Thiamine is associated with carbohydrate utilization, oxygen uptake, steroid synthesis, and fatty acid synthesis. Thiaminase, an enzyme present in the viscera of some raw fish, destroys thiamine. The cat requires 5 times as much dietary thiamine as the dog (5 mg/kg dry matter versus 1 mg/kg dry matter) and because cats are occassionally fed raw fish, they are more commonly affected.[19]

Increased susceptibility to insects and fleas has been reported in thiamine-deficient animals. Deficiency also produces anxorexia, vomiting, weight loss, and convulsions.[20] Its effects on the skin are indirect. Cutaneous edema and cyanosis have been reported in beriberi.[4]

Riboflavin (Vitamin B_2) Deficiency

Riboflavin is utilized in a number of metabolic processes, especially those involving skin, eyes, and the mucous membranes of the mouth and digestive tract. Meat and dairy products contain a large amount of riboflavin that is not destroyed by cooking. A high-carbohydrate diet protects against deficiency by promoting intestinal synthesis.

Experimentally, riboflavin deficiency is characterized by erythema and a dry, flaky dermatitis (seborrhea) of the rear legs, chest, and abdomen.[3,4,21] Long-term deficiency may produce fissuring and dry scaling of the lips and commissures of the mouth (cheilosis). Mucous membranes, including those of the genital tract, become inflammed and inflammation of the digestive tract results in difficulty swallowing, malabsorption, and diarrhea.

Acute deficiency in the cat is characterized by alopecia about the head and occassionally on the chest and forelegs, with anorexia and emaciation.[21]

Riboflavin deficiency is prevented by feeding the dog a diet that contains 2.2 mg/kg dry matter or 5.0 mg/kg dry matter to a cat.[1,2,3]

Niacin (Vitamin B_3) Deficiency

Niacin (nicotinic acid) and riboflavin deficiencies result in similar clinical symptoms as both are constituents of coenzymes needed for electron transfer. Niacin is important for the maintenance of normal tissue integrity, particularly of the skin, gastrointestinal tract, and the nervous system.[4]

A deficiency of niacin is manifested in many mammalian species as pellagara (black tongue). There is sensitivity and reddening of the oral mucosa and lips and later, the cheeks and floor of the buccal cavity. Patches of superficial necrosis may occur in these areas as well as the tongue, which becomes sore and purplish black. Mucous membranes of the digestive tract are also inflammed with ulceration and bleeding of the large intestines and cecum resulting in hemorrhagic diarrhea and emaciation.[3] The hair coat becomes rough and a scaly pruritic dermatitis of the rear legs and abdomen develops. In the cat, niacin deficiency is mainly characterized by diarrhea, emaciation, and death. Oral lesions may or may not be present.

A deficiency of niacin is rare in animals fed commercial pet foods as these usually contain sufficient amounts. To produce a deficiency, diets must be of low quality and contain a large proportion of corn. Corn, as with other cereal grains, is low in tryptophan. Except for the cat, most animals are able to convert tryptophan to niacin. A diet containing 11.4 mg/kg of dry matter of niacin for the dog and 45 mg/kg of dry matter for the cat is sufficient to prevent a deficiency.[1,2]

Pyridoxine (Vitamin B_6) Deficiency

Pyridoxine is an essential growth factor and may be involved in the transport of amino acids. A deficiency causes anorexia, poor utilization of food, weight loss or poor weight gain, and some vomiting and diarrhea. In dogs, dermal edema with accompanying swelling, hyperkeratosis, and necrosis of the ears, paws, nose, and lips have been reported experimentally. Progressive degeneration of peripheral nerves with ataxia and paralysis has been reported. A brown secretion may form around the eyes and microcytic, hypochromic anemia may occur. The signs and symptoms of this condition appear to be identical to that due to a lack of certain unsaturated fatty acids.[4]

Histopathology of the skin reveals atrophy of the epidermis, hair follicles, and sebaceous glands with loose hyperkeratosis, alopecia, and inflammation.[4] In the dog, 1.0 mg/kg of dry matter and in the cat 4.0 mg/kg of dry matter of pyridoxine is recommended to prevent deficiency.[1,2]

Biotin Deficiency

Like all B-vitamins, biotin is produced by many microorganisms present in the intestinal tract of all normal animals. It is essential for normal metabolism. Biotin is a coenzyme necessary for fatty acid and amino acid synthesis.

Biotin deficiency may occur from either a prolonged administration of oral antibiotics that sterilize the gut or from excessive ingestion of raw egg whites that contain a heat labile protein called avidin that binds biotin thus rendering it unavailable for intestinal absorption.[3]

Experimental deficiency results in a thin hair coat and dry skin with diminished sebaceous secretion.[4] A greasy, scaly dermatitis develops in advanced cases. Lesions appear on the ears and ventral neck and spread to the lips, shoulders, thorax, abdomen, and eventually the entire body. In fur-bearing animals, depigmentation and partial alopecia around the eyes results in a condition known as spectacle eye. Lethargy, diarrhea, emaciation, and progressive paralysis may develop.[3] In cats, a "miliary dermatitis-like" condition has been reported secondary to biotin deficiency.[22,23]

Treatment involves cessation of raw egg whites in the diet, withdrawal of oral antibiotics, if they produced a sterilization of the gut, and/or 100 μg of biotin/kg body weight 2 to 3 times per week until the signs of the deficiency are corrected.[3,16]

Pantothenic Acid Deficiency

Pantothenic acid is necessary for several metabolic processes. Experimental deficiency in dogs has been associated with depigmentation or discoloration of hair, hemorrhage, and poor health. Inflammation of the skin and mucous membranes at the mucocutaneous junctions has been reported as an early sign of deficiency.[4] Most commercial pet foods contain adequate levels of pantothenic acid.

Vitamin C (Ascorbic Acid) Deficiency

Ascorbic acid is involved in the oxidation of tyrosine and phenylalanine, the conversion of folic acid to folinic acid, production of intercellular cement substance, increasing phagocytic activity of leukocytes, hydroxylation of steroid hormones in the adrenal cortex, and other metabolic processes.[4]

In ascorbic acid deficiency (scurvy), there is weakening of collagen resulting in diffuse petechial hemorrhages in many tissues, including skin and mucous membranes, and deficient wound healing. Broken "corkscrew" hairs develop along with surface and follicular hyperkeratosis. Even though dogs and cats can synthesize vitamin C, deficiency may develop during stress or disease such as diuresis or diarrhea. Fifty milligrams of ascorbic acid daily is usually adequate supplementation. This can be administered either by providing a diet high in vitamin C (fresh fruit) or via a proprietary preparation administered parenterally or orally.[3,10]

Vitamin E (Alpha-Tocopherol) Deficiency

Vitamin E, selenium, and fatty acids have a balanced relationship. In cats, the combination of high dietary levels of unsaturated fatty acids, such as is found in fish-based foods, with low levels of the antioxidant vitamin E leads to the deposition of ceroid pigment in adipose tissue with fat cell necrosis and a subsequent inflammatory reaction.[16,24–27] Food processing or fat oxidation can also inactivate vitamin E resulting in signs of imbalance. The condition, known as pansteatitis ("yellow fat disease"), produces pyrexia, anorexia, lethargy, and discomfort and hyperesthesia on gentle handling and abdominal palpation. Abdominal radiographs show a mottled or irregular radiodensity of the subcutaneous, falciform and inguinal fat, and poor radiographic contrast within the abdomen. If untreated, cats may die within several months. Postmortem examination reveals large, firm lumps in the subcutaneous tissues and abdominal cavity, and yellow fat.

In dogs, excessive dietary fat or a vitamin E deficiency has been shown experimentally to produce a seborrheic syndrome characterized by partial alopecia of the head and limbs, skin that is pale, wrinkled, cold to the touch, and lifeless with open sores over pressure points.[28] Other data on experimental vitamin E deficiency in dogs has shown a severe suppression of lymphocyte blastogenesis.[29]

Treatment with vitamin E (d-alpha-tocopherol acetate), 10 mg/kg body weight daily will reverse the signs of vitamin E deficiency and pansteatitis.[10] In cats, it is also helpful to use systemic corticosteroids during the initial painful period (2 to 3 weeks). Prednisone, at 1 mg/kg b.i.d. orally, may be helpful in stimulating the appetite and decreasing inflammation. A diet change is mandatory but it is often difficult to induce cats to eat other types of food once they have become accustomed to canned seafood diets. Some of the affected cats appear to be almost addicted to the food and change dietary habits only with great reluctance.

Vitamin E-Responsive Dermatoses

Vitamin E in doses of 400 IU orally twice daily has been used successfully in the treatment of discoid lupus erythematosus, systemic lupus erythematosus and in disorders involving the basement membrane.[10] Evidence suggests that the damage in these diseases results from the release of hydrolytic enzymes from lysosomes that denature tissue proteins and in effect convert them into a foreign protein to which the body reacts by producing antibodies.[30,31] Since vitamin E is a physiologic stabilizer of cellular and lysosomal membranes it has been suggested that a relative deficiency leads to damage of the lysosomal membrane, thus initiating the autoimmune process.[31]

MINERAL IMBALANCES

Minerals make up less than 0.7 percent of the body's weight, nearly all being macrominerals: calcium, phosphorus, potassium, sodium, and magnesium. These function mainly to maintain acid-base balance, osmotic pressures necessary for maintenance of body fluid balance, membrane potentials necessary for nerve conduction and muscle contraction, and structural functions. The microminerals, with the exception of iodine, which is a necessary constituent of thyroid hormones, are all necessary primarily as components of metallo-enzymes. These enzymes control the rate of the body's many chemical reactions that constitute all metabolic functions.[20]

Dietary minerals should be regarded as a group rather than individually. If more of one mineral is consumed than needed, the increased amount may bind other minerals preventing their absorption and resulting in a relative deficiency. It is, therefore, the balance of all minerals in the diet that is important.[20]

Copper Deficiency

Copper deficiency most commonly results from an excess of zinc added to the diet as the two compete for absorption in the gut.[20] Copper is needed by enzymes that convert L-tyrosine to melanin and is required by epidermal cells for the conversion of prekeratin to keratin. Experimental deficiency results in lack of pigmentation and faulty keratinization of the skin and hair follicles with the coat becoming dull and rough. Diets providing 7.3 mg/kg of dry matter for the adult dog (twice that for the growing dog) and 5.0 mg/kg of dry matter for the adult cat should be adequate.

Zinc Deficiency

Zinc is a component of over 70 metallo-enzymes that affect carbohydrate, lipid, protein, and nucleic acid synthesis or degradation.[32] It must be supplied continuously because there are only small amounts of readily available zinc stored in the body. The possibility of zinc deficiency occurring in dogs fed commercial dog foods is not great, but certain substances have been shown to act as metabolic antagonists to zinc and to produce a relative deficiency when present in sufficient quantities (e.g., calcium, phytic acid, copper, and cadmium.)[33] Phytic acid is a major component of whole meal wheat and when consumed in high amounts can cause a negative zinc balance. Vitamin D and protein may favorably influence the metabolism of zinc.

Experimental zinc deficiency in dogs produces emaciation, emesis, conjunctivitus, keratitis, and retarded growth.[34,35] Cutaneous changes usually develop on the extremities, over areas of stretch and friction, and at the mucocutaneous junctions (Figs. 8-2, 8-3). Lesions consist initially of small

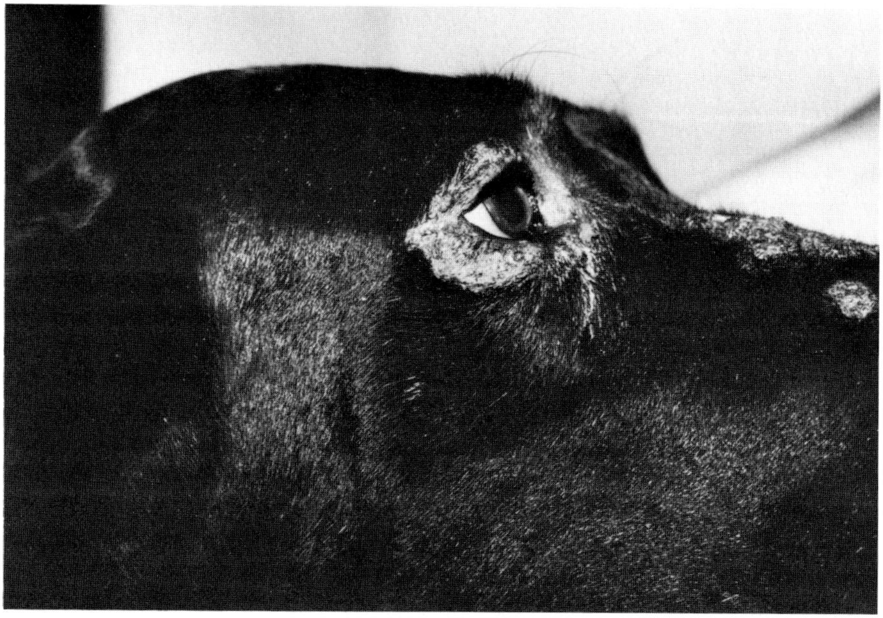

Fig. 8-2. Six-year-old male Labrador retriever with alopecia and hyperkeratosis around the eyes and on the nasal planum. This is a result of a zinc deficiency due to the ingestion of a poor-quality generic dry dog food.

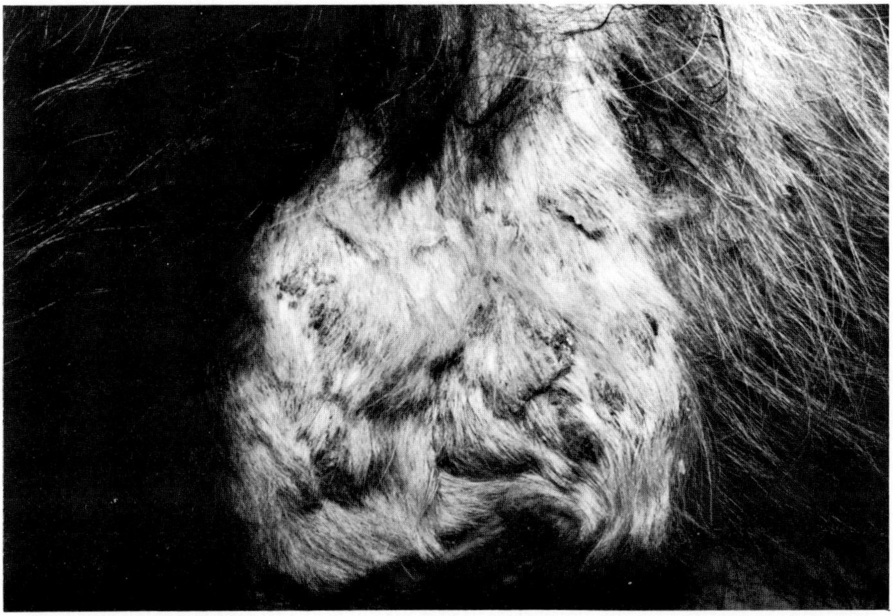

Fig. 8-3. Zinc deficiency due to the ingestion of a poor quality generic dry dog food. Thick crusts are attached to the hair over the elbow of a 3-month-old male malamute-mix.

erythematous plaques. These produce an excessive sebaceous secretion followed by an accumulation of keratinous crusts, which may become quite thick. The perilesional skin is erythematous, wrinkled, dry, and scaly. The hair coat in general will become thin. Secondary infections may occur as a result of a decrease in chemotaxis for monocytes and neutrophils and impaired cell mediated immunity. In clinical situations, rapidly growing puppies that are often over-supplemented with vitamins and minerals are more commonly affected.

Histopathology of affected skin reveals a hyperplastic superficial perivascular dermatitis with marked surface and follicular hyperkeratosis. Intraepidermal pustules and a suppurative folliculitis reflect secondary bacterial infection.[10]

In cats fed a diet deficient in zinc, thinning and slow growth of the hair coat, scaliness of the skin, and ulcerations of the buccal margins develop.[36]

The NRC recommends that a diet contain at least 50 mg/kg of dry matter (0.11 mg/kg of body weight) for the dog and 30 mg/kg of dry matter for the cat.[1,2] Zinc deficiency is treated by giving zinc sulfate (100 to 220 mg of zinc sulfate twice daily) or zinc gluconate 10 mg/kg of body weight per day. Excessive amounts of zinc interfere with copper and iron absorption.[10] If given over a long period of time, excessive zinc results in a decreased growth rate and feed efficiency, anorexia and possibly diarrhea, drowsiness, and paralysis.[3]

Suspected zinc deficiency has been seen by the author in a series of 13 dogs fed generic dry dog foods containing low amounts of zinc. Clinical and histologic changes were identical to those seen in dogs with experimental zinc deficiency. All animals responded promptly to a change in diet.

Zinc-Responsive Dermatosis

Zinc-responsive dermatosis is a condition that occurs primarily in Siberian huskies and Alaskan malamutes but has also been reported in other breeds.[37,38] Lesions usually develop during puberty, although older dogs may be affected. Thick crusts, scale, and suppuration develop around the mouth, chin, eyes, and ears (Fig. 8-4). Crusting may also form on the elbows and pressure points. The prepuce, scrotum and other body openings may be affected. In chronic cases, hyperpigmentation may develop.

Research has shown that some Alaskan malamutes have a genetic defect that results in a decreased capability of zinc absorption from the gut.[39] This, combined with factors that might slightly increase their daily requirements (e.g., reproduction), may alter the body zinc levels enough to cause clinical signs. Therapy is the same as for treatment of zinc deficiency.

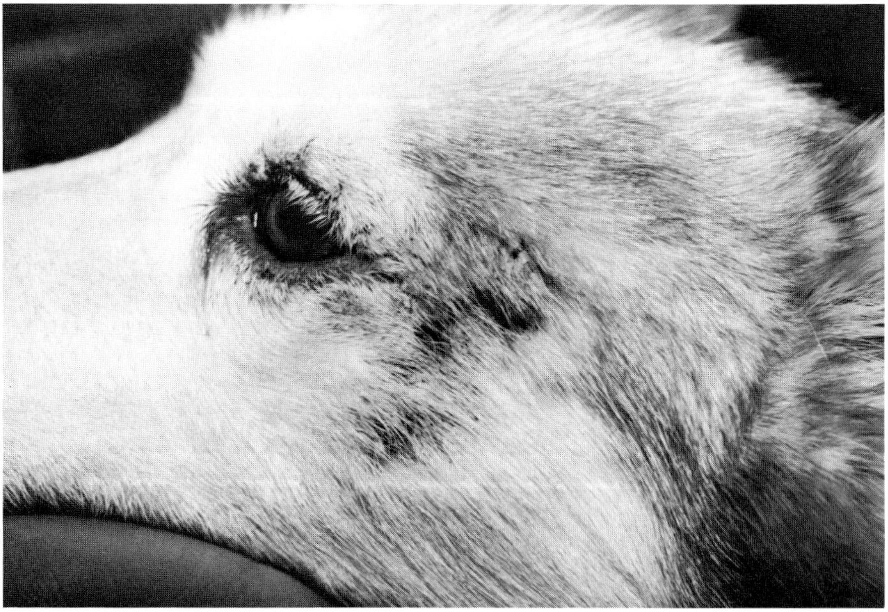

Fig. 8-4. Zinc responsive dermatosis. Periocular crusting in a 4-year-old female Siberian husky.

FOOD ALLERGY

Hypersensitivity reactions to a variety of antigenic materials in the diet can cause a nonseasonal, pruritic dermatosis that may be poorly responsive to glucocorticoids.[40–45] Concurrent gastrointestinal disturbances are present in only about 10 to 15 percent of the cases.[40] The exact pathomechanism is unclear but type I hypersensitivity reactions have been documented in man and are felt by some to be responsible for 80 to 85 percent of all food allergies in domestic animals.[46] Type II, III, and IV reactions have been suspected, but cannot usually be positively identified.

No age, breed, or sex predilections have been reported for food hypersensitivity in the dog or the cat. Reactions may develop slowly or suddenly, and in about 70 percent of the cases the animals have been eating the offending diet for over 2 years.[43]

Clinical signs of food hypersensitivity are extremely variable. In dogs, clinical syndromes may mimic (1) atopy, (2) flea allergy dermatitis (FAD), (3) generalized pruritic folliculitis, (4) seborrhea, (5) recurrent acute moist dermatitis ("hot spots"), (6) urticaria and angioedema, (7) otitis externa, or (8) pruritus without lesions.[10,44] Cats may be presented with (1) miliary dermatitis, (2) ulcerative dermatitis of the head and axillae (due to self-trauma), (3) generalized pruritus without skin lesions, (4) urticaria and angioedema, (5) seborrhea, (6) eosinophilic plaque, or (7) psychogenic alopecia (Fig. 8-5).

The differential diagnosis in dogs includes atopy, FAD, drug hypersensitivity reaction, intestinal parasite hypersensitivity, contact allergic or irritant dermatitis, scabies, pediculosis, idiopathic seborrhea, and folliculitis.[10] In the cat, the differential diagnosis includes atopy, FAD, drug hypersensitivity reaction, intestinal parasite hypersensitivity, cheyletiellosis, pediculosis, dermatophytosis, notoedric mange, and idiopathic miliary dermatitis.[10]

Diagnosis is made by history, physical examination, and on the basis of elimination diets and test meal investigations. Up to 10 percent of the dogs and 5 percent of the cats referred to the author's practice with a pruritic dermatosis respond to a hypoallergenic diet. Routine laboratory tests are not useful. Blood or tissue eosinophilia is rare. Histopathologic examination of the skin reveals a nonspecific, subacute to chronic, nonsuppurative dermatitis.[44] Prick, scratch, and intradermal skin testing with food allergens are felt to be unreliable.[47] There are several possible explanations including the fact that some food allergens may not be formed until after digestion or that some food allergens may exist as haptens and do not become allergenic until they combine with a body protein. The Radio Allergosorbant Test (RAST) and cytotoxicity examinations are being employed experimentally in human medicine. Recently, a RAST test for food allergens in the dog has been introduced.

The elimination diet is chosen on the basis of avoiding food items to which the animal is routinely exposed. Switching from one commercial diet to another is not satisfactory as it will not eliminate many common ingredients including colorings, flavorings, and preservatives. The author feeds a diet of lamb and

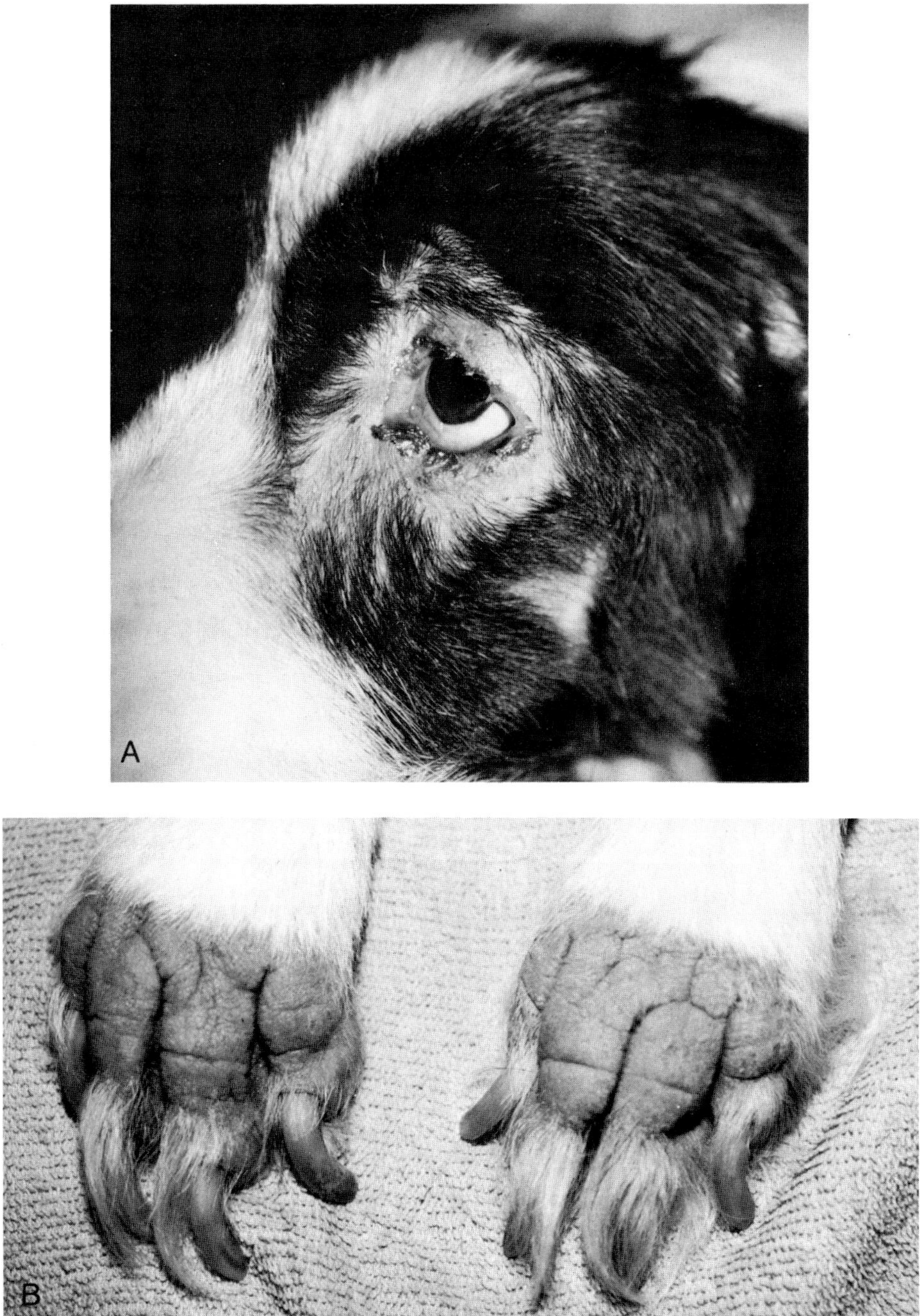

Fig. 8-5. (A) Food allergy in a 3-year-old female springer spaniel. Periocular alopecia, erythema, and lichenification. (B) Alopecia, erythema, and lichenification in a well-demarcated pattern on the dorsum of the forepaws. (*Figure continues.*)

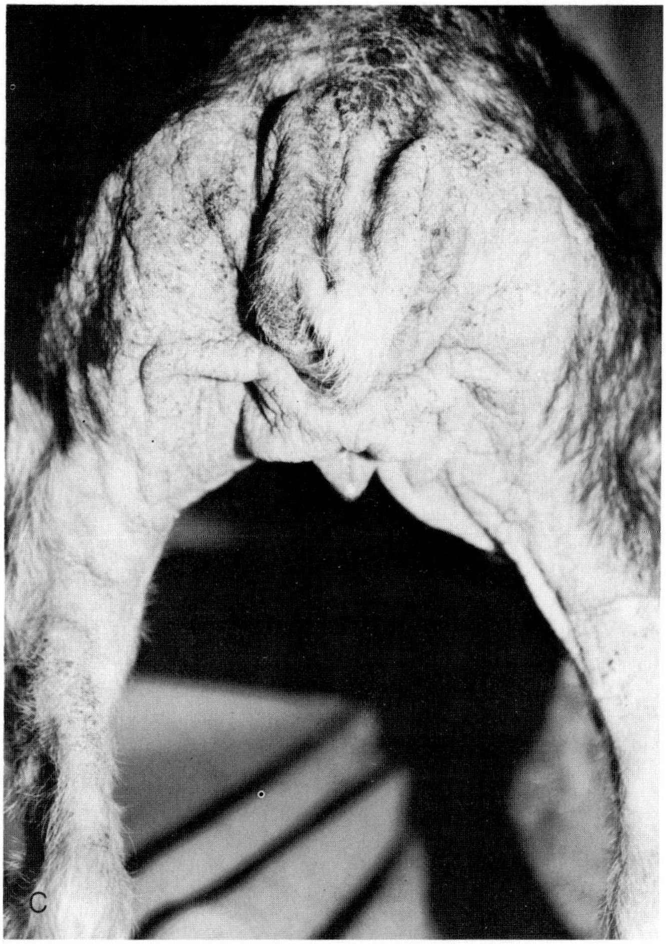

Fig. 8-5. (*Continued*). (C) Alopecia, lichenification, and crusting over the caudal dorsum, hips and rear legs.

brown rice for the dog (Table 8-1) or baby-food lamb or chicken for the cat for 14 to 21 days. The client is also instructed to discontinue vitamin supplements, table scraps, and other snacks. If a food allergy is present the level of pruritus should markedly decrease, often within the first 3 to 7 days, but occasionally not until 10 to 14 days or longer.[10] The cutaneous lesions will gradually resolve (Fig. 8-6).

Once the animal's condition is improved or the level of pruritus has markedly subsided, a challenge or provocation test should be done by feeding the animal its regular diet once again. If the elimination diet was the reason for the improvement then an increase in the level of pruritus will be noted, usually within 1 to 5 days. If the animal is fed its regular diet for 1 week and no increase in pruritus is seen then the cause for the condition was most likely not in the

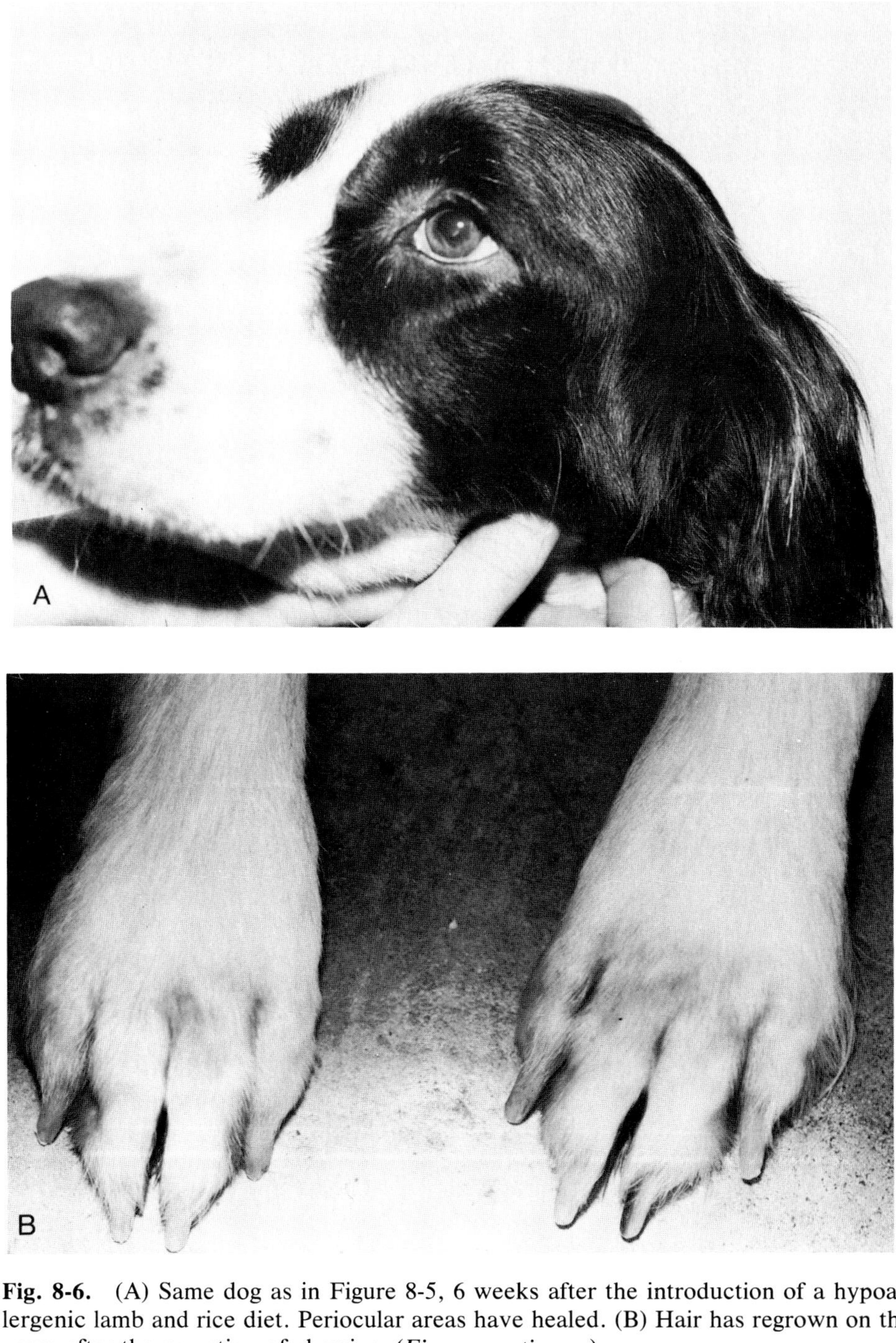

Fig. 8-6. (A) Same dog as in Figure 8-5, 6 weeks after the introduction of a hypoallergenic lamb and rice diet. Periocular areas have healed. (B) Hair has regrown on the paws after the cessation of chewing. (*Figure continues.*)

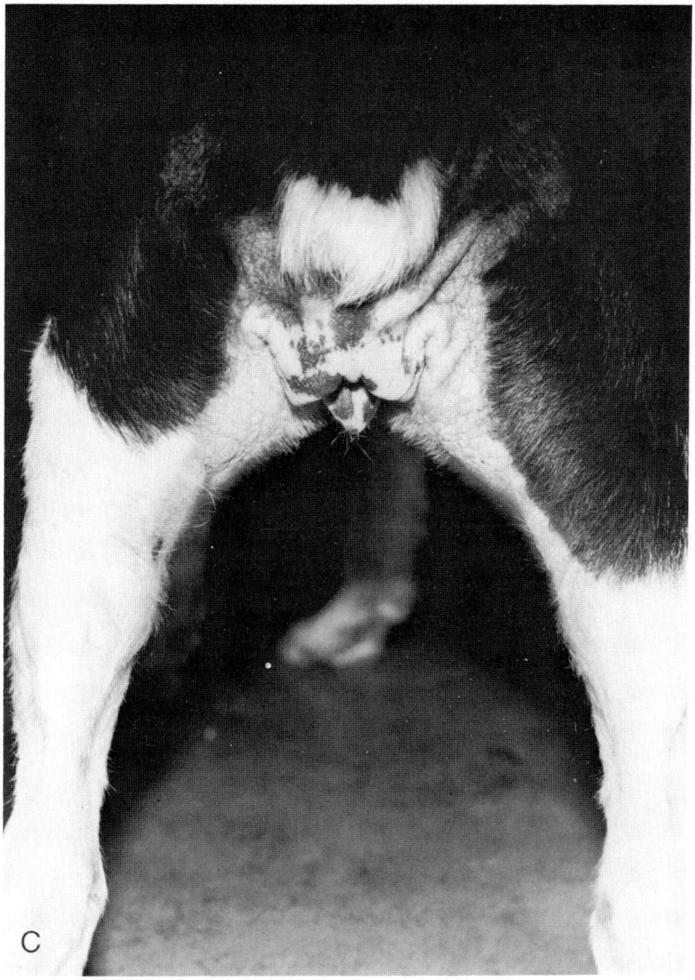

Fig. 8-6. (*Continued*). (C) Note almost complete healing of the caudal trunk with hair regrowth and resolution of the pyoderma.

diet and the clinician must look elsewhere (e.g., change of shampoos, seasonal changes in pollen levels, improved flea control, use of antibiotics, etc.).

Therapy consists of dietary avoidance. Corticosteroids are often of minimal benefit. Single items are added to the patient's diet on a weekly basis, evaluating the animal's response, and gradually accumulating a list of foodstuffs the animal can tolerate without exacerbating the allergy. A daily vitamin-mineral and fatty acid supplement should also be provided. Occasionally a limited ingredient commercial pet food (e.g., chicken and soy-based, lamb and rice-based) that meets the NRC requirements for nutrition can be found that the animal can tolerate. Otherwise, the client must be instructed in the preparation of a nutritionally balanced home-cooked hypoallergenic diet.

Table 8-1. Hypoallergenic Lamb and Brown Rice Diet

1 lb diced or ground lamb
6 cups of cooked brown rice

Cook rice according to package directions.
Brown lamb in a frying pan or microwave oven.
Combine lamb and all cooking juices with rice.
Do not season the meat during cooking.

Yield: approximately 4 lbs

Mixture can be kept refrigerated for 3 days or can be frozen. It can then be brought to room temperature or warmed (e.g., microwave oven) before serving. Quantities can be doubled, halved, or quartered depending on the size of the dog.

Feeding Guide

Body Weight	Approximate Daily Feeding
5 lb	$\frac{1}{3}$ lb
10 lb	$\frac{1}{2}$ lb
20 lb	1lb
40 lb	$1\frac{1}{2}$ lb
60 lb	2 lb
80 lb	$2\frac{1}{2}$ lb
100 lb	3 lb

Some animals prefer that the diet be divided into two meals.
Acceptable snacks are rice cakes (unseasoned) or lamb chunks that have been boiled or broiled.

REFERENCES

1. NRC: Nutrient requirements of cats, No. 13. National Research Council, National Academy of Sciences, Washington, DC 1978
2. NRC: Nutrient requirements of dogs, No. 8. National Research Council, National Academy of Sciences, Washington, DC 1982
3. Lewis, LD: Cutaneous manifestations of nutritional imbalances. Proc Am Anim Hosp Assoc 48:263, 1981
4. Mosier JE: Relationships of nutrition and skin problems. Mod Vet Prac 105, 1978
5. Lowe NJ, DeQuoy PR: Linoleic acid effects on epidermal DNA synthesis and cutaneous prostaglandin levels in essential fatty acid deficiency. J Invest Dermatol 70:200, 1978
6. Fulco AJ, Mead JF: Metabolism of essential fatty acids. J Biol Chem 234:1411, 1959
7. Rivers JPW, Frankel TL: Fat in the diet of cats and dogs. p. 67. In Anderson RW (ed): Nutrition of the Dog and Cat: Proceedings of an International Symposium. Pergamon Press, Elmsford, NY 1980
8. Hansen AE, Wiese HF: Fat in the diet in relation to nutrition of the dog. I. Characteristic appearance and gross changes of animals fed diets with and without fat. Tex Rep Biol Med 9:491, 1951
9. Hansen AE, Wiese HF: Studies with dogs maintained on diets low in fat. Proc Soc Exp Biol Med 52:205, 1943
10. Muller GH, Kirk RW, Scott DW: Small Animal Dermatology. 3rd Ed. WB Saunders, Philadelphia, 1983
11. Brewer NR: Nutrition of the cat. J Am Vet Med Assoc 180:1179, 1982
12. Olson JA: The biological role of vitamin A in maintaining epithelial tissues. Isr J Med Sci 8:1170, 1972

13. Logan WS: Vitamin A and keratinization. Arch Dermatol 105:748, 1972
14. Prutkin L: The effect of vitamin A acid on keratinization and the keratoacanthoma. J Invest Dermatol 49:165, 1967
15. Gershoff SN, Andrus SB, Hegsted DM, Fentini EA: Vitamin A deficiency in cats. Lab Invest 6:227, 1957
16. Sousa CA, Ihrke PJ: Nutritional skin diseases. p. 592. In Pratt PW (ed): Feline Medicine. 1st Ed. American Veterinary Publications, Santa Barbara, CA 1983
17. Ihrke PJ, Goldschmidt MH: Vitamin A-responsive dermatosis in the dog. J Am Vet Med Assoc 182:687, 1983
18. Parker W, Yager-Johnson JA, Hardy MH: Vitamin A responsive seborrheic dermatosis in the dog: a case report. J Am Anim Hosp Assoc 19:548, 1983
19. Kendall P: Some nutritional differences between the dog and cat. Kal-Kan Forum, Summer:28, 1982
20. Scott PP: Nutrition and Disease. p. 137. In Catcott EJ (ed): Feline Medicine and Surgery. 2nd Ed. American Veterinary Publications, Santa Barbara, CA, 1978
21. Leahy JS, Shillam WG, Waterhouse, CE: Studies of the riboflavin requirements of the kitten. J Small Anim Pract 8:351, 1967
22. Carey CJ, Morris JG: Biotin deficiency in the cat and the effect on hepatic propionial CoA carboxylase. J Nutr 107:330, 1977
23. Joshua JO: The use of biotin in certain skin diseases of the cat. Vet Rec 71:201, 1959
24. Cordy DR: Experimental production of steatitis (yellow fat disease) in kittens fed a commercial canned food and prevention of the condition by vitamin E. Cornell Vet 44:310, 1954
25. Griffiths RC, Thorton GW, Willson JE: Pansteatitis (''Yellow Fat'') in cats. J Am Vet Med Assoc 137:126, 1960
26. Marder MW: Clinico-pathologic conference. J Am Vet Med Assoc 142:1133, 1963
27. Gaskell CJ, Leedale AH, Douglas SW: Pansteatitis in the cat: a report of four cases. J Small Anim Prac 16:117, 1975
28. Anderson HD, Elvehjem CA, Gonce JE: Vitamin E deficiency in dogs. Proc Soc Exp Biol Med 42:750, 1939
29. Langweiler M, Schulz RD, Sheffy BE: Effect of vitamin E deficiency on the proliferative response of canine lymphocytes. Am J Vet Res 42:1681, 1981
30. Ayres S Jr, Mihan R: Lupus erythematosus and vitamin E: an effective and nontoxic therapy. Cutis 23:49, 1979
31. Ayres S Jr, Mihan R: Is vitamin E involved in the autoimmune mechanism? Cutis 21:321, 1978
32. Riordan JF: Biochemistry of zinc. Med Clin North Am 60:661, 1976
33. Davies GK: Factors influencing zinc availability in animals. p. 378. In Prasad AS (ed): Zinc Metabolism. Charles C. Thomas, Springfield, IL 1966
34. Robertson BT, Burns MJ: Zinc metabolism and the zinc deficiency syndrome in the dog. Am J Vet Res 24:997, 1963
35. Sanecki RK, Corbin JG, Forbes RM: Tissue changes in dogs fed a zinc-deficient ration. Am J Vet Res 43:1642, 1982
36. Kane E, Morris JG, Rogers QR, et al: Zinc deficiency in the cat. J Nutr 111:488, 1981
37. Kunkle GA: Zinc-responsive dermatoses in dogs. p. 472. In Kirk RW (ed): Current Veterinary Therapy VII. WB Saunders, Philadelphia, 1980
38. Fadok VA: Zinc responsive dermatosis in a great dane: a case report. J Am Anim Hosp Assoc 18:409, 1982

39. Brown RG, Hoag GN, Smart ME, Mitchell LH: Alaskan malamute chondroplasia. V. Decreased gut zinc absorption. Growth 42:1, 1978
40. Walton GS: Skin responses in the dog and cat to ingested allergens. Observations on one hundred confirmed cases. Vet Rec 81:709, 1967
41. Baker E: Food allergy. p. 79. In Chamberlain KW (ed): The Veterinary Clinics of North America. Vol. 4. WB Saunders, Philadelphia, 1974
42. Baker E: Food allergy in the cat. Fel Prac 5:18, 1975
43. Walton GS: Allergic responses to ingested allergens. p. 576. In Kirk RW (ed): Current Veterinary Therapy VI. WB Saunders, Philadelphia, 1977
44. Scott DW: Immunologic skin disorders in the dog and cat. p. 641. In Schultz RD (ed): The Veterinary Clinics of North America. Vol. 8 WB Saunders, Philadelphia, 1978
45. Stogdale L, Bomzon L, van den Berg PB: Food allergy in cats. J Am Anim Hosp Assoc 18:188, 1982
46. Collins R: Allergy, a review for the practitioner—part I. VM/SAC 61:679, 1966
47. Leitze A: Laboratory research in food allergy. I. Food allergens. J Asthma Res 7:25, 1969

9 Feline Dermatoses

Gene H. Nesbitt

Feline dermatoses have received much attention in the literature during the last decade, however, the understanding of the specific etiology and the pathogenesis of many of the commonly recognized dermatoses remains unknown.[1] Classification of feline dermatoses is most commonly based upon etiology. A suggested general classification is found in Table 9-1.

APPROACH TO FELINE DISEASES:

It is recognized that feline skin has a limited spectrum of primary eruptive processes; therefore manifesting with similar clinical findings with many different causes.[2] Thus, a good history and thorough physical and dermatologic examinations are necessary in order to make a definitive diagnosis. The systematic approach discussed in Chapter 1 is very applicable to feline dermatoses. This includes history taking, comprehensive physical and dermatologic examinations, and diagnostic tests. The initial list of differential diagnoses is often longer than those for dogs because of the lack of specificity of clinical signs. An algorithm for feline dermatoses is often helpful to direct the clinician to pertinent history, clinical signs and diagnostic tests. (Figs. 9-1, 9-2) The history and clinical findings as well as the common histopathologic findings of feline diseases reported to be pruritic are summarized in Tables 9-2 and 9-3 respectively. It is apparent from this summary that the majority of recognized dermatoses may have a pruritic history. Included in this chapter are those feline diseases not discussed in other chapters.

Table 9-1. Major Causative Classifications of Feline Skin Disease

Infectious
Bacterial
Fungal
Parasitic
Viral
Immunologic (immune-mediated)
Allergic
Autoimmune (immune-mediated bullous)
Hormonal (endocrine)
Feline endocrine alopecia
Physiochemical
Contact irritant dermatitis
Solar dermatitis
Keratinization defects (seborrheic syndromes)
Congenital and hereditary
Nutritional
Neoplastic
Diseases of multiple or unknown causes
Miliary dermatitis (eczema)
Eosinophilic granuloma complex
Indolent ulcer (eosinophilic ulcer)
Eosinophilic plaque
Linear granuloma
Psychogenic alopecia and dermatitis (neurodermatitis)
Plasma cell pododermatitis
Nodular panniculitis

(Nesbitt GH, Kedan GS: Differential diagnosis of feline pruritus. Compend Contin Educ Pract Vet 7:163, 1985)

INFECTIOUS DISEASES

Parasitic

Fleas

Flea dermatitis or flea allergy dermatitis (FAD) ranks as one of the most common dermatoses in cats[1,3,4] (see Chapter 2).

Notoedric Mange (Feline Scabies)

Notoedres cati, a sarcoptid mite, is an uncommon disease but should be included in the initial differential diagnoses for the pruritic cat.

Notoedric mange is characterized by intense pruritus of the head and neck. Contagion among rabbits, dogs, and humans is reported. As in the dog the pinnae margins are commonly alopecic, crusty, and erythematous as are the head and neck. The perineum and feet are less commonly involved. Occasionally, a more generalized distribution is observed.

The definitive diagnostic test is the finding of the mites on skin scrapings. Mites may also be found in biopsies of affected skin.

Table 9-2. Summary of Historical and Clinical Factors Associated with Feline Pruritic Disease

Disease	Historical and Clinical Factors[a]								
	Age[b] (years)	Breed[b]	Sex[b]	Location of Lesion	Erythema	Pruritus	Crusts/ Scales	Alopecia	Expected Incidence[c]
Bacterial folliculitis	–	–	–	Chin++, face+, trunk+	+–	+–	+–	+–	R
Fungus (dermatophytosis)	<1++, >1+	–	–	Multifocal+, head++, feet++	+–	+–	+–	+	C
Parasites									
Notoedric mange	<1	–	–	Head, ears, neck, legs	+	+	+	+	R
Cheyletiella mange	Young	Long-haired	–	Dorsum	–	+–	+	–	V
Otodectic mange	<1++, >1+	–	–	Ear canal++, head	+–	+–	+–	+–	C
Demodectic mange	–	–	–	Neck, head, ears	+	+–	+–	+	R
Fleas	–	–	–	Dorsum	+–	+–	+–	+–	C
Trombiculiasis	–	–	–	Head, ears, feet	+–	+–	+	+	V
Pediculosis	–	–	–	Generalized	+–	+–	+	+–	R
Immunologic disorders									
Food allergy	>2	–	–	Head, neck	+	+	+	+	C
Contact allergy	>2	–	–	Contact surfaces	+	+	+–	+	R

Table continues

Table 9-2. Summary of Historical and Clinical Factors Associated with Feline Pruritic Disease (*continued*)

	Historical and Clinical Factors[a]								
Disease	Age[b] (years)	Breed[b]	Sex[b]	Location of Lesion	Erythema	Pruritus	Crusts/ Scales	Alopecia	Expected Incidence[c]
Fleabite allergy	3–6	–	–	Neck++, dorsum++, ventrum+	+–	+	+	+	V
Drug eruption	–	–	–	Multifocal	+–	+–	+–	+–	U
Urticaria/angioedema	–	–	–	Localized/ generalized	+–	+–	–	–	R
Inhalant allergy (atopy)	>1	–	–	Multifocal	+	+	+–	+–	U
Intestinal parasites	–	–	–	Generalized	+–	+	+–	–	R
Autoimmune disorders									
Pemphigus foliaceus	2–13 (average 6)	–	–	Head, ears, feet	+	+–	+	+	R
Pemphigus erythematosus	>5	–	–	Head, ears	+–	+–	+	+	R
Pemphigus vulgaris	>5	–	–	Oral mucosa, lip, pinnae, feet, nares	+	+–	+–	–	R
Systemic lupus erythematosus	–	–	–	Generalized	+–	+–	+–	+–	R
Physiochemical disorders									
Solar dermatitis	>3	White skinned	–	Ears++, eyelids+, nose, lips+	+	+	+	+	V

Irritant contact dermatitis	–	–	–	Contact surfaces	+	+ –	+ –	+ –	C
Diseases of unknown/multiple causes									
Eosinophilic granuloma complex									
Eosinophilic (indolent) ulcer (rodent ulcer)	5–6	–	F	Upper lip, mouth	+ –	–	+ –	+ –	O
Eosinophilic plaque	2–6	–	–	Abdomen, medial thigh	+	+	+ –	+	O
Linear granuloma	1–5 (average 1)	–	F	Posterior hindleg, oral	+ –	+ –	+ –	+ –	O
Neurodermatitis	–	Siamese, Burmese, Himalayan, Abyssinian	–	Local or multifocal	+ –	+	–	+	O
Miliary eczema (dermatitis complex)	–	–	–	Dorsum	+ –	+ –	+	+ –	C
Nodular panniculitis	5–9	–	–	Trunk, multifocal	+ –	+ –	+ –	+ –	R
Neoplastic diseases									
Mast cell tumor	–	–	–	Solitary or multifocal	+	+ –	+ –	+	O
Cutaneous lymphosarcoma	>5	–	–	Multifocal	+ –	+ –	+ –	+ –	R

[a] **Key:** – = not reported to be a consistent historical or clinical observation, + = reported to be a common observation, + + = reported to be the most common observation, and + – = reported to have variable historical and clinical observations.

[b] Predilection but not absolute.

[c] **Key:** R = rarely observed, O = occasionally observed, C = commonly observed, V = variable incidence depending on geographic location, and U = unknown incidence.

(Nesbitt GH, Kedan GS: Differential diagnosis of feline pruritus. Compen Contin Educ Pract Vet 7:163, 1985.)

Fig. 9-1. Diagnostic algorithm for the pruritic cat.

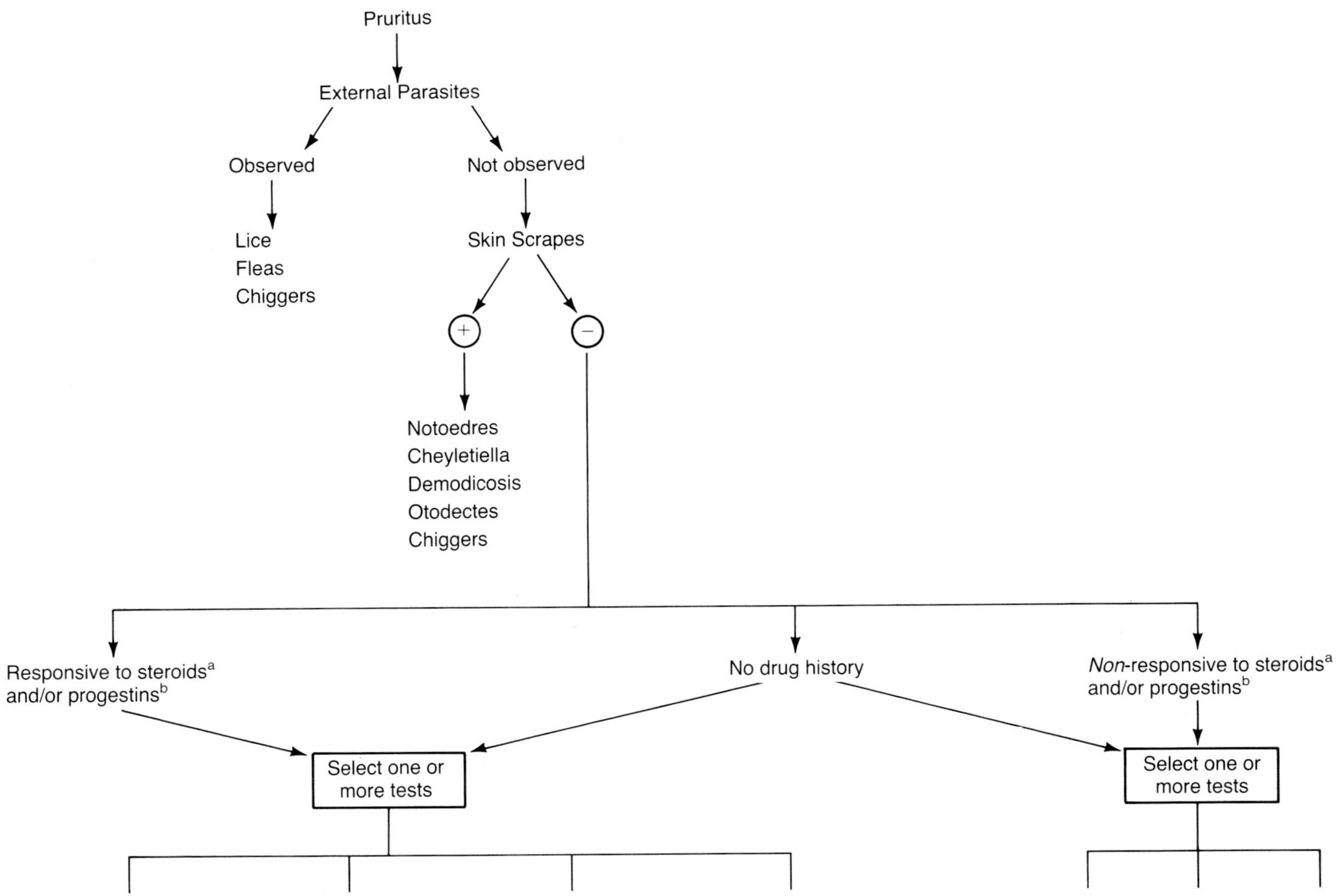

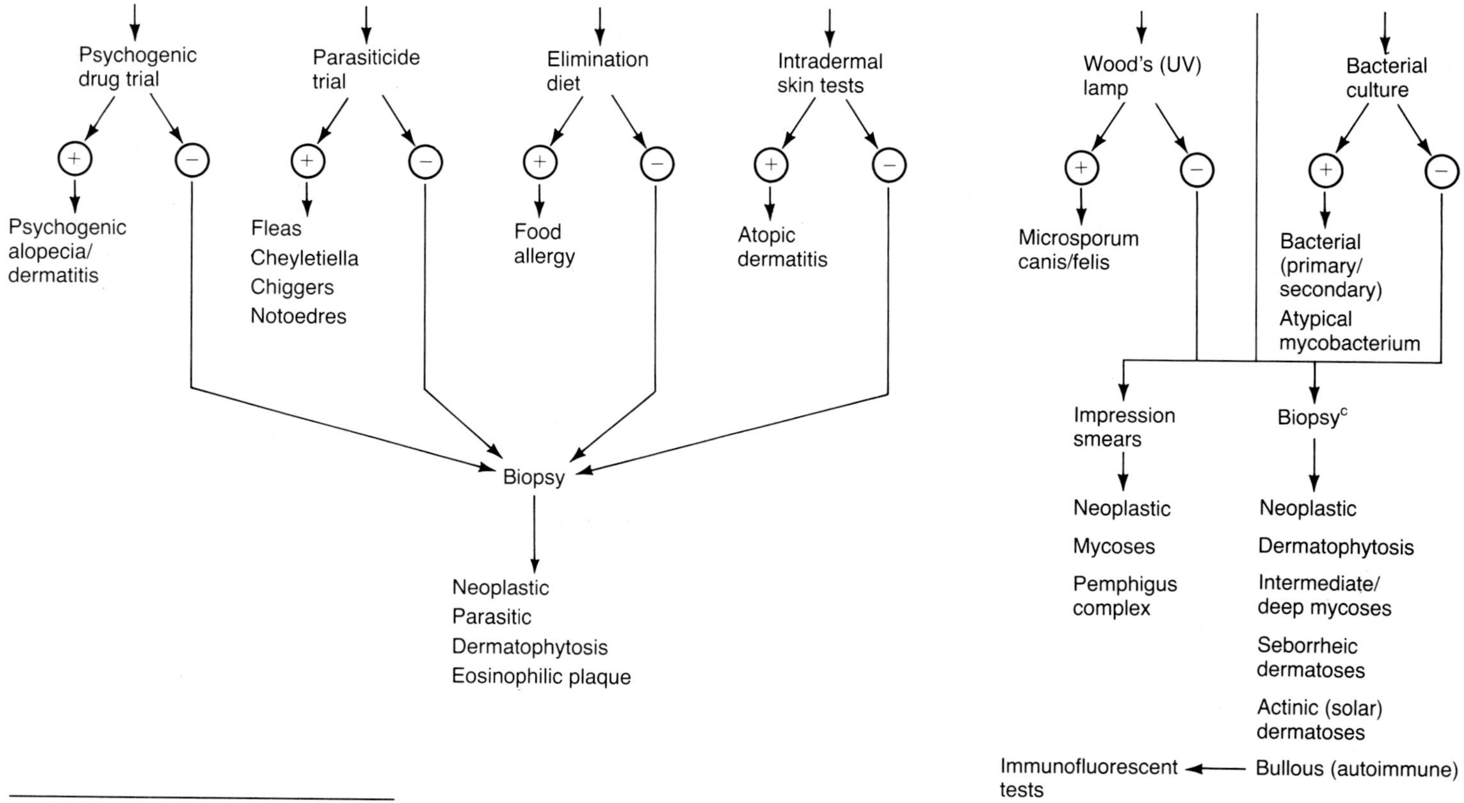

[a] Steroids include methylprednisolone acetate (Depo-Medrol, Upjohn) at a dosage of 20 mg/cat administered subcutaneously and prednisone and prednisolone at a dosage of 2 to 4 mg/kg orally

[b] Progestins include megestrol acetate (Ovaban, Schering) and repository progesterone at a dosage of 2.2 to 22 mg/kg administered subcutaneously or intramuscularly.

[c] Biopsies include needle aspiration, excisional, and/or punch techniques.

Table 9-3. Summary of Histopathologic Data in Feline Pruritic Disease

Disease	Histopathologic Observations
Bacterial folliculitis	Folliculitis and furunculosis. Bacteria may be observed.
Superficial dermatophytosis	Subacute to chronic nonsuppurative mild or moderate perifolliculitis, furunculosis, pyogranulomatous dermatitis, or perivascular dermatitis, or perivascular dermatitis (spongiotic or hyperplastic) with hyperkeratosis and occasional parakeratosis. Intraepidermal vesicular or pustular dermatitis is occasionally observed. Fungal hyphae and spores are observed in 80% of cases.
Parasites	
Notoedric mange	Perivascular (hyperplastic, spongiotic), chronic, nonsuppurative dermatitis. Mite segments are occasionally found in the corneal layer. Tissue eosinophil numbers vary.
Cheyletiella mange	Subacute to chronic, nonsuppurative, perivascular (hyperplastic, spongiotic) dermatitis. Mite segments are occasionally seen. Tissue eosinophil numbers vary.
Demodectic mange	Varying degrees of folliculitis and perifolliculitis with segments of mites in the follicle or superficial epidermis.
Trombiculiasis	Variable superficial perivascular (spongiotic, hyperplastic) dermatitis with many tissue eosinophils.
Pediculosis	Subacute to chronic, nonsuppurative dermatitis with numerous eosinophils.
Immunologic disorders	
Food allergy	Subacute to chronic, nonsuppurative, perivascular (spongiotic, hyperplastic) dermatitis with neutrophils predominating in the superficial dermis followed by plasma cells, lymphocytes, and mast cells. Secondary suppurative changes are frequently observed.
Contact allergy	Perivascular dermatitis (spongiotic, hyperplastic). Lymphocytes and histiocytes predominate in the dermis.
Flea allergy	Subacute to chronic nonsuppurative perivascular (spongiotic, hyperplastic) dermatitis with numerous eosinophils. Intraepidermal eosinophilic microabscesses and suppurative folliculitis and intraepidermal pustular dermatitis are common.
Drug eruption	Perivascular (spongiotic, hyperplastic), interface (hydropic, lichenoid) dermatitis, intraepidermal vesiculopustular or subepidermal vesicular dermatitis.
Urticaria/angioedema	Ranging from vesicular dilatation and edema in the superficial and middle dermis to perivascular dermatitis with variable mixed cellular infiltration.
Intestinal parasites	Variable degrees of perivascular (hyperplastic, spongiotic) dermatitis with a small to large number of tissue eosinophils.

Table continues

Table 9-3. Summary of Histopathologic Data in Feline Pruritic Disease (*continued*)

Disease	Histopathologic Observations
Autoimmune disorders	
Pemphigus erythematosus	Intragranular or subcorneal acantholysis with cleft and vesicle or pustule formation. Either neutrophils or eosinophils predominate within the vesicle.
Pemphigus foliaceus	Same as pemphigus erythematosus. Neutrophils predominate.
Pemphigus vulgaris	Suprabasilar acantholysis with cleft and vesicle formation.
Systemic erythematosus	Subcorneal vesicle, liquefaction degeneration of the basal cell layer.
Physiochemical disorders	
Solar dermatitis	Chronic suppurative dermatitis to squamous cell carcinoma.
Diseases of unknown/multiple causes	
Eosinophilic (indolent) ulcer (rodent ulcer)	Chronic, hyperplastic, ulcerated perivascular dermatitis with neutrophils, plasma cells, and mononuclear cells predominating.
Eosinophilic plaque	Hyperplastic or spongiotic superficial and deep nonsuppurative perivascular dermatitis. A diffuse dermatitis with epidermal microvesicle formation is often observed. Large numbers of eosinophils with fewer mast cells are common.
Linear granuloma	Nodular to diffuse dermatitis due to granulomatous inflammation with marked collagen degeneration. Tissue eosinophilia is present in about 50% of cases.
Neurodermatitis (psychogenic alopecia and dermatitis)	Subacute to chronic nonsuppurative dermatitis (dermatitic form) or normal skin (alopecic form).
Miliary eczema (dermatitis) complex	Subacute to chronic superficial perivascular dermatitis (spongiotic, hyperplastic) with variable numbers of eosinophils, mast cells, mononuclear cells, neutrophils, and plasma cells. Intraepidermal pustular dermatitis, perifolliculitis, folliculitis, and furunculosis may be associated with bacteria or fungi.
Nodular panniculitis	Varying degrees of fat necrosis, acute inflammation with neutrophils, pyogranulomatous to granulomatous inflammation with foamy macrophages, and foreign body giant cells and fibroplasia.
Neoplastic diseases	
Mast cell tumor	Diffuse to multinodular proliferation of mast cells.
Cutaneous lymphosarcoma	Diffuse dermal and subcutaneous infiltration by malignant lymphocytes. Occasionally neoplastic lymphocytes will be observed in the epidermis.

Nesbitt GH, Kedan GS: Differential diagnosis of feline pruritus. Compend Contin Educ Pract Vet 7:163, 1985.

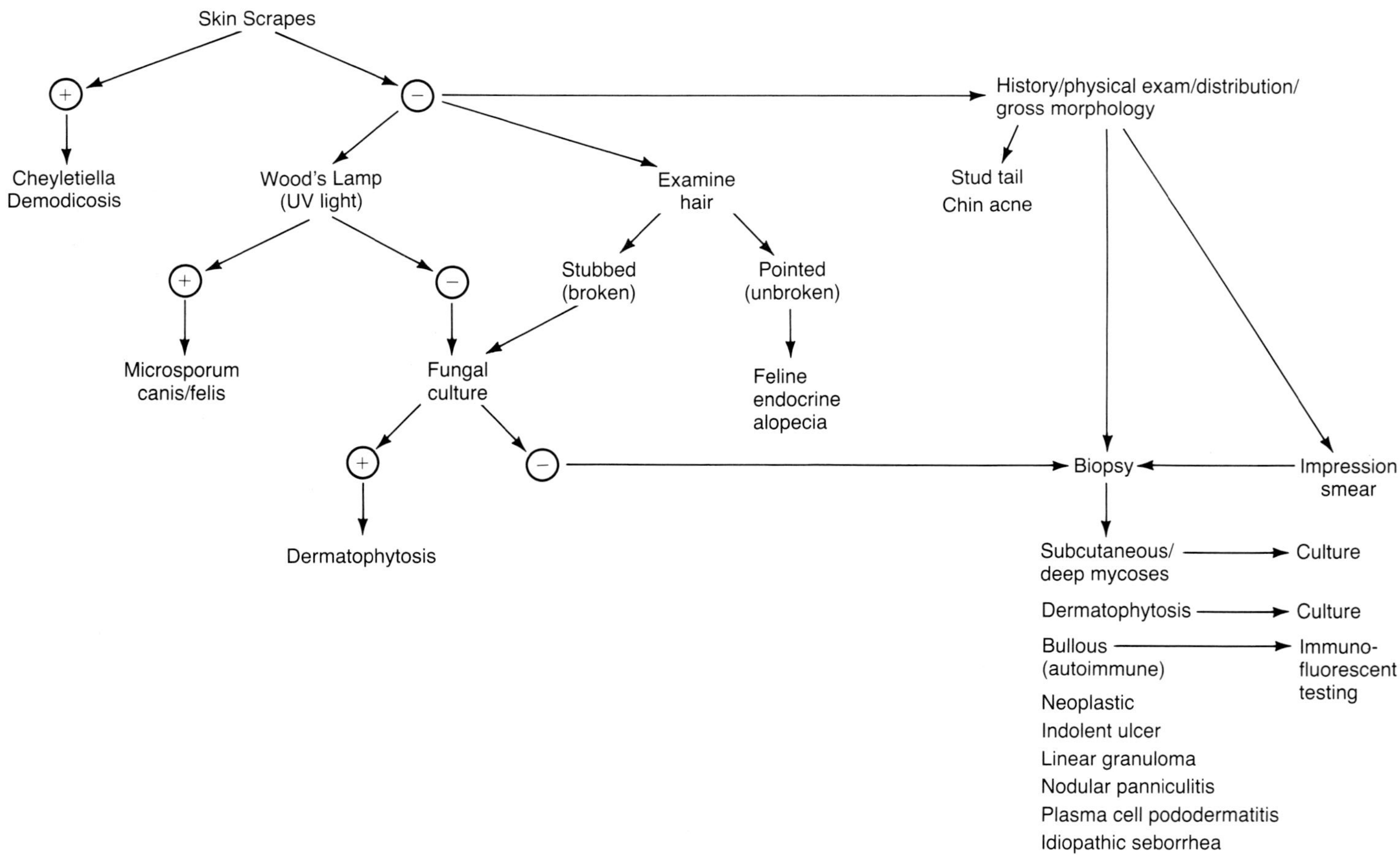

Fig. 9-2. Diagnostic algorithm for the nonpruritic cat.

Recommended treatment includes clipping hair from affected areas, removing crusts with soap and water, and applying a lime-sulfur dip. The dip is repeated at weekly intervals until resolved. Amitraz (Mitaban, Upjohn) has been used in a 0.025 percent concentration although it is not approved for cats in the United States.[5].

Cheyletiellosis

Cheyletiella blakei is the most common species affecting cats although *C. yasguri* and *C. parasitovorax* are reported to also infect cats.

Infested cats often have a history of mild pruritus. Human contagion is common and may be the reason for the cat being presented for examination. Transmission to humans and other cats is by either direct or indirect contact. Scaling on the dorsum, either generalized or localized, is the most common finding. Focal excoriation is occasionally observed as is a miliary dermatitis. Some cats are asymptomatic.

Cheyletiella spp is referred to as the "walking dandruff" mite. It lives in the keratin layer of the epidermis moving through pseudotunnels in the dermal debri. The entire life cycle is spent on the host. However, the adults may survive off the host for several days.

Diagnosis is made by identifying the mite in skin scrapings. Mites are usually found in superficial scrapings with the dandruff being removed. A very effective technique is to use clear cellophane tape to collect hair and scale from the surface of the skin, and with subsequent examination of the specimens under the microscope. The large mites with hooks on the accessory mouth parts are readily observed. Large eggs attached to the hair shafts with fine strands from one end of the egg may also be observed.

Cheyletiellosis is treated with any of the topical parasiticidal agents used for fleas in cats. Pyrethrins, carbamates, malathion, methoxychlor, and lime-sulfur are used. Treatment should be continued for at least 1 week beyond clinical remission, usually a minimum of 3 weeks. All animals in the household must be treated. Since the mites can survive off the host, it is necessary to thoroughly clean the environment including vacuuming, disinfection of hard surfaces, and the use of an insecticidal premise spray. Occasionally, fumigation is necessary to break the life cycle.[6]

Demodicosis

Clinical signs associated with *Demodex cati* are rare although they are considered normal residents of feline skin.[5] A new feline demodectic mite species has been described, but as yet unnamed.[7]

The reported clinical signs associated with feline demodicosis are variable including solitary or multifocal patches of alopecia, scale, erythema, crusting, papules, and excoriation.[8,9] The localized form usually involves the head and neck. It has also been associated with a ceruminous otitis. Generalized feline demodicosis has been seen with concurrent diabetes mellitus.[5].

Diagnosis is made by identifying *D. cati* on skin scrapings. *D. cati* mites are very similar in appearance to *D. canis*. The adults of the new species of Demodex described are shorter than *D. cati* and have broad, blunted abdomens.

Other Cutaneous Parasites of Cats

Trombiculidiasis is a rare disease caused by several species of chigger mites including *Eutrombicula alfreduggesi, E. autumnalis,*[10] *Walchia americana,*[11] *Bryobia praetiosa*,[10] and *Leewenhoekia australiensis*.[12]

Clinical signs of papules and pustules of the head, ears, and feet are observed. Pruritus is variable. A seasonal occurrence in the summer and fall is most common. A definitive diagnosis is based on the finding of larvae in skin scrapings. Treatment with lime-sulfur, pyrethrins, and/or carbamates is usually effective if reinfestation does not occur.[5]

Otodectes cyanotis will occasionally be associated with a nonpruritic alopecia or pruritic dermatitis of the head and neck, caudal back, or feet. These lesions are usually seen concurrently with otitis externa. Diagnosis is based on identifying the mite in scrapings of the lesions. Treatment consists of insecticidal preparations such as lime-sulfur, pyrethrins, and carbamates on the body as well as local treatment of the ears.

Pediculosis (lice) is uncommon but reported to be increasing in incidence.[2] The biting louse, *Felicola subrostratus*, is associated with variable clinical signs from asymptomatic to scales, papules, crusts, and severe pruritus. White, glistening nits may be observed attached to the hair. The lice nits must be differentiated from Cheyletiella eggs. Cheyletiella eggs are smaller and attach to the hair by filaments on one end of the egg while the larger louse nit is attached most of its length. Lice are susceptible to most parasiticides including pyrethrins, carbamate, and methoxychlor.

Viral

Viral infections associated with feline dermatoses are reported. The role of the feline leukemia virus in pyodermas, eosinophilic ulcers, seborrheic disorders, pruritus, and some neoplastic diseases has not been determined.[13] Cat pox virus (cow pox) has been identified in ulcerated nodules.[13,14] The herpes virus is reported to be the cause of an ulcerative dermatitis and stomatitis.[12] Erosive/ulcerative lesions of the feet, tongue, and lips are associated with a calici virus.[15] Definitive diagnosis of viral infections is based on viral isolation and the presence of viral inclusion bodies on microscopic examination of lesional tissue.

Fungal and Bacterial

Dermatophytosis is a common dermatosis of cats. The intermediate and deep mycoses are less common. Refer to Chapter 6 for an indepth discussion of fungal infections. Other than cat bite predisposed abscesses, bacterial infections in cats are uncommon. Feline bacterial diseases are discussed in Chapter 5.

IMMUNOLOGIC DISORDERS

Among the immunologic dermatoses of cats, flea-bite hypersensitivity and food allergies have been most widely reported. (See Chapters 2 and 8). Drug eruptions[16] and allergic contact dermatitis are rarely recognized.[17] Feline atopy has recently been recognized as an important clinical entity in cats.[2,12,17,18] The autoimmune dermatoses are uncommon, but increasing in reported incidence. (See Chapter 4.)

Feline Atopy

The existence of feline atopy as a clinical entity is based on the many similarities to canine atopy. These similarities include a seasonal or nonseasonal pruritus, a distribution of lesions including the head, extremities, and trunk, positive intradermal skin tests, and clinical response to hyposensitization. The specific pathogenesis of feline atopy has not been verified since feline IgE has not been isolated.

Reedy found that 15 (75 percent) of 20 cats had positive reactions to one or more skin test antigens.[18] The positive cats included seven with miliary dermatitis, seven with psychogenic alopecia, and one with eosinophilic ulcer. The author has observed similar results (GH Nesbitt, unpublished data). Three cats with eosinophilic plaques, two with eosinophilic ulcers, two with linear granulomas, four with seasonal pruritus, and five with idiopathic pruritus based on history, lesions, and other diagnostic tests had one or more positive skin test reactions. Nine cats with idiopathic pruritus were negative. In addition, two pruritic cats with dermatophytosis and one pruritic feline leukemia-positive cat tested positive. In total, 19 (67.9 percent) of 28 cats had positive skin tests.

These studies accentuate the diversity of history and clinical signs associated with feline atopy. Most of the cats would fall into the unknown or multiple etiology disease classification based on history and negative diagnostic test results excluding intradermal skin testing. A true feline asthmatic condition may coexist with the atopic dermatitis.[2]

Intradermal skin testing is the definitive test for feline atopy. The techniques described in Chapter 3 for intradermal testing in dogs is followed for cats. Some cats do resist physical restraint, and ketamine, 10 mg/kg IM, may be given if needed.[12] The wheals associated with intradermal tests in cats tend to be flatter, poorly circumscribed, and less erythemic as compared to canine ID test reactions. Thus, feline ID test reactions are generally more difficult to interpret.

As in the dog, effects of immunosuppressive drugs may result in false-negative test reactions. Approximately 48 percent (10 of 21) of the cats which had received megestrol acetate 6 weeks to 3 months prior to the ACTH stimulation test had below average basal cortisol levels while two-thirds of the poststimulation cortisol values were lower than normal controls (GH Nesbitt, unpublished data). However, there was a poor correlation between suppressed ACTH stimulation tests and positive intradermal reactions, suggesting that the ACTH stimulation test can not be used to accurately predict the degree of immunosuppression and therefore skin testing blockade. Glucocorticosteroids and tranquilizers should also be avoided.

Feline atopy was controlled by hyposensitization with alum-precipitated allergens in approximately two-thirds of 20 cats.[18] Methylprednisolone acetate (Depo-Medrol, Upjohn) at a dose of 20 mg/cat SC at monthly or longer intervals is often effective. Prednisone or prednisolone administered at a dose of 1 to 2 mg/kg/day loading dose and then alternate day dose as needed for maintenance may also be tried. In the author's experience most cats respond rather poorly to the oral short-acting corticosteroids.

PHYSIOCHEMICAL DISORDERS

This disease classification includes several different entities. Irritant contact dermatitis and solar dermatitis are the most common. Other reported physiochemical disorders include temperature-dependent hair color changes, burns, frostbite, hair mats, thallotoxicosis,[20] chlorinated naphthalene,[21] and quartenary ammonium poisonings.[12]

Irritant Contact Dermatitis

Most contact dermatitis reactions in cats are primary irritant rather than allergic or immune-mediated. Primary irritants reported to cause contact dermatitis in cats include flea collars, insecticides, kerosene, turpentine, paint, tars, phenols, cresols, soaps, oils, greases, chlorine, iodine and quartenary ammonium compounds, naphthols, fertilizers, acids, salt, benzoyl peroxide, and various topical medicaments.[17]

Primary irritant contact reactions can occur on the first exposure. The history will often reveal recent exposure to a potentially irritant substance. Clinical signs are variable. The hairless or thinly haired areas of the body are predominantly affected unless a liquid has been applied. An acute irritant contact dermatitis is characterized by an erythematous, moist lesion. If pruritic, these lesions progress rapidly to excoriation, ulceration, crusting, and alopecia.

In less severe or chronic reactions, scaling, hyperpigmentation, and occasionally lichenification and scarring will be observed.

The diagnosis of an irritant contact dermatitis is based on history of exposure, isolation from suspect contactants, and elimination of other differential diagnoses. Treatment is symptomatic and supportive.

Solar Dermatitis

In white cats, solar or actinic dermatitis occurs most commonly on areas exposed to sunlight, especially the eartips and eyelids. Ultraviolet light waves of 3,000 Ångstrom unit band and genetic predisposition are thought to play major roles in the pathogenesis of solar dermatitis. Evidence suggests that the ultraviolet rays alter deoxyribonucleic acid (DNA) synthesis and replication in the epidermis.[22] Porphyrin metabolism was reported to be normal in cats with solar dermatitis.[23] There usually is a history of progressive lesions in the involved areas starting with mild erythema and scaling and becoming more severe with alopecia, crusting, pruritus, and curling of the ear margins. There may be seasonal exacerbations and remissions since there is a direct correlation between length of exposure to intense sunlight and clinical signs. Squamous cell carcinoma is a common sequela to solar dermatitis of several years duration.[22] Squamous cell carcinomas manifest as persistent, ulcerative, locally invasive lesions. Diagnosis of solar dermatitis is based on history and clinical signs. Biopsies are indicated to differentiate between inflammation associated with solar dermatitis and squamous cell carcinoma. Treatment of solar dermatitis consists of avoidance of direct sunlight, topical sun screens, and topical or systemic glucocorticosteroids. Cats with nonulcerative solar dermatitis have been treated successfully with a carotenoid (110 mg betacarotene and 150 mg canthaxanthin) administered orally.[23] Surgical excision of the pinna is the treatment of choice for early squamous cell carcinoma. Radiotherapy has also been used for early lesions.

DISORDERS OF KERATINIZATION

Disorders of keratinization include those diseases and cutaneous reactions manifested by abnormal keratinocyte maturation including mitosis, differentiation, and exfoliation. Feline acne, stud tail, and seborrheic syndromes are associated with keratinization abnormalities.

There are many factors which influence keratinization. Intrinsic factors include prostaglandins and probably an epidermal chalone. Extrinsic factors include the dermis, epidermal growth factors, vitamin A, corticosteroids, estrogens, zinc, minor trauma, and humidity.[24]

Feline Acne

Feline acne is a relatively common disorder of unknown etiology.[25] It has no sex, breed, or age predilection. Failure to clean the chin during normal grooming with subsequent accumulation of sebum and debri on the surface may predispose to plugging of hair follicles and comedone formation. Another proposed predisposition is the failure of telogen hairs to force keratosebaceous plugs out of the follicular opening.

Clinically, the cat has comedones on the chin and lower lips. These are usually asymptomatic with no inflammation or pruritus. Occasionally they become infected resulting in papules, pustules, edema, and abscessation. Pruritus may accompany the more severe lesions.

Diagnosis is usually based on clinical signs. Skin scrapings are always indicated. If the lesions fail to respond to symptomatic treatment other diagnostic tests should be performed including culture and biopsy if indicated.

Treatment in mild cases is usually unnecessary. If the lesions are more severe or treatment is requested by the client for aesthetic reasons, manual evacuation of the comedones, gentle cleansing of the chin with keratolytic shampoo, and the topical application of a keratolytic agent such as benzoyl peroxide or an astringent is indicated.

When infection is present, clipping the area, cleaning with an antibacterial soap, hot packs, and systemic antibiotics are recommended. Because feline acne is often relapsing, maintenance of local treatment with washing and topical keratolytic astringents may be needed every few days for life.

Stud Tail

Feline stud tail is a syndrome most frequently observed in intact males, but may occur in females or castrated males. Persian, Siamese, and rex cats are reported to have a higher incidence.[25]

Stud tail is characterized by comedones and yellow to black accumulation of debri on the dorsum of the tail. These clinical findings are associated with hyperactivity of the supracaudal organ (preen gland). The specific cause is unknown. It has been postulated that inadequate grooming associated with confinement predisposes to the condition.

Treatment of a mild lesion is usually not needed. Keratolytic shampoos as needed to control the lesions may be indicated. Megestrol acetate has been used with variable success. Changing the cat's environment, especially to provide outdoor exposure, has been recommended. Castration is not helpful in controlling clinical signs.

Seborrheic Syndromes

Idiopathic generalized seborrhea, either seborrhea sicca or seborrhea oleosa, is uncommon. Most seborrheic syndromes in cats are secondary to other diseases.[25] Primary diseases to consider include cheyletiellosis, pediculosis, endoparasitism, dermatophytosis, nutritional disorders, systemic diseases such as feline leukemia, cardiomyopathy, liver disease, and neoplasia as well as environmental factors including high temperature and low humidity.

All possible primary etiologies must be ruled out before a diagnosis of idiopathic feline seborrhea is made. In addition to the treatment of the primary cause, symptomatic treatment with antiseborrheic shampoos which do not contain coal tar is indicated.

CONGENITAL AND HEREDITARY DISORDERS

Congentital and hereditary disorders in the cat are uncommon.[26] The most widely recognized disease is cutaneous asthenia (Ehlers-Danlos Syndrome). This is characterized by increased fragility and hyperextensibility of the skin accompanied by extensive scarring. The history and clinical findings are usually diagnostic.

Other diseases in this classification include epitheliogenesis imperfecta characterized by a congenital absence of epidermis and associated adnexa, alopecia universalis, and hypotrichosis characterized by a downy hair coat at birth and then progressive irreversible alopecia.

NEOPLASTIC DISEASES

Skin tumors in cats are reported to represent 15 to 47 percent of all feline neoplasia.[27] Epithelial tumors occur slightly more often than mesenchymal tumors. Melanocytic tumors are rare. Skin tumors are malignant in 60 to 80 percent of the cats.[28]

Basal Cell Tumor

Basal cell tumors are a common epithelial tumor representing 15 to 18 percent of all skin tumors.[29] The distribution is usually on the head, back, or shoulders. They are usually solitary, but may be multiple. The characteristic appearance is a well-circumscribed, firm, dome-shaped nodule. They may be heavily pigmented and occasionally will be ulcerative. Basal cell tumors are benign.

A presumptive diagnosis of basal cell tumor can be made on the basis of history and clinical findings. An excision biopsy is indicated to confirm the diagnosis since early surgical excision is the treatment of choice. Incomplete excision of the tumor may result in recurrence.[29]

Squamous Cell Carcinoma

Squamous cell carcinomas are a common epithelial tumor. The pinna, nasal planum, external nares, lips, and eyelids are most commonly affected. Cats with nonpigmented skin are at higher risk. A solar dermatitis is the most common predisposing factor.

Squamous cell carcinomas are characterized as solitary, broad based, locally invasive tumors. They are poorly demarcated and are often erosive. Biopsy and histopathologic examination are necessary to make a definitive diagnosis although the history and clinical signs are often suggestive.

Several therapeutic modalities have been used to treat squamous cell carcinomas. The treatment of choice is aggressive surgical excision. Radiation therapy is reported to be a successful treatment.[30] Cryosurgery can be tried when excision and radiation are not possible. Hyperthermia has also been used with some success.[31]

Adnexal Gland Tumors

Collectively, adnexal gland tumors represent the third most common epithelial feline tumor. This group includes apocrine, ceruminous and sebaceous gland tumors, hair matrix tumors, trichoepithelioma, and perianal gland tumors.[27]

The treatment of choice of adnexal gland tumors is surgical excision. Histopathologic examination is recommended for prognostic purposes.

Fibrosarcoma and Fibroma

Fibrosarcomas and fibromas are mesenchymal tumors accounting for 20 to 33 percent of feline skin tumors.[27] In young cats multiple fibrosarcoma tumors are associated with the feline sarcoma virus and feline leukemia virus. In older cats, lesions are usually solitary and not associated with the feline sarcoma virus.

Since fibrosarcomas are extremely locally invasive, aggressive surgical excision is recommended. Recurrence is common. Chemotherapy and radiation may be tried, but results are often unsatisfactory. The prognosis is guarded.

Fibromas are uncommon solitary tumors. Surgical excision usually results in a cure.

Mast Cell Tumors

Mast cell is the second most common mesenchymal tumor in the cat.[27] The cutaneous manifestations occur in 38 to 50 percent of the affected cats. The clinical manifestations of cutaneous mast cell tumors are variable. Most are multiple, firm, raised, dermal masses. The borders may be well demarcated or have nondiscrete borders. Most are erythematous and ulceration is common. Plaque lesions may predominate. Most multiple cutaneous feline mast cell tumors are malignant and thus have a poor prognosis. Solitary tumors often have a long-term survivial rate.[12]

All lesions in which mast cell tumor is suspected should be biopsied. Fine needle aspirate cytology may be diagnostic. Smears of the buffy coat and radiographic studies should be completed to detect evidence of a systemic mastocytosis. Recommended treatment of primary cutaneous mast cell tumor is surgical excision if possible. Since many cats have multiple lesions, immunosuppressive doses of corticosteroids are used, but with relative poor response. Chemotherapy has not been effective. Radiation therapy may be considered.

Other Feline Tumors

Several skin tumors occur rarely. These include lipomas, liposarcomas, giant cell tumors, myxomas, myxosarcomas, hemangiomas,[27] and lymphosarcomas[32]. Needle aspirates and biopsies are indicated to obtain a diagnosis and prognosis.

DISEASES OF UNKNOWN OR MULTIPLE ETIOLOGY

In feline dermatology several common diseases are recognized in which the specific cause is unknown. These include the eosinophilic granuloma complex, miliary dermatitis, psychogenic alopecia and dermatitis, feline acne, and feline endocrine alopecia. Seborrheic dermatoses, plasma cell pododermatitis, and nodular panniculitis are other uncommon diseases with an unknown etiology. Feline acne and seborrheic dermatoses are discussed under the heading of Diseases of Keratinization elsewhere in this chapter. Feline endocrine alopecia is discussed in Chapter 7.

Eosinophilic Granuloma Complex

The eosinophilic granuloma complex remains a frustrating clinical entity for the clinician. Three distinct morphologic lesions, including the eosinophilic plaque, indolent ulcer (eosinophilic ulcer, rodent ulcer) and the linear granuloma remain grouped under the same clinical diagnosis. All three entities are treated similarly. Some cats will have more than one type of lesion.

Although a specific cause has not been identified, there are several theories. There is some evidence of an infectious agent being involved. Lesions have been transmitted from one area to another on the same cat with autologous tissue.[33] Scott reported that 90 percent of cats with indolent ulcers were positive for the feline leukemia virus (FeLV). The author has not identified a similar correlation. There is also a clustering of cats with similar lesions, suggesting the possibility of a contagious or hereditary factor.[34] Virus particles resembling calicivirus in size and shape were observed in tissue from an eosinophilic granuloma lesion.[12]

As was discussed under feline atopy, immunologic factors are thought to be involved in some cases with the eosinophilic granuloma complex. Reedy reported positive intradermal skin tests in one cat with an eosinophilic ulcer.[18] This author found positive skin test reactions in eight cats including three with ulcers, three with plaques, and two with linear granulomas (GH Nesbitt, unpublished data). Cats manifesting seasonal clinical signs and microscopic lesions resembling those reported for the eosinophilic granuloma complex have been observed in Australia.[35]

History and Clinical Signs

Eosinophilic Plaque. The eosinophilic plaque has no breed or sex predilections. Pruritus manifested as intense licking is usually reported. The lesions are well-circumscribed, raised, ulcerated, exudative, erythemic, and alopecic. Size is variable.[34] The majority of lesions are found on the abdomen and medial thigh although other areas of the skin and oral cavity are sometimes involved. Blood and tissue eosinophilia are common. Histopathologic findings are not specific for a definitive diagnosis since microscopic findings of food and flea allergies are similar.

Indolent Ulcer. The indolent (eosinophlic) ulcer is reported to occur three times more frequently in females than males.[34] They are usually not pruritic or painful. Hemograms are usually normal. Lesions are characterized by well-circumscribed, ulcerated lesions with raised borders and a central necrotic crater. They are of variable size located most commonly on the upper lip margin. It may be unilateral or bilateral. Indolent ulcers are occasionally observed on the lower lip, nose, oral cavity, and on the skin of the trunk. Lip ulcers may progress to squamous cell carcinomas.

Linear Granuloma. The linear granuloma occurs in the younger cat with an average age of 1 year. There is a predilection for females.[34] Most cats are asymptomatic. Spontaneous regression may occur. The lesions are characterized by well-circumscribed, raised, firm, yellow-pink, dermal masses arranged in a narrow linear pattern most commonly occurring on the posterior aspects of the rear legs. Lesions may be seen in the oral cavity as well as on other areas of the body. Histopathologic findings are that of a granulomatous reaction including collagen degeneration, along with histiocytes and giant cells. Eosinophilia, both tissue and blood, are commonly associated with oral eosinophilic granulomatous lesions.[34] Oral lesions are not reported to spontaneously regress.

Diagnosis

The history and clinical signs are very suggestive of this complex. Skin scrapings as well as fungal cultures are often indicated. Complete blood counts may help support a diagnosis. Biopsies are needed to differentiate mast cell tumor from eosinophilic plaque. Likewise, to differentiate an early squamous cell carcinoma from an indolent ulcer, a biopsy is needed. If allergies are suspected, diet testing and intradermal skin testing are indicated.

Therapy

The two most commonly used drugs in the treatment of eosinophilic plaques, indolent ulcers and linear granulomas are megestrol acetate (Ovaban, Schering) and methyl prednisolone acetate (Depo-Medrol, Upjohn). Megestrol acetate is administered at a rate of 2.5 to 5 mg daily or every other day until lesions are in remission and are then tapered to once or twice weekly if needed to control recurrence of lesions. Megestrol acetate, which is not approved for use in the cat in the United States, must be used with caution. Potential side effects, especially with long-term administration, include polyphagia and obesity, polydipsia, temperament changes, mammary gland hyperplasia, and rarely neoplasia, diabetes mellitus (usually transient), endometritis, pyometra, and uterine stump abscesses.[2] The author has seen cats with signs similar to iatrogenic Cushing's disease including trunkal alopecia. Post-ACTH cortisol levels are depressed. Repositol progesterone at a dose of 2.2 to 22.0 mg/kg IM or SC every 2 weeks is also used.

Methylprednisolone acetate is administered subcutaneously at a dose of 20 mg every 2 to 3 weeks until lesions are in remission.[34] Cats appear to tolerate this therapy well on a long-term basis if not administered more frequently than every 4 weeks. Other therapeutic modalities include radiation therapy,[33] cryosurgery,[36] levaminisole, and thiabendazole.[33] Surgical excision or curettage have not been widely recommended.[34]

Regardless of which method of therapy is used, recurrences are common. It is predictable that some lesions, regardless of type, will not respond to one therapeutic agent, yet will respond to another. All types of lesions must be treated continuously until they are in total remission. It should be noted that both linear granulomas and indolent ulcers have been reported to clear spontaneously.

Miliary Dermatitis (Miliary Eczema)

Miliary dermatitis is strictly a clinical diagnosis. The symptoms of miliary dermatitis should initiate the search for one or more primary etiologies. Among the most common causes of miliary dermatitis are allergies, parasites, and infections.[34,37] The most common cause of allergy is fleas although food and atopic dermatitis are sometimes initiating factors. Among parasitic diseases fleas, cheyletiellosis, notoedric and otodectic mange, and rarely trombiculidiasis and demodicosis are considered to cause miliary lesions. In addition, endoparasitism has been associated with miliary dermatitis. The major infectious agents are dermatophytes. Bacterial infections associated with a folliculitis are infrequently associated with feline miliary dermatitis. Other entities which should be considered in a list of differential diagnoses include drug eruptions and fatty acid deficiencies. Only when all possible specific etiologies are ruled out should a diagnosis of idiopathic feline miliary dermatitis be made.

Clinical signs are characterized by a crusting, papular eruption on the dorsum, especially on the neck, shoulders, or tail regions although it may be generalized. In the earlier stages erythema may be present. Pruritus and alopecia are variable. Because the etiologies are many, there is no age, sex, or breed predilection for the clinical entity.

Diagnosis is based on the thorough history and dermatologic examination and the completion of indicated diagnostic tests including skin scrapings, fungal cultures, therapeutic trials with insecticides, diet testing, intradermal skin tests, biopsies, and a dietary trial with fatty acid supplements.

The treatment should be based on the definitive diagnosis. In the case of idiopathic feline miliary dermatitis megestrol acetate at a dosage of 2.5 to 5.0 mg is given daily or preferably every other day until lesions are resolved. If the problem is relapsing, a maintenance dose of weekly or biweekly megestrol acetate may be indicated.

Psychogenic Alopecia and Dermatitis (Neurodermatitis)

Psychogenic dermatoses are self-inflicted skin disorders initiated or intensified by nonorganic causes.[38] Feline psychogenic alopecia is characterized by continued mild licking of an area of skin until hair is removed from it. The continued licking may become more vigorous progressing from alopecia to abrasion, ulceration, and secondary infection.

The initiating cause or causes of this syndrome may be otitis or external parasites. Other causes may be fear or tension as a result of territorial intrusion by man or animal and anxiety as a result of a separation from a favorite location or from a human or animal companion.

There is no sex or age predisposition. Breeds most commonly affected are the Siamese, Burmese, Himalayan, and Abbyssinian.[34] Clinical signs are variable. In the alopecic form noninflammed areas of complete alopecia or solitary patches of slowly progressive alopecia are observed. In the dermatitic form, solitary lesions associated with erythema, ulceration, variable size and distribution are observed. Multiple lesions are present in some cats. In either form, the lesions are always associated with excessive grooming and licking.

Diagnosis is based on history, clinical signs, exclusion of other diagnoses, and the identification of broken hair shafts or stubbed hairs in the involved areas. The intact hairs or stubs do not epilate easily. Several diagnostic tests including skin scrapings and fungal cultures are routinely performed to rule out other primary causes.

Treatment of psychogenic alopecia and dermatitis must be oriented towards resolving the underlying problems. The major treatment modalities include topical treatment of the lesion, manipulation using psychotropic drugs, and nonpharmacologic behavior modification. Usually, a combination of several different modalities is most effective.[38]

The psychotropic drugs used to treat psychogenic dermatoses include phenobarbital (2.2 to 6.6 mg/kg orally b.i.d.), diazepam (1.25 to 2.5 mg orally b.i.d.), and megestrol acetate (2.5 to 5.0 mg daily) until licking ceases and then every other day, gradually tapering over a minimum of 1 month. Some cats will respond to one drug and not to another.

The prognosis for psychogenic alopecia and dermatitis is variable. If the predisposing cause can be identified and eliminated, the prognosis is good. A relapse is common when the predisposing factor reappears. Some cats require long-term or life-time maintenance therapy.

Plasma Cell Pododermatitis

Plasma cell pododermatitis is an uncommon condition of cats of unknown etiology. No age, breed, or sex predilection has been noted. It is characterized by swelling and softening of multiple foot pads, most commonly the metatarsal and metacarpal, on multiple paws.[34] Ulceration of the affected pads is a variable finding. Pruritus is not usually associated with plasma cell pododermatitis. Similar lesions, referred to as plasma cell stomatitis have been observed in the commissures of the mouth.[12] Diagnosis is based on a history of poor response to antibiotics and antiinflammatory doses of glucocorticoids, clinical signs, and characteristic histopathologic findings from biopsied tissue.[12]

The two recommended modalities of treatment are immunosuppressive doses of glucocorticoids (2 to 4 mg/kg) and aurothioglucose (Solganol, Schering).[34] Some cats undergo spontaneous remission.

Nodular Panniculitis

Nodular panniculitis is a rare disease of unknown etiology of middle aged cats with no breed or sex predilection. Lesions are characterized as well-demarcated, firm, and occasionally painful nodules. The nodules become fluctuant and rupture. A thick, blood-tinged exudate is discharged. Ulceration and fistulous tracts follow the rupture. The lesions are usually multiple on the trunk. Scarring is a common sequela. The cats usually are pyrexic, lethargic, and anorectic prior to onset of skin lesions.[33]

Diagnosis is based on a history of poor response to antibiotics and anti-inflammatory doses of glucocorticoids, clinical signs, and laboratory tests. A leukocytosis with a left shift is often observed. The exudate is usually sterile. Biopsies reveal a panniculitis.

Treatment with large doses of prednisone or prednisolone (4 mg/kg) is recommended until the lesions resolve. The dose is then gradually tapered and maintained if needed on a minimum alternate-day dosage. Relapses may occur.

REFERENCES

1. Proceedings of the Meeting of the American Academy of Veterinary Dermatology. Las Vega, NV, April, 1982
2. Halliwell REW: Alopecia and pruritus in the cat. Proc Am Anim Hosp Assoc, March, 150, 1985
3. Scott DW: Feline dermatology 1900–1978: A monograph. J Am Anim Hosp Assoc 16:331, 1980
4. Ihrke PJ: Clinical evaluation of skin disease. p. 555. In Pratt PW (ed): Feline Medicine. American Veterinary Publication, Inc., 1983
5. Scott DW: Feline Dermatology: A monograph 1900–1978. J Am Anim Hosp Assoc 16:365, 1980
6. Alexander MM, Ihrke PJ: Cheyletiella dermatitis in small animal practice. A Review: Calif Vet 36:9, 1982
7. Conroy JD, Healey M, Bane AG: New Demodex sp. infesting a cat: A case report. J Am Anim Hosp Assoc 18:405, 1982
8. Nutting WB: Hair follicle mites (Demodex sp) of medical and veterinary concern. Cornell Vet 66:214, 1976
9. Stogdale L, Moore DJ: Feline demodicosis. J Am Anim Hosp Assoc 18:427, 1982
10. Fadok VA: Miscellaneous parasites of the skin (Part II). Compend Contin Educ Pract Vet 21:707, 1980
11. Comenstine LJ, Carpenter JL, O'Conner BM: Trombiculosis in a cat. J Am Vet Med Assoc 1275:289, 1979
12. Scott DW: Feline Dermatology 1979–1982: Introspective retrospection. J Am Anim Hosp Assoc 20:537, 1984
13. Scott DW: Feline Dermatology: A monograph 1900–1978. J Am Anim Hosp Assoc 16:375, 1980
14. Scott FW: Catpox virus infection. Cornell Feline Health Center Veterinary News. Summer, 1983
15. Cooper LM, Sabin M: Paw and mouth disease in a cat. Aust Vet J 48:644, 1972
16. Nesbitt GH: Cutaneous drug reactions in small animals. p 190. In Fellner MJ, Zeide DA (eds): Clinics in Dermatology. Vol. 4. JB Lippincott, 1986
17. Scott DW: Feline Dermatology: A monograph 1900–1978. J Am Anim Hosp Assoc 16:377, 1980
18. Reedy LM: Results of allergy testing and hyposensitization in selected feline skin diseases. J Am Anim Hosp Assoc 18:618, 1982
19. Nesbitt GH: Feline and Canine Dermatology: A systematic approach. Lea & Febiger, Philadelphia, 1983
20. Scott DW: Feline Dermatology 1900–1978: A monograph. J Am Anim Hosp Assoc 16:395, 1980
21. Wegener K: Possible effects of German wood preservative on cats and dogs, with special reference to hyperkeratosis. J Am Vet Med Assoc 120:145, 1952
22. Hargis AM: A review of solar-induced lesions in domestic animals. Compen Contin Educ Pract Vet 3:287, 1981
23. Irving RA, Day RS, Eoles L: Porphyrin values and treatment of feline solar dermatitis. Am J Vet Res 43:2067, 1982
24. Montagna JW, Parakkal PF: The Structure and Function of Skin. 3rd Ed. Academic Press, New York, 1974
25. Scott DW: Feline Dermatology 1900–1978: A monograph. J Am Anim Hosp Assoc 16:406, 1980

26. Scott DW: Feline Dermatology 1900–1978: A monograph. J Am Anim Hosp Assoc 16:403, 1980
27. Susaneck SJ: Feline skin tumors. Compend Contin Educ Pract Vet 5:1251, 1983
28. Scott DW: Feline Dermatology 1900–1978: A monograph. J Am Anim Hosp Assoc 16:419, 1980
29. Macy DW, Reynolds HA: The incidence, characteristics and clinical management of skin tumors in cats. J Am Anim Assoc 17:1020, 1981
30. Carlisle CH, Gould S: Response of squamous cell carcinoma of the nose of the cat to treatment with x-rays. Vet Radiol 23:186, 1982
31. Grier RL, Brewer WG, Thielen GH: Hyperthermic treatment of superficial tumors in cats and dogs. J Am Vet Med Assoc 177:227, 1980
32. Caciolo PL, Nesbitt GH, Patnaik AK, Hayes AA: Cutaneous lymphosarcoma in the cat: A report of nine cases. J Am Anim Hosp Assoc 20:491, 1984
33. Hess PW, MacEwen EG: Feline eosinophilic granuloma. p. 103. In Kirk RW (ed): Current Veterinary Therapy VI. WB Saunders, Philadelphia, 1977
34. Scott DW: Feline Dermatology 1900–1978: A monograph. J Am Anim Hosp Assoc 16:406, 1980
35. Wilkinson GT, Bate MJ: A possible further clinical manifestation of the feline eosinophilic granuloma complex. J Am Anim Hosp Assoc 20:325, 1984
36. Willemse TA: Cryotherapy in small animal dermatology. p 495. In Kirk RW (ed): Current Veterinary Therapy VII. WB Saunders, Philadelphia, 1980
37. Kunkle GA: Feline miliary dermatitis. Carnation Research Digest 18:1, 1982
38. Young MS: Psychogenic dermatoses. Dermatology Reports. Veterinary Learning Systems, Inc., Princeton Jct., NJ 3:1, 1984

10 Dermatologic Disorders of Common Small Nondomestic Animals

Bobby R. Collins

MAMMALS

Clinical abnormalities of the cutis and subcutis are common reasons for the presentation of rodents, rabbits, and ferrets for veterinary care. The client is usually observant enough to identify or palpate abnormalities that are readily confirmed by his practitioner. Although the average practitioner does not have an intimate understanding of the common diseases of these species, basic knowledge of the principals of veterinary medicine and dermatology should enable him to diagnose and treat the vast majority of the clinical conditions.

The Mongolian Gerbil (*Meriones unquiculatus*)

Bacterial Diseases

Staphylococcus aureus and *Staphylococcus epidermidis* are the bacteria most frequently isolated from the skin of animals, but rarely are these organisms a primary cause of skin disease in small nondomestic species. Most of the time they are secondary to other less obvious etiologies, e.g., dermatitis secondary to mites or lice. Once a lesion develops, other bacterial species, such as *Proteus vulgaris, E. coli,* and *Streptococcus* spp., may colonize the wound and contribute to the morbidity and mortality observed.

Staphylococcal dermatitis has been reported in weanling gerbils (21 to 27 days of age) after their arrival at a research facility.[1] The initial lesions were erythema and localized alopecia, but eventually progressed to an extensive moist dermatitis. The lesions began around the external nares and spread to the feet, legs, and ventral surface of the thorax and abdomen. After 2 to 3 weeks, 75 percent of the animals were affected. A chronic condition persisted in the affected animals for 3 to 4 months, but rarely did the condition result in debilitation and death. Of the older animals in the colony only 25 percent were ever affected at any one time. Trauma associated with blood sampling or fighting and periods of high relative humidity (80 percent) dramatically increased the severity of the disease and the occurrence of death.

Bacterial identification was completed using standard microbiological media and techniques. White-to-yellowish opaque colonies that produced beta hemolysis on 4 percent bovine blood agar displayed the typical positive Gram's stain and morphology consistent with *Staphylococcus*. These same isolates fermented mannitol salt agar and were coagulase positive. Phage typing indicated that 4 different types were present among the 10 isolates tested. Only one of the phage types (WH1) would reproduce the disease when inoculated into the abraded skin of experimental animals.

Histologically, a variable suppurative inflammatory response extended into the epidermis, superficial dermis, and hair follicles. In 54 percent of the animals so examined, the neutrophilic infiltrates were mild, and were accompanied by acanthosis and hyperkeratosis. Fifteen percent of the gerbils also had microabcesses in the liver.

Antibiotic sensitivity testing indicated that the staphylococci were sensitive to nitrofurazone, lincomycin, neomycin, novabiocin, erythromycin, and chloramphenicol.[1] Gerbils medicated via the water for 14 days with chloramphenicol succinate (0.083 g/100 ml) or tetracycline hydrochloride (0.3 g/100 ml) recovered completely. However, 25 percent experienced a recurrence which began to appear in as few as 30 days or more. Topical treatment with 0.02 percent nitrofurazone aqueous dip or topical nitrofurazone dressing resulted in a regression of the lesions, but few animals completely recovered.

Recommendations for treating staphylococcal dermatitis should include localized topical treatment with providone-iodine surgical scrub, systemic antibiotics, (Table 10-1) and isolation of the affected animals. When using topical compounds about the face, an ophthalmic ointment should be utilized to minimize the risk of ocular irritation. Also, all visible traces of the providone-iodine scrub should be removed to reduce the scaliness of the skin due to the irritating effects of topical iodine. Care should be taken to prevent hypothermia in these small animals when using external heat sources, such as heat lamps, to dry the animals. The cages, water bottles, and other caging accessories may be disinfected with a 1:30 dilution of 5 percent sodium hypochlorite solution.

The fact that these lesions started about the face and nares may indicate

Table 10-1. Antibiotic Dosages for Mammals[a,b]

Drug	Species	Dosage/Unit of Body Weight or Water	Route of Administration
Ampicillin	Gerbil, mouse, rat	2–10 mg/100 g t.i.d.	PO
	Rabbit, ferret	22–44 mg/kg divided doses, t.i.d.	PO
Cepholathin	Rabbit	12.5 mg/kg q.i.d.	IM
Cephaloridine	Guinea pig	10 mg/kg s.i.d.	IM
Chloromphenicol succinate	Gerbil	83 mg/100 ml of water	PO
Chloramphenicol palmatate	Mouse, rat, hamster, guinea pig	50 mg/kg t.i.d.	PO
	Rabbit, ferret	50 mg/kg t.i.d.	SC, IM, IV
Furazolidine	Rabbit	200 mg/pint of water	PO
Gentamicin	Gerbil, mouse, rat, hamster	5 mg/100 gm s.i.d.	SC
	Rabbit, ferret	4 mg/kg s.i.d.	SC
Neomycin	Gerbil, hamster, mouse, rat	5 cc Biosol/100 ml water for 5 days; then half this dose for 5 more days	PO
Penicillin (without procaine or streptomycin)	Gerbil, mouse, rat	100,000 IU/kg b.i.d.	IM
	Rabbit, ferret	60,000 IU/kg b.i.d.	IM
Tetracycline or Oxytetracycline	Gerbil, mouse, rat, guinea pig, rabbit, ferret	50 mg/kg q.i.d.	PO
Sulfamethazine	Gerbil, rat, hamster, mouse, rabbit	5 ml of 12.5% solution/ pint of water	PO
	Mouse	1 ml of 12.5% solution plus 49 ml of water. Give 0.5 ml to an adult mouse b.i.d.	PO
	Rabbit, guinea pig	10 ml of 12.5% solution plus 40 ml water. 10 ml b.i.d. to 5 kg rabbit and 1 ml b.i.d. to an adult 0.5 ml guinea pig.	PO
Trimethoprim/sulfa	Gerbil, rat, hamster, mouse, rabbit, guinea pig, ferret	30 mg/kg s.i.d. or b.i.d.	PO, SC
Tylosin	Gerbil, rat, mouse, hamster, rabbit	0.2–0.8 mg/100 g b.i.d. or 10 mg/100 g b.i.d.	IM PO

[a] Data from Russell RJ, Johnson DK, Stunkard JA: A Guide to Diagnosis, Treatment, and Husbandry of Pet Rabbits and Rodents. Veterinary Medicine Publishing, Lenexa, Kansas, 1981.

[b] Data from Jacobson ER, Kollias GV, Peters LJ: Dosages for antibiotics and parasiticides used in exotic animals. Compend Contin Educ Pract Vet 5:315, 1983.

that the accumulation of Hardian gland secretions may be involved in the pathogenesis of the condition.

Ectoparasites

A dermatitis characterized by alopecia, serous exudate, scales, crust, and secondary bacterial infection was diagnosed in a group of 25 gerbils purchased from a local breeder.[2] The lesions were confined to the face, thorax, abdomen, and extremities. Four of the animals yielded a demodectic mange mite upon microscopic examination of skin scrapings. The name *Demodex merioni* was proposed for this mite.

A similar clinical picture was observed in a dead 4-year-old pet gerbil submitted to a necropsy laboratory for examination.[3] Demodectic mites were isolated from a lesion about the tailhead.

Except for the two preceeding reports, no other clinicians have reported their experiences with *Demodex* mites in gerbils. Demodectic mites usually reside in hair follicles and sebaceous glands and have been reported in mice, rats, hamsters, guinea pigs, and rabbits.[4] Since *Demodex* infestations are believed to be species specific, it is most likely that the mites reported on the gerbil are a separate species.

Clinical signs commonly occur when the health of the host is compromised by old age, dietary deficiencies, or chronic infections.[3] Although the programs of colony management and nutrition were not described for the first report, it is quite possible that poor sanitation, ventilation, or nutrition contributed to the clinical problem observed in those gerbils. Small, local producers of animals are usually more likely to follow lower standards of animal care than the larger commercial facilities. In the case of the second report, the animal was at the extreme of the maximum life span reported for gerbils (4 years). Aging and the presence of concurrent age-related diseases, such as chronic interstitial nephritis, undoubtly contributed to the development of clinical demodicosis.

Neoplasia

Previous investigators have reported that most of the neoplasms observed in gerbils occurred in aged animals (2 to 4 years of age), especially in the reproductive tract of the female where the incidence of ovarian tumors was high.[5] The skin was the second most frequently reported organ system where masses were observed.

Both pigmented and nonpigmented masses occur in the Mongolian gerbil.[5–9] To date, no naturally occuring mesenchymal tumors of the skin and subcutis have been reported. The types of masses reported from the skin of the gerbil are summarized in Table 10-2.

The most commonly observed site for neoplasia to occur is the ventral marking gland or scent gland. In addition to its chemocommunication function

Table 10-2. Spontaneous Neoplastic and Nonneoplastic Masses of the Skin of the Mongolian Gerbil

Type of Mass	Location	Age (Months)	Sex	Metastasis Present	Reference
Amelanotic melanoblastoma	Perianal region, root of the tail, and abdominal wall	24	M	Yes (fat tissue of abdominal wall, mammary gland, peribronchial lymph nodes and lungs)	Benit & Kramer[5]
Melanoma	Ventrum of right hind foot	24	M	No	Cramlet, Toft & Olsen[6]
	Inner aspect of pinna of right ear	38	M	No	Vincent, Porter & Ash[7]
	Canthus of left eye	23	F	No	Vincent & Ash[8]
	Dorsal extremity of left forelimb	*	M	No	Vincent & Ash[8]
Pigmented nevus	Proximal to calcaneous of left hind foot	26	F	No	Benit & Kramer[5]
Malignant blue nevus	Dorsum of left hind foot	18	M	No	Benit & Kramer[5]
	Behind left ear	12	F	No	Vincent, Porter, & Ash[7]
Sebaceous gland adenoma	Ventral scent gland	20	M	No	Benit & Kramer[5]
		41	F	No	Vincent, Porter, & Ash[7]
		22	M	No	Vincent, Porter, & Ash[7]
		23	F	No	Vincent & Ash[8]
		23	F	No	Vincent & Ash[8]
Sebaceous gland carcinoma	Ventral scent gland	29	M	No	Vincent & Ash[8]
Squamous cell carcinoma	Pinna of right ear and chest	23	M	Yes (lungs)	Vincent, Porter & Ash[7]
	Base of left ear	45	F	No	Vincent, Porter & Ash[7]
	Ventral scent gland	39	M	No	Vincent, Porter & Ash[7]
	Ventral scent gland	31	M	No	Vincent & Ash[8]
			M	No	Vincent & Ash[8]
	*	33	M	No	Vincent & Ash[8]
	*	38	M	No	Vincent & Ash[8]
Papilloma	Ventral scent gland	24	F	No	Meckley & Zwicker[9]

* Not described in the reference cited.

(species identification and individual recognition), it also functions as a heat source in the female, important in the normal development of neonatal behavior, such as ultrasounding and righting reflex.[10] This unique structure is composed of 200 to 300 holocrine glands.[7] The glandular portion of this specialized sebaceous gland is more prominently developed than the associated hair follicles. The gland is highly vascularized and increases in size in response to gonadal steroids.[11]

Gerbils presenting with an adenoma of the ventral marking gland exhibit a reddened or red nodular pad.[7] Crust, occasional ulceration, and the presence of secondary infection frequently result in the owner complaining of an abscess on their pet's abdomen. Scent glands with squamous cell carcinomas usually present as circular, encrusted ulcers.[7] The appearance of the once-reported papilloma was typical of that type of mass.[9]

Other frequent sites for masses to occur are the ear and foot. Squamous cell carcinomas and melanomas both appear as ulcerated masses, but the melanomas and nevi are usually black.

The treatment for cutaneous masses is biopsy and/or total excision as soon as they are diagnosed. Cutaneous masses in small animals such as the gerbil are substantial relative to the size of the animal. The early surgical removal of small masses generally results in less morbidity and mortality.

Since the vast majority of the gerbils with cutaneous masses are aged animals, the overall health of the animal must be evaluated prior to anesthesia. A urine sample can be collected by placing the animal in a wire bottom cage or by picking the animal up and restraining it by the nape of the neck. Rodents generally urinate and defecate at the time of restraint. Depending on the volume collected, the urine should be evaluated for the presence of protein, the presence of cast and cells in the sediment and the specific gravity. Animals judged healthy may be anesthetized with ketamine (40 mg/kg) or diazepam (10 mg/kg) via the intraperitoneal route, followed by methoxyflurane via a nose cone or syringe casing for more precise control of the anesthetic episode.[12]

All biopsies or masses should be evaluated histologically. Although infrequent, metastases have been reported for a squamous cell carcinoma of the ear[7] and a melanoblastoma of the tailhead.[5]

Behavioral Induced Diseases

Barbering or Hair Chewing. Although gerbils tolerate crowded conditions better than most other rodents, they will chew or "barber" the hair of cagemates. The affected areas appear to have been shaved, and rarely are there any gross lesions on the skin. The dorsum of the tail and the crown of the head are most often involved.[12]

Aggression. Rodents are prone to bite each other on the tail and perianal area. Therefore, crust, abscesses, and fistulous tracts may be common in these areas. Extreme overcrowding of gerbils may lead to cagemates biting each other about the tail and sacrum.[12] The introduction of new animals into established cages may result in their injury and death, especially when males are paired with other males who will defend their territory against an "invader."[13] The pairing of sexually mature males and females, especially in the female's cage, may also lead to injury or death for the male. All pairings of mature males and females should take place in the male's cage, and should be observed closely for aggressive behavior on the part of each animal. Sexually mature gerbils are monogamous and may never fully accept a new mate after pair-bonding has occured.

The treatment for injured gerbils involves separation from the aggressor(s), topical treatment of the wounds, and systemic antibiotics as described earlier.

Bald Nose and Nasal Dermatitis. "Bald nose" describes a clinical condition common to the gerbil which is characterized by the loss of hair about the dorsum of the nose and muzzle. The area is usually void of lesions. It has been attributed to mechanical trauma associated with feed containers[14] and burrowing in the bedding.[12] Placing the animals in a smooth-sided enclosure or aquarium with soft bedding such as shredded paper has been suggested as a possible treatment.[15]

Bald nose may be an early form of nasal dermatitis, since animals with this condition often develop a staphylococcal infection in the inflammed area.[15] In a recent study, beta-hemolytic *Staphylococcus aureus* of several phage types was cultured from the nasal area of both affected and normal animals.[16] The presence of *Staphylococcus saprophyticus* was associated with the development of early nasal lesions.

The accumulation of the Harderian gland secretions about the nasal and facial areas apparently leads to the development of nasal dermatitis. The animal's failure to groom the area and thus clean the accumulated secretions from the face leads to further irritation and self-inflicted trauma.

While placing the gerbils on clean sand instead of pine shavings can result in partial recovery of nasal dermatitis, surgical removal of the Harderian gland will eliminate the condition.[17]

Treatment for nasal dermatitis involves the use of topical therapy and systemic antibiotics as previously described. Keeping the animals on clean sand is easy to do and may be helpful. Although surgical removal of the Harderian gland is easily performed[18], the long-term effects of the removal of this gland on the overall health of the eye and the gerbil has not been assessed. Thus far, no adverse effects have been reported.

Miscellaneous Diseases

Abnormal Hair Pigmentation and Growth of the Newborn Gerbil. An occasional litter will be born showing abnormalities of hair growth and pigmentation in all the young.[13,14] The back may be completely naked, and the surrounding fur scant or patchy. The color of the hair is almost white. The majority of the affected pups fail to thrive and die at the time of weaning (3 weeks). Surviving gerbils develop a normal coat as they approach maturity. The etiology of this condition is unknown, and none of the affected animals have been evaluated histologically. Animals exhibiting abnormal hair growth should not be selected for breeding.

The Golden or Syrian Hamster (*Mesocricetus auratus*)

Bacterial Diseases

Staphylococcus. A primary staphylococcal dermatitis has not been reported for the golden hamster. However, staphylococci may be recovered from isolated cases of cutaneous abscesses and bite wounds.[12]

The treatment of bite wounds and abscesses involves both topical and systemic therapy as previously described.

Antibiotic therapy for the hamster, guinea pig, and rabbit should be approached with caution due to the possibility of antibiotic-associated colitis. A fatal diarrhea within 3 to 6 days after the initiation of therapy has been attributed to an antibiotic-induced alteration of the intestinal flora and the proliferation of *Clostridium difficile* and other clostridial species.[12] The toxins produced by these organisms are responsible for a fatal enterotoxemia. This situation can be avoided for the hamster by administering only those antibiotics that suppress both gram-negative and gram-positive bacteria (neomycin, chloramphenicol palmatate, and oxytetracycline or tetracycline HC1.)

Streptococcus. A beta-hemolytic Streptococcus has been reported as the etiologic agent involved in acute mastitis in lactating females 7 to 10 days after parturition.[19] One of the hamsters was sacrificed for necropsy examination. The affected glands were dark red, firm, and contained suppurative exudate. The presence of hemorrhage and edema within the abdominal subcutis indicated that the inflammation extended beyond the mammary gland. Microscopically, polymorphonuclear inflammatory cells were present throughout the ducts, alveoli, and glandular tissue.

Bacterial identification was based upon the colony morphology on blood agar and the Gram's stain reaction. Both cultures taken from the affected gland at necropsy and the specimens expressed from the mastitic gland of another female were positive for a beta-hemolytic *Streptococcus*.

No attempt was made to treat the hamsters. One female fully recovered and subsequently raised several litters. The relative frequency with which mastitis is reported, coupled with the ability of hamsters to fully recover from the infection without treatment, probably indicates that these animals are quite able to resolve this type of infection without the necessity of antibiotic therapy.

Pasturella. *Pasturella pneumotropica* is a short, pleomorphic, gram-negative, nonsporeforming, nonmotile rod. It has been recognized as a latent bacterial infection of the rodent respiratory tract, which particularly affects mice. In the hamster, *P. pneumotropica* has been reported to be a cause of pneumonia.[20] Cutaneous abscesses midway between the eye and ear have also been observed in hamsters 2 to 3 weeks after receiving 500 to 2,500 rads of whole body x-irradiation.[21] This infection eventually proved fatal in all hamsters developing abscesses. Occassionally, this organism will be isolated from localized abscesses resulting from bite wounds.

Identification of the organism was accomplished using trypticase soy agar plates containing 5 percent sheep blood incubated at 37°C. After 48 hours, small, convex, gray colonies appeared on the agar. Although the organism was not hemolytic, occassional greening of the agar occurred under the colonies.

Treatment of *Pasturella* abscesses should include surgical drainage and topical therapy with povidone-iodine surgical scrub. Antibiotic sensitivity testing has indicated that tetracycline (50 mg/kg b.i.d.) and chloromycetin (20 mg/1,000 gm body weight) result in the largest zones of inhibition.[21] Combined topical and systemic therapy should prevent the development of fulminating pneumonia and death.

Ectoparasites

The golden hamster is one of the few animals colonized by two different species of demodectic mites, *Demodex criceti* and *Demodex aurati*.[22] The *D. aurati* are elongated mites which live within the hair follicles, whereas *D. criceti* are stout and inhabit the pits in the surface epidermis. In a study of the differential distribution of both species of mites no gross preferential site was observed on hamsters 20 to 80 days of age. In hamsters older than 2 years, *D. aurati* far outnumbered *D. criceti*, especially on the dorsum.[22,23]

The incidence in breeding colonies had been reported to range from 66 to 100 percent.[24] *D. aurati* was found in 60 percent and *D. criceti* in 33 percent of the hamsters. No pathology has been reported with the presence of mites in young hamsters. However, clinical disease has been observed in a colony of aged male hamsters exposed to low-level carcinogens.[25] Alopecia was evident at 30 weeks of age, but was less severe in the control animals. Grossly, the skin exhibited a moderate-to-severe alopecia, which was especially prominent over the lumbosacral area. Scales and small crusts were present in the affected area. Microscopically, numerous follicles were dilated and distended with mites and debris present. The corneum was slightly thickened, and the crust was located in the uppermost superficial corneum. There was little evidence of an inflammatory response around the hair follicles. Skin scrapings from the affected areas were warmed in 10 percent sodium hydroxide (NaOH), and yielded mites consistent with *D. aurati*.

Malnutrition, concurrent disease and age have been mentioned as common predisposing factors toward clinical manifestation of the disease.[25] In a study of the diseases of the aging hamster, the most common abnormality of the skin was parasitic infestation.[26]

A diagnosis of demodicosis is confirmed on the basis of finding mites in skin scrapings from the affected sites. When clinical disease is evident, numerous mites should be present in the specimens collected for microscopic examination.

The treatment of demodectic mange in the hamster has not been extensively evaluated. Successful treatments have been reported with weekly bathings in Canolene (Pitman-Moore) and a once only injection of dexamethasone (1 mg SC) in those animals exhibiting pruritis.[27] An immediate clinical response was noted. After 2 months of therapy the pruritis was absent, but areas of alopecia were still present. A 1:5.5 dilution of ronnel concentrate in propylene glycol mixture applied daily for 5 weeks has also been reported to be effective,[12] but ronnel is difficult to obtain. (*Note: no longer available.*)

Endocrine Related Disease

Confirmation of a clinical diagnosis of endocrine related skin disease in the hamster has been a rare occurrence. Only a single report documents the occurrence of hyperadrenocorticism in teddy bear hamsters, which are long-haired mutants of the golden hamster.[28] The clinical signs included bilateral symmetrical alopecia, hyperpigmentation, and thinning of the skin. The plasma cortisol for one of the affected hamsters was 110.4 ηmol/L verses 49.7 ηmol/L in a normal animal.

One of the hamsters, a 2½-year old female, was submitted for necropsy. A firm white mass 1 centimeter in diameter was present in one adrenal gland while the other adrenal gland was atrophic. Histologically, an adenocarcinoma was present in the adrenal cortex.

Two treatment regimens were instituted. One hamster received o,p′-DDD(1,1-dichloro-2,2-bis(p-chlorophenyl)ethane) orally at a dose of 5 mg per day for 1 month. The other hamster received metyrapone at dose of 8 mg daily for 1 month. In both instances the drugs were mixed in a corn syrup and water base given directly in divided doses. The animal receiving metyrapone responded rapidly with new hair growth that was complete after 12 weeks. No improvement was noted in the hamster receiving the o,p′-DDD. Changing the hamster to metyrapone did not result in any clinical improvement; therefore, the client elected to euthanitize the animal. A diagnosis of chromophobe adenoma of the pituitary gland with adrenal cortical hyperplasia was made.

Pituitary tumors are exceedingly rare in the hamster.[29] On the contrary, neoplasia of the adrenal cortex is relatively high. Incidence rates of 1 to 50 percent have been reported for certain colonies or inbred lines. Nodular hyperplasia of the cortex is also a common finding in 46 percent of the older hamsters. With frequency rates approaching those recorded above, the clinician should see clinical cases among his population of older hamster patients.

Neoplasms of the adrenal gland are more common in the male than the female.[30] Castration of the male hamster commonly results in a shortened survival time and a significantly higher incidence of benign adrenal neoplasms and nodular hyperplasia. Ovariohysterectomy apparently had no effect on the adrenal gland of females. This should be taken into consideration when clients request that the male animals be castrated.

Laboratory confirmation of a diagnosis of an endocrine disease requires the collection of whole blood for the determination of serum hormone values. This can be accomplished via anesthesia with ketamine (80 mg/kg) plus xylazine (5 to 10 mg/kg) injected intramuscularly, or fentanyl-droperidal (0.15 ml/100 g) intramuscularly.[12] For more fragile animals requiring greater control of the anesthetic episode, methoxyflurane and air via a nose cone are a ready alternative. While anesthetized, blood may be collected via a clipped tail[28] or via the intracardiac route. One milliliter or less of whole blood is usually sufficient to perform the assay using radioimmunoassay technology.

Based on the response to therapy as reported above, metyrapone is the recommended therapeutic agent to use. The clinical signs, plus clinical specimens negative for mites, pathogenic bacteria, or fungal agents, help support a diagnosis of Cushing's disease in the hamster, and may be sufficient to institute therapy without laboratory confirmation. A positive response to therapy within 2 weeks would add further support for the clinical diagnosis.

Neoplasia

The incidence of spontaneous neoplasia in the hamster is low, and tumors of the skin are rare. Except for a few types of tumors, such as melanomas and tumors of the lymphoreticular system, the biology, pathology, and histology of spontaneously occurring masses of the skin are poorly described. The various types of spontaneously arising masses involving the cutis and subcutis of the hamster are summarized in Table 10-3.

Melanomas are not uncommon in some colonies of hamsters.[31–35] The mean incidence of those tumors is 0.4 percent, with a reported range of 0.1 to 2.76 percent.[35] The tumors characteristically appear in aged animals, and occur in males much more frequently than females.

Grossly, the masses may be found anywhere on the skin, but the back, head, neck, and the flank gland are the most frequent sites of primary tumor. The masses are usually firm or nodular on palpation, and may be covered with skin or exhibit ulceration with crust or bleeding. The surrounding skin is usually hairless. The color of the mass varies from bluish-black (melanotic) to gray-white (amelanotic). For the hamster, the color of the mass is of prognostic value. The pigmented tumors are more innocuous-appearing histologically and are less likely to undergo rapid growth with metastasis to other organs.

Cellular blue nevi (melanocytomas) are apparently rare in the hamster. An overall incidence rate of 0.2 percent has been observed.[36,37] Nevi may be observed at any time throughout life, whereas true melanomas are usually observed in older animals.

One survey of the literature indicated that lymphosarcomas represented 57 percent of the reported neoplasms of the Syrian hamster.[38] Occassional reports have indicated that cutaneous involvement was a common form of lymphosarcoma among hamsters within the colonies evaluated.[38,39]

Table 10-3. Spontaneous Neoplastic Masses of the Skin of the Syrian Hamster

Type of Mass	Location	Age (Months)	Sex	Metastasis Present	Reference
Melanoma	Thigh, foreleg	37	5M	almost all organs involved in some cases	Fortner & Allen[31]
	Dorsum of neck, lower abdomen, mid-ventrum, and vagina	114	2F		
	Flank organ	130	M	throughout the viscera	Green[32]
	Face	*	M	cervical lymph nodes	Bomirski, Dominiczak, & Nowinska[33]
	Eyelid	104	M	lymph nodes, liver, lung	Mangkoewidjoyo & Kim[34]
Cellular nevi (Melanocytomas)	*	*	21M F	N/A	Kirkman[36] Kirkman & Algard[37]
Lymphoma	Skin	89	F	Lymph node, skin, liver	Yabe, Kataoka, & Kogama[38]
	Skin	76–114	M	Lymph node, spleen, liver, kidney	
	Skin	125	M	Superficial lymph nodes, spleen	Toth[39]
	Skin	83, 122	2F	Lymph nodes, spleen	
Reticulum cell sarcoma	Upper lip	105	M	None	Brindley & Banfield[41]
Plasmacytoma	Subcutis of cervical area	83	M	None	Garcia, Bahroni, & Rappaport[42]
Sarcoma	Subcutis	*	F	*	Lee, Toth, & Shubik[43]
	Subcutis	94	M	*	Van Hoosier, Spjut, & Trentin[44]
Fibrosarcoma	Subcutis of dorsal neck	*	M	Lungs, thoracic wall, diaphragm, liver, spleen, kidney	Kelin[45]
Fibroma	Subcutis of face	*	*	N/A	Van Hoosier & Trentin[35]
Squamous cell carcinoma	Skin	80	M	Lymph node	
Basal cell carcinoma	Skin	*	*	*	Kirkman[36]
Carcinoma	Skin	*	*	*	Kirkman[36]
Keratoacanthoma	Skin	*	*	*	Kirkman[36]
Papilloma	Skin	*	*	N/A	Kirkman[36]

*-Not described in the reference cited.
N/A-Not applicable.

In the studies, hamsters affected with cutaneous lymphoma, especially animals with advanced disease, exhibited fatigue, limited movement, or biting and scratching of the skin.[38] When touched they became nervous and reacted as if in pain. Early, the skin exhibited epilation, hyperkeratosis, and acanthosis primarily on the dorsal and ventral sides of the body. Occassionally, superficial ulcerations and crusts were present. With advancing disease the inguinal lymph nodes were consistently enlarged.

On gross necropsy examination tumor cells could be recognized in the lymph node and skin, but rarely in the spleen, liver, or kidney. The findings were confirmed with histopathologic examination.

Microscopically, the early skin lesions exhibited hyperkeratosis with a few infiltrative cells beneath the epidermis. In more advanced cases the invading neoplastic cells in some areas intermingled with inflammatory cells extending downward halfway into the cutis. The occassional formation of abscess-like lesions in the superficial epidermis prompted some investigators to diagnosis mycosis fungoides in the hamster.[36] However, the results of electron microscopic studies have suggested that the lymphoblastic cells are more typical of cutaneous lymhosarcoma than mycosis fungoides.[39]

The reticulum cell carcinoma appeared as a firm mass on the upper lip of an aged hamster.[40] On cut surface the mass was firm and white in color. Histologically, the mass was confined to the dermis. Neither the epidermis nor the hair follicle was invaded by the neoplasm. Uniform rounded mononuclear cells with poorly defined cytoplasm were closely packed throughout the mass. Relatively clear macrophages were scattered throughout the mass, some of which were degenerating cells and cellular debris.

A plasmacytoma was observed in the subcutis of the cervical area in an aged male hamster. The mass was surrounded by a capsule of varying thickness, consistent with the capsule of a lymph node.[41] The tumor was composed of relatively small cells with eccentrically located nuclei and abundant cytoplasm. Only a few nuclei exhibited the "spoke wheel" arrangement characteristic of mature plasma cells. The number of binucleated cells and mitotic figures was consistent with a poorly differentiated plasmacytoma.

Several other spontaneous malignant and nonmalignant neoplasms of the skin have been reported for the hamster, but only rarely. Among these are the sarcoma, fibrosarcoma, fibroma, squamous cell carcinoma, basal cell carcinoma, carcinoma, keratoacanthoma, and papilloma.[42–45]

The treatment for cutaneous neoplasia is surgical excision at the earliest possible date. Metastases have been reported for most of the malignant neoplasms. All masses should be examined histologically for confirmation of the diagnosis, for the adequacy of surgical excision, and the rendering of a prognosis. Animals with suspected neoplasms of the lymphoreticular system should be isolated from their cagemates.

The reticular cell sarcoma has been transferred by the bite of mosquitoes or by cannibalism,[41] while lymphoma has been horizontally transmitted to other hamsters.[36–40]

Behavioral-Induced Diseases

Aggression. Female hamsters are generally more aggressive than males, yet different females display different levels of aggression toward intact males.[46] Except when the female is in estrus and paired with an animal of equal body weight, most females are very aggressive and keep the subordinate males at a distance. However, when a male outweighs the female by 20 grams or more, the male may dominate an aggressive female.

A minority of females are tolerant of males and these nonagressor females maintain this behavior even when lactating and caring for a litter. The males are usually permitted to share the nest with the female and litter, as well as retrieve the young without eliciting aggression from the female. Placement of nonagressor females with castrated males and other females results in aggression.

Aggressive behavior on the part of male hamsters is testosterone dependent.[47] Castration significantly reduces fighting during male to male encounters between adult hamsters. Ovariohysterectomy of the female has no such effect.

Aggression in hamsters can be reduced if the animals are housed together before reaching sexual maturity, generally prior to 4 to 5 weeks of age.[15] Also, anesthesia followed by simultaneous recovery in a neutral cage or aquarium can reduce the level of aggression between two known cagemates. In situations where two or more animals are housed together, enclosed containers should be available for individuals to escape and hide from an aggressor. The ceramic caves and logs utilized by tropical fish hobbyist are excellent for this purpose.

Bite wounds should be treated topically as previously described. Systemic therapy should be instituted with caution due to the potential occurrence of antibiotic-associated colitis in the hamster.

Miscellaneous

The Scent Gland, Flank Gland, or Hip Gland. The Syrian hamster possesses a circumscribed pigmented structure on each side of the flank. Costovertebral in location, it is slightly thickened and consists of epidermis, hair follicles, sebaceous glands, and the supporting connective tissue. The glands are more prominent in the males, expressing themselves most fully under the effects of androgens. The secretions from these glands are used to mark territorial boundaries and provide stimuli that help initiate breeding behavior.

Occasionally, clients mistake these glands for abnormal structures and present their pet for evaluation because of the copious nature of the secretions or the gland's size (suspected neoplasm.) On rare occasions melanomas have been observed to arise spontaneously from these structures. No other type of spontaneous neoplasms have been reported.

Guinea Pig (*Cavia porcellus*)

Bacterial Diseases

Staphylococcus. *Staphylococcus aureus* has been associated with a variety of sporadic infections in the guinea pig. It has been recovered from abscesses of the foot following foot pad injections with inactivated foot-and-mouth disease virus. This occurrence probably represents the introduction of skin-dwelling staphylococci into the subcutis during the injection procedure.[48]

Beta-hemolytic staphylococci have been isolated from the nasal passages of 42 percent of the normal guinea pigs in a colony.[49] Phage typing indicated that the strains isolated were species-specific for the guinea pig.

Staphylococcus sp have also been infrequently identified from cases of acute necrotizing mastitis.[50] A necrotizing *S. aureus* was isolated from the oral cavity of nursing pups, and was suggested as the source of the infection.

An outbreak of exfoliative skin disease has been observed in a guinea pig colony, chiefly among the females in the late stages of pregnancy.[51] Bacterial contamination of the rusty cage floors was suggested as the etiology of the initial lesion. The lesions began as an alopecia of the ventral abdomen. Suddenly, the skin was erythematous, rough and thick. The animals squealed with pain when handled. After 1 to 2 days fissures appeared in the skin folds. Large thick flakes of dried skin desquamated over the following 4 to 7 days. The skin was completely healed 10 to 14 days after the onset of erythema. None of the adults died, but the mortality was extremely high among the suckling animals. The females were reluctant to allow the young to nurse due to the pain.

S. aureus was isolated from the skin, pharynx, trachea, and nasal washings of affected animals. Histologic sections showed intraepidermal cleavages through the stratum granulosum with occassional cellular debris, clusters of cocci, and rare microabscesses.

An exfoliative toxin produced by the staphylococci has been reported to be the cause of the lesions of exfoliative dermatitis. Desquamation resulted in the disappearance of the bacteria and the healing process could then begin. No course of treatment was offered.

A cheilitis evidenced by the thickening of the lips and hyperkeratosis of the commissures of the mouth has been reported following the feeding of tough, fibrous hay.[52] A coagulase-positive *S. aureus* was isolated from the lesions. Oral tetracylines (55 mg/kg) in 250 ml of fresh drinking water daily resulted in a resolution of the condition.

The most frequent disease associated with staphylococcal infection in the guinea pig involves the foot pad (pododermatitis) and osteoarthritis of the phalanges and metacarpal joints. The condition has been observed in 1- to 4-year-old animals maintained on both solid bottom cages with contact bedding as well as wire-bottom cages. This disease has been attributed to trauma of the foot pad, poor sanitation, obesity, and aging.[53,54]

The animals react vigorously when the feet are palpated. Grossly, the foot pad and dermis are markedly enlarged and erythematous. Crust, ulcers, and hemorrhages may be present on the volar surfaces. On cut surface a firm mass of white glistening tissue extends from the ventral surface of the foot pad to the skeletal components of the foot. The joints may be edematous and distended with turbid, yellow exudate.

Soft tissue swelling and bony proliferation may be observed radiographically, in advanced cases.[54] Periosteal proliferation with partial or complete destruction of the bony architecture of the metacarpal and phalangeal joints are suggestive of osteomyelitis and sepsis.

The microscopic soft tissue lesions are those of hyperkeratosis, ulceration, hemorrhage, necrosis, and chronic inflammation. Neutrophils were the primary inflammatory cell, with evidence of newly joined vascular structures, fibroblasts and collagen. Dense connective tissue was present deep within the lesion. The joints were characterized by synovial hypertrophy, villous hyperplasia, congestion, and fibrinopurulent exudate. Proliferation of the periosteum and necrosis of the bone were constant features in advanced cases.

The diagnosis was confirmed with the isolation of staphylococci from the inflamed foot pad. Impression smears stained with Wright's stain and Gram's stain revealed numerous gram-positive cocci. The inocculation of blood agar plates with exudate or swabs collected from the foot lead to the isolation of organisms with the characteristics typical for a coagulase-positive *Staphylococcus aureus*.

Most guinea pigs presenting with this condition have a poor prognosis. Amyloidosis involving the kidney, spleen, liver, and lymph nodes is a frequent consequence of this long-standing bacterial infection.[53]

Pododermatitis can be prevented by frequent cleaning of soiled cages, changing soiled bedding, replacement of irregular wire surfaces with smooth surfaced material, individual weight control, and routine foot care. Guinea pigs need to be checked frequently for overgrown toenails, horny callouses, and ulcers. Early pad lesions can be treated with topical cleaning with povidine-iodine surgical scrub, topical povidine-iodine ointment under a bandage, and placement on soft bedding. More advanced cases may be treated as described above with the addition of an occlusive hydroactive dressing under a bandage. In both cases the bandages should be removed every 2 to 3 days for reevaluation and topical treatment.

Systemic antibiotics are indicated when the infection has extended into the dermis. Antibiotics such as chloramphenicol palmitate (50 mg/kg t.i.d. for 10 days) and trimethoprim-sulfa (30 mg/kg b.i.d. for 10 days) are among the safer antibiotics to use. Both of these compounds may be used for 10 days in succession where prolonged therapy is needed. However, the animals must be monitored for anorexia, a not uncommon consequence of antibiotic therapy lasting approximately 10 days. In the event of anorexia the antibiotics should be suspended. Antibiotic-associated colitis is a possibility any time guinea pigs are treated with antibiotics.

A nonsteroidal anti-inflammatory agent such as flunixin meglumine (2 to 3 mg/kg b.i.d.) may be given intermittently for 5-day periods to reduce the pain and discomfort.

Like humans and nonhuman primates, the guinea pig requires vitamin C daily (30 mg/kg) or clinical signs of scurvy may become evident within 11 to 14 days. Guinea pigs with a deficient intake become more susceptible to bacterial infections. Therefore, all sick guinea pigs should be treated with oral or parenteral vitamin C (30 to 50 mg/kg) daily until its oral intake has returned to normal. Oral vitamin C is extremely bitter and should be mixed with fruit juice to increase its palatability. A handful of fresh greens such as kale, spinach, cabbage, or a quarter orange per day will meet the daily vitamin C requirement of a healthy adult guinea pig.[12]

Streptococcus. Streptococci are infrequently associated with primary skin disease in the guinea pig. They form the dominant flora of the oral cavity and may be a frequent cause of respiratory disease, myocarditis, and septicemia.

Both alpha and beta hemolytic streptococci have been recovered from the mammary gland of normal postparturient guinea pigs, and are considered part of the normal flora.[55] However, both alpha hemolytic streptococci and *Streptococcus zooepidemicus* have been reported to be a cause of mastitis in lactating guinea pigs.[56,57]

Members of Lancefield Group C (beta-hemolytic *Streptococcus* and *Streptococcus zooepidemicus*) are the most prevalent cause of streptococcosis in the guinea pig.[58] The most commonly recognized form is the chronic condition known as "lumps" or submandibular (cervical) lymphadenitis. The affected animals usually appear normal except for a variable-sized subcutaneous enlargement in the ventral cervical area at the angle of the jaw. The masses are ovoid, firm on palpation, and may be unilateral or bilateral in occurrence.

Grossly, the swollen nodes are irregular, round to ovoid, and fluctuant.[59] Incision of the nodes yields a yellow-white purulent material that is occasionally inspissated and caseous. Fibrous tracts may be observed leading from the lymph node to the oral cavity or skin surface. When bacteremia occurs a fibrinopurulent exudate may adhere to the pleural and peritoneal surfaces. Foci of purulent material may be present in the heart, liver, and kidney.

Microscopically, the cervical lymph nodes are surrounded by a well-vascularized collagenous capsule. The center of the lymph nodes become necrotic with numerous neutrophils and debris. A zone of fibrin, macrophages, and lymphocytes extends from the necrotic center to the capsule. Histologic evidence of pericarditis, peritonitis, pleuritis, and chronic nephritis may be present. Streptococci may be observed in sections of the lymph nodes and heart.

Clinically, the affected lymph nodes may rupture to the skin surface causing a localized dermatitis at the site of the drainage. Spontaneous drainage is usually followed by healing with granulation tissue.[58]

The method of spread appears to be via the abraded skin or mucosa.[58] The removal of affected animals helps control the spread of streptococci, but will not eradicate it from a colony.

A diagnosis of streptococcosis is rendered on the basis of bacterial isolation on agar plates and the Gram's stain. On blood agar media streptococci are round, smooth, glistening colonies surrounded by a clear zone of hemolysis.

Chains of gram-positive cocci are seen in stained smears of exudate or colonies isolated from agar plates.

Antibiotic therapy alone has been reported to be an effective treatment for this condition. Cephaloridine (20 mg/kg IM) daily for 14 days resulted in the disappearance of the enlarged cervical lymph nodes and a return to normal.[60] The affected lymph nodes were sterile when cultured at a later date.

Prior to drainage, the fur should be clipped from the affected surgical site and the site then cleansed with povidine-iodine surgical soap. After the skin is sprayed with povidine-iodine solution the localized lymph node may be incised and drained. The wound should be irrigated and cleaned daily until it is healed. Cephaloridine may be administered to treat streptococci involving other organs.

During treatment the guinea pig should be isolated from other guinea pigs. The cage and its accessories should be disinfected with a povidine-iodine soap solution at least weekly. This regimen should continue until the lesion has resolved.

Regardless of the type of treatment instituted, the exudate from the enlarged lymph nodes should be submitted for culture, sensitivity, and Gram's stain. In addition to the streptococci, *Streptobacillus moniliformis, Bacteriodes caviae, Yersinia pseudotuberculosis, Salmonella limete* and *Mucor* sp have been recovered from the enlarged cervical lymph nodes of the guinea pig.[61] The absence of streptococci in smears of the exudate would suggest that one of the other organisms should be considered. Except for *Mucor*, a fungus, the other organisms are gram-negative. *Streptobacillus moniliformis* will grow only on media containing 30 percent serum in an anaerobic environment. *Bacteriodes cavial* also requires anaerobic conditions for isolation. *Yersina* and *Salmonella* can be recovered with standard media and aerobic incubation. Sabouraud agar must be utilized to culture for *Mucor* sp.

Viral Diseases

Guinea Pig Pox-Like Virus. A single report in the literature documents the occurrence of a cutaneous viral disease of the guinea pig. Several 8-month old guinea pigs spontaneously developed a large fibrovascular proliferation in the thigh muscle[62]. Both basophilic and eosinophilic cytoplasmic inclusions were present in tissue culture-adapted cells. The presence of large particles consistent with a pox virus was confirmed by electron microscopy. The presence of lesions on several animals suggests an infectious process and should be treated as such.

Mycotic Diseases

Dermatomycosis, or ringworm, is one of the most common skin diseases of the guinea pig. However, invasion of the hair or skin must be demonstrated before a positive diagnosis is rendered. The carriage rate for *Trichophyton mentagrophytes* from the skin of clinical normal guinea pigs has been reported to range from 6 to 13.3 percent.[63,64]

Ringworm in the guinea pig is almost always caused by *Trichophyton mentagrophytes*.[65] A single report documents an infection due to *Microsporum audouinii*.[66] The distribution and clinical signs were similar to infections described for *Trichophyton*.

The circumscribed lesions usually appear only on the nose as scales. The fungus then spreads to the areas above and below the eyes, forehead, and ears. If allowed to progress, the lesions can eventually cover the dorsal lumbar area. The limbs and dorsal thorax are usually spared.

As the hyperkeratotic lesions progress, the fungus extends through the hair follicle into the hair cuticle, solubilizing the hard keratin of the shaft. This results in the loosening of the hair papilla. The loosened hair either falls out or is broken off, leaving a patchy baldness or folliculitis. When severe inflammation develops, patches of hair epilate easily.

Fungal by-products often diffuse into the tissues, resulting in a type I allergic reaction. Type IV delayed reactions may also occur, and are associated with severe inflammation.

Diagnosis depends on demonstration of the hyphae in the skin and/or ectothrix spores in the infected hair treated with 10 to 40 percent potassium hydroxide (KOH). Samples of the hair and scales can be grown on Sabouraud's agar with chloramphenicol and cycloheximide added to inhibit the growth of bacteria and nonpathogenic fungi. The colonial morphology for *Trichophyton mentagrophytes* consists of a white granular variety with a tan or mahogany reverse pigment. Microscopic examination of the colonies with lactophenol reveals the unique characteristics of *Trichophyton* in the guinea pig: The microconidia are irregular in size and have a grape-like arrangement with spiral hyphae.[65]

Treatment can be accomplished with oral griseofulvin at a dosage of 25 mg/kg daily for 14 days, or 25 mg/100 g/bw every 10 days for 3 treatments. Pediatric oral solutions are available for ease of medicating the animal. A single local application of 10 percent polyvinyl iodine solution or 1.5 percent griseofulvin in dimethylsulfoxide applied once or twice daily for 5 to 7 days may be effective topical treatments.[67,68] Griseofulvin is a teratogen and should be avoided in pregnant or breeding animals.

Ectoparasites

Lice. The guinea pig may become infested by two species of lice from the family Gyropidae, a family limited in nature to neotropical animals originating in South America.[69] *Gliricola porcelli* will be observed much more frequently than *Gyropus ovalis*.

The life cycle of these two biting or chewing lice is largely unknown. Transmission occurs by direct contact with an infested host or bedding, but lice rarely leave the host. *Gliricola* has been observed to abrade the skin with its mouthparts and to ingest the fluids from the lesion.

Most infestations by gryopid lice occur without clinical signs. However, heavy infestations may result in a roughened hair coat, alopecia, excoriations, and crust due to excessive scratching, especially around the ears.[12]

A diagnosis of pediculosis can be made by examining the fur directly with a hand lens or dissecting microscope. The margin of the lesions should be observed for parasites. Indirect examination of the fur can be accomplished by holding the guinea pig over a sheet of black construction paper and combing the animal from head to tail with a sterile surgical scrub-brush. Any lice that are dislodged will usually be mobile and whitish-yellow in color. Dead animals can be placed under refrigeration for 30 minutes and then rewarmed to room temperature. Lice that remain alive will migrate from the cold skin to the warmer tips of the hair shaft.[12]

The lice can be eliminated by dusting the animals and bedding with 0.5 percent pyrethrin powder. A sponge bath with 0.5 percent malathion is also effective.[70] Preweanling animals (less than 3 to 4 weeks of age) should not be bathed with malathion. Silica dust alone or with pyrethrins may be mixed with the bedding material to kill the lice by abrading their cuticle.[12] This results in dessication and death.

Two-inch squares of resin strips impregnated with dichlorvos may be placed on or near a cage-top out of reach of the animal for 48 hours. This procedure should be repeated at weekly intervals for at least three applications to insure killing of all ectoparasites. This method of control is dependent upon building a vapor of sufficient concentration to be lethal to the ectoparasites. Therefore air flow in the room must be restricted during the 48-hour period.[12] Animals that are not under treatment should be removed from the room. Also, open water containers and moist foods, such as fruits and vegetables, should not be allowed long-term exposure to the vapors. The use of water bottles and several 10 to 15 minute feeding periods throughout the day would be advisable.

Ivermectin (22,23-dihydroavermectin B_1), either orally or subcutaneously at dosage rates of 300 to 500 μg/kg body weight is also an effective treatment. Two treatments 10 days apart are required to ensure complete elimination of the lice.

All cages and accessories should be sanitized. Any bedding materials or supplies that could potentially harbor the ectoparasites should be sanitized or discarded.

Mites. The guinea pig has been reported to be infested with several species of mites. Among these are *Demodex caviae*, *Myocoptes musculinus*, *Sarcoptes scabiei*, *Notedres muris*, *Trixacarus caviae*, and *Chirodiscoides caviae*.[69] Only the latter two species are likely to be encountered in clinical practice.

Chirodiscoides caviae is a member of the family Listrophoridae, a family of mites commonly found on fur-bearing animals. They may be widely distributed throughout the fur with the heaviest concentrations around the perineal and hip area.[71] These small, barely visible mites are generally found clinging to the hair shaft. Large numbers of mites may be present without any harmful effect. In some instances of heavy infestation pruritus, alopecia, and dermatitis may result.[72]

Most stages of the life cycle are spent on the hair shaft well away from the skin surface. Apparently 50 percent of the parasites are frequently observed joined in pairs with a mature male being carried by a nymphal female.[72] Eggs are deposited midway along the hair shaft. The larvae and three subsequent nymphal stages result in sexual maturity in approximately 14 days.

The diagnosis and treatment for *Chirodiscoides* is as previously described for lice.

Trixacarus caviae is a burrowing sarcoptiform mite similar enough in appearance to *Sarcoptes scabiei* to be mistaken for it. *Sarcoptes* are larger in size, and the anus is terminal rather than dorsal in position as in the case of *Trixacarus*.[73]

The severity of the clinical disease is proportional to the duration of the infestation.[74] Early cases exhibit mild alopecia, erythema, and pruritus. Longer-standing cases exhibit severe dermatitis and pruritus with almost total hair loss over the affected areas. The skin becomes lichenified and hyperpigmented. Any hairs remaining in affected areas are brittle and easily epilated. The areas most commonly involved are the dorsal cervical and thoracic areas. The distal extremities and the head are not commonly involved, but in severe cases the entire skin surface may be affected. A variable amount of scale is commonly observed. Occasionally, the scale accumulations form masses or ridges around the neck and face that are difficult to remove.

The resulting irritation causes lethargy, inappetance and, progressive emaciation. Unless treated at the earliest possible date the affected animals become debilitated and die due to bacterial infection or immune mediated renal disease. Hyperesthesia, seizures, and death have also been observed. Resorption of fetuses and abortion have also been reported in breeding animals.[75]

The diagnosis is confirmed by examination of skin scrapings in 10 percent KOH. With light infestations the mites may be too few to recover with the scraping. In severe cases large numbers of mites and eggs are usually observed.

Lime sulfur diluted 1:40 with water and applied with a sponge over the entire body has been a successful treatment regimen.[74] Treatments were repeated at weekly intervals for 6 weeks. Three weekly applications of 1 percent lindane in a bath have also been reported to be effective.[75] These animals should also be treated with antibiotics and vitamin C daily until recovery is complete.

Trixacarus will temporarily infest man, causing pruritus and erythema of the skin. Clients should be warned about the potential for the zoonosis to occur.

Fleas. Fleas of the genus *Ctenocephalides* are the genus most likely to infest the guinea pig. They represent the species carried by cats and dogs, which may share the home with small nondomestic mammals. *Ctenocephalides felis* has been recovered from hamsters, rats, guinea pigs, rabbits, and ferrets.

Animals with infestations or exhibiting signs of anemia (lethargy, pale mucous membranes, etc) should have the packed cell volume evaluated as a minimum evaluation. If a sufficient volume of blood can be collected, a CBC would be indicated.

Removal of the fleas requires treatment of the pet and the environment using standard eradication procedures. Commercially available canned sprays containing 0.045 percent pyrethrins are available for small rodents. The spray may be repeated 2 or 3 times per week until the fleas are eradicated. Aqueous base pyrethrin sprays suitable for cats are less likely to cause dry skin and scales.

Neoplasia

The occurrence of spontaneous neoplasia in the guinea pig has been reported to be a rare event. This conclusion is biased by the fact that most guinea pigs in research colonies are relatively young animals. This statement is substantiated by several studies that have found little or no neoplasia in animals less than 3 years of age (0.4 to 1.7 percent), whereas animals greater than 3 years exhibited a significant incidence of neoplasia (14.4 percent). One colony of guinea pigs exhibited a 29.4 percent incidence rate for animals over 27 months of age.[76] Since guinea pigs maintained in private households routinely live 4 to 5 years,[12] clinicians should carefully examine older animals for evidence of neoplasia.

A recent literature review of neoplasia in the guinea pig indicated that 15.4 percent of all spontaneous tumors ever reported involve the skin and subcutis.[76] Only tumors of the lung were more common. This figure is biased by the large number of trichofolliculomas reported in the review.[76]

The histology, biology, and pathology of the spontaneous neoplasms of the skin of the guinea pig are poorly described in the literature when compared to those experimentally induced with chemicals. The various types of neoplasms occurring spontaneously reported for the skin and subcutis of the guinea pig are summarized in Table 10-4.[76–87]

Trichofolliculomas are the most commonly reported type of neoplasm.[76] These masses appear clinically as solitary nodules that elevate the skin. Almost all of these tumors are located in the hypodermis. The dorsal lumbar region is most frequently mentioned as the site for occurrence.

On gross observation the neoplasm is nonencapsulated and consists of a central cyst surrounded by a stroma that supports numerous smaller cysts.[77,78] The cyst, which sometimes contains hair, is filled with a white-to-yellow caseous material. Those trichofolliculomas that penetrate the epidermis possess a papillary projection or central pore that connects the cyst to the skin surface.

Histologically, the tumors are multiloculated cystic structures. The walls of the cyst are lined with stratified squamous epithelium, abortive hair follicles, and sebaceous glands. Some abortive hair follicles produce the cortical components of hair while others produce the soft keratin components consistent with the medullary portion or inner root sheath of the hair. The stratum granulosum of the latter type contain prominent trichohyaline granules. The sebaceous glands are mature and produce secretions that add to the contents of the cyst.

Table 10-4. Spontaneous Neoplastic Masses of the Skin of the Guinea Pig

Type of Mass	Location	Age (Months)	Sex	Metastasis Present	Reference
Trichofolliculoma	17 dorsal lumbar area 3 lateral femoral area 1 cranial aspect of shoulder	1.5–32	9 Males 12 Females	N/A	Ediger, Dill, & Kovatch[77]
	1 dorsal lumbar area	96	Male	N/A	Zwart, Mander Hoge, Mullink, et al[78]
	1 flank region	24	*	N/A	
	1 right flank	30	Female	N/A	Kitcen, Carlton, & Bickford[79]
	1 back	24	Female	N/A	
	1 *	*	*	N/A	
Trichoepithelioma (epithelioma adenoids cysticum)	*	*	*	N/A	Manning[76]
Sebaceous adenoma	Flank region	24	Male	N/A	Zwart, Mander Hoge, Mullink, et al[78]
Adenocarcinoma	Ventral neck region	34	Female	None	Heston & Deringer[80]
Undifferentiated carcinoma	Medial side of the metatarsal region	*	*	*	Kitcen, Carlton, & Bickford[79]
Fibroma	*	18.5	*	N/A	Stenback[81]
Fibrolipoma	Subcutaneous abdominal area	*	*	N/A	Dickson[82]
Fibrosarcoma	Midline of ventral neck	*	Male	Right axillary area	Murray[83]
Fibrosarcoma neurogenic	Angle of right jaw	*	*	*	Haagensen & Krehbiel[84]
Lipoma	Subcutaneous thoracic wall	36	Female	N/A	Warren & Gates[85]
	Left cervical area	54	Male	N/A	Rogers & Blumenthal[86]
Liposarcoma	Left mammary gland	*	Female	None	Blumenthal & Rogers[87]
	*	*	*		Rogers & Blumenthal[86]
Schwannoma	Lumbar area	84	Male	*	Kitcen, Carlton, & Bickford[79]
Undifferentiated sarcoma	*	*	*		Manning[76]

*-Not described
N/A-Not applicable

One report describes three cases of trichoepithelioma in guinea pigs that are histologically indistinguishable from the trichofolliculomas above and can be considered as such.[78,79] In one instance a black, fatty substance could be expressed from a mass with a central pore.[78]

The other types of epithelial tumors of the skin are rarely reported. Among these are the trichoepithelioma,[76] sebaceous adenoma,[78] undifferentiated carcinoma,[79] and an adenocarcinoma.[80]

Mesenchymal tumors involving the subcutis are more frequently observed than tumors of the cutis. They also present a more varied array of neoplasms. Among these are the fibroma,[81] lipoma,[79] fibrolipoma,[82] fibrosarcoma,[83,84] liposarcoma,[85,86] undifferentiated sarcoma,[86] and the schwannoma.[79] They usually appear as discrete tumors, either yellow or gray in color, depending on the amount of fat present.[87]

The treatment for cutaneous neoplasia in the guinea pig involves surgical excision and histologic classification of the tumor type. Although few metastases have been reported for malignant tumors of the guinea pig, all neoplasms should be removed at the earliest possible date.

Miscellaneous Conditions

Alopecia Occurring In Intensively Bred Females. An alopecia of a variable intensity develops in most guinea pigs during the last trimester of pregnancy. This condition is reported due to reduced anabolism of maternal skin associated with fetal growth.[88] Constantly pregnant or lactating females will develop a more intense alopecia. The alopecia is most prominent over the lumbrosacral area. In addition to the metabolic demands of pregnancy and lactation, genetic factors have also been suggested as part of the etiology.

Alopecia of Weanling Animals. A thinning of the hair is common around the time of weaning (2 to 4 weeks of age). The alopecia has been associated with the period of transition in which more coarse guard hairs typical of adult fur begin to appear among the fine hairs that make up the guinea pig undercoat.[88]

Barbering. Guinea pigs establish male-dominated stable social hierarchies, and animals of low social ranking and young animals may lose considerable amounts of hair due to barbering by adult animals.

A diagnosis of barbering is based on observing the irregular stepwise manner in which the hair has been bitten off.[88] The skin will usually be free of lesions.

Animals may also be guilty of self-barbering. These animals that self-barber will exhibit hair loss only in those areas that they can reach with their mouth. The fur on the head, neck, and anterior shoulders will be intact.

The addition of long-stem hay has been reported to prevent the development of barbering within a guinea pig colony.[89] This suggests that barbering results from a need for fiber or boredom. The hay may fulfil a need for oral activity that is not met by commercial hard pelleted rations.

Circumanal Sebaceous Accumulations. Sebaceous glands are especially abundant around the anal orifice and the folds of the circumanal and genital region of sexually mature male guinea pigs.[88,90] Excessive accumulations of sebaceous secretions, and occasionally bedding material and feces, may become entrapped in the folds.[88] These folds should be cleansed periodically with saline or povidine-iodine surgical scrub to prevent infections and unpleasant odors. Isolated males and old males are more susceptible to developing this condition than sexually active young males.[88] The postejaculatory genital groom and the habit of dragging the perineum along the bottom of the cage before and after coitus promote the natural cleansing of this area.[91]

Seborrhea of the Sacral Sebaceous Glands. The dorsal surface of the guinea pig is well endowed with sebaceous glands.[90] At the posterior of the dorsal sacral area these abundant glands produce secretions that collect to give the fur a matted, yellow appearance. Occasionally, a localized seborrhea develops in this area. The seborrhea can be treated locally by removing the fur, bathing the skin with a mild keratolytic shampoo and the topical applications of an astringent 3 to 4 times daily until the condition resolves.

Hyperkeratosis of the Foot Pads. Heavy guinea pigs maintained in wire-bottom caging for long periods of time frequently develop horny growths projecting from the ventral surface of the foot pad epithelium.[88] These areas of hyperkeratosis are usually observed on the front feet, and are probably the result of long-term irritation asociated with standing on an uneven wire surface. The horny projections or callouses can be removed with manicuring scissors and an emery file. Replacement of the cage surfaces with smoother materials will retard or prevent the callouses from developing.

Aggression

Hair Pulling. Hair pulling is a common behavior in guinea pig pups, and it is usually directed toward the dam, especially during or shortly after the end of lactation.[91] A mouthful of hair is grasped in the teeth, pulling it out and ingesting it. The hair pulling may persist into adulthood where it takes on an element of aggression under conditions of crowding or stress. Alopecia develops in some guinea pigs as aggressor animals attempt to displace others at water bottles, feed bowls, or other desirable sites in the cage.

Ear Chewing. Chewing of the pinnae of the ears is believed to be associated with excessive male aggressiveness.[88] An ear subjected to constant bouts of chewing will exhibit notches along the margin, or will be cropped close to the head.[91]

Fighting. Bite wounds, scratches, alopecia, and dermatitis are evidence of excessive aggression or fighting.[88] A single animal can frequently be identified as being responsible for most of the fighting, and removal of the aggressor animal can significantly reduce or terminate the problem. Castration and placement in a new cage will probably reduce intermale aggression.[92] The effects of castration on territorial defense are unknown.

The placement of new males into the cage of another male, especially in crowded cages or cages in which females in estrus are present will normally result in a fight. Females are less aggressive than males. The housing of animals together as adolescents (1 to 3 months of age) will reduce the amount of aggression within a group of guinea pigs.[88]

A dermatitis of the preputial and perineal area secondary to fighting has been reported as a colony-wide problem.[93] Twelve percent of the males developed an ulcerative dermatitis that became contaminated with excreta from the bottom of the cage. Involvement of the prepuce usually prevent the animal from retracting the glans penis. Four of the animals died. The survivors were successfully treated by frequent cleaning with warm water and soap, followed by topical zinc-oxide ointment.

The Rabbit (*Oryctologus cuniculus*)

Bacterial Diseases

Pasturella. Pasteurellosis is the most common bacterial disease of the rabbit. Induced by *Pasteurella multocida*, a gram-negative nonsporeforming, short, bipolar staining rod, it presents in a variety of clinical forms. Among these are rhinitis, pneumonia, conjunctivitis, pneumonia, orchitis, septicemia, and subcutaneous abscesses.[94] Most rabbits carry the bacteria asymptomatically in the nasal cavity. Under conditions of stress, the bacteria multiply, leading to overt clinical disease.

Subcutaneous abscesses develop in the rabbit as a result of septicemia, external wound contamination, or direct extension from deeper sites. The abscesses are of variable size and are usually firm on palpation.

The abscesses are filled with thick, white-to-tan exudate surrounded by fibrous capsule. Due to the consistency of the exudate, aspiration of the contents of the abscess may be difficult.

Isolation of *Pasteurella multocida* requires the use of media enriched with whole blood or serum. The organism will not grow on MacConkey agar. After 24 to 48 hours at 37°C, smooth or mucoid gray colonies without hemolysis are present. Also, the bacteria are nonmotile, indole-positive, and oxidase-positive. Gram's stains reveal small, gram-negative rods, and coccobacilli.

Frequently, the thickness of exudate from a subcutaneous abscess in the rabbit precludes the actual drainage of the abscess. This requires that the exudate be flushed out or surgically removed. The wound should be treated topically with Lugol's solution or povidine-iodine surgical ointment. Systemic antibiotics such as intramuscular procaine penicillin G (60,000 IU/kg b.i.d.) or oral oxytetracycline (50 mg/kg b.i.d.) are appropriate to prevent septicemia and further spreading of the disease. The use of antibiotics should be approached with caution in the rabbit due to the possibility of inducing antibiotic-associated colitis (see Table 10-1).

Staphylococcus. Staphylococcosis is a common disease entity in the domestic rabbit. This disease is caused by *Staphylococcus aureus*, and has been identified as a cause of subcutaneous abscesses, septicemia, mastitis, and osteomyelitis.[94] The septicemic form is more common in young rabbits and rabbits under stressful conditions. Normal rabbits have been reported to carry staphylococci without evidence of disease. The sites most often mentioned are the ear, skin, nasal passages, and upper respiratory tract.

The clinical signs of subcutaneous abscesses are redness, swelling, and induration of the overlying skin. In chronic infections the abscesses may be firm or fluctuant upon palpation. Purulent material and suppurative inflammation are typical of cutaneous staphylococcosis.

Diagnosis depends on the results of culture and sensitivity testing. On blood agar both alpha-hemolytic and beta-hemolytic coagulase-positive *S. aureus* have been recovered from lesions.

Topical treatment of subcutaneous abscesses follows the same procedures as previously described for *Pasteurella* abscesses.

Staphylococcus aureus is frequently recovered from the foot lesions of ulcerative pododermatitis or "sore hocks" of the rabbit.[95] The lesions are typically found on the plantar surface of the metatarsal area, and less commonly on the volar surface of the metacarpal-phalangeal area.

The disease occurs due to pressure necrosis of the skin as a result of unsanitary cage conditions, rough cage surfaces, or obesity. A genetic predisposition may also be present in those animals who are poorly furred on the bottom of their feet. Staphylococci invade the ulcerated areas of the bottom of the foot and form abscesses. In severe infections the disease may extend to the bony structures of the foot and result in septicemia.

Topical treatment of these lesions is similar to the procedures previously described for guinea pigs with pododermatitis. The animals should be moved to soft bedding to lessen the trauma to the feet.

Pseudomonas. *Pseudomonas aeruginosa* is a widely distributed gram-negative bacillus commonly found as a saphrophyte in water bowls, water lines, drains, soil, the intestinal tract, and the skin. Under appropriate conditions, *Pseudomonas* may occasionally cause subcutaneous abscesses and more frequently, a localized moist dermatitis in areas that are continuously wet.[94,95] The skin of the muzzle, the dewlap, the flank, and the haunches are the most frequently mentioned areas. If left untreated the dermatitis may spread to cover the entire body and result in the death of the animal.

The most striking clinical feature of the disease is the blue-green color of the fur in animals with white fur. The bacteria produces a water soluble pigment called pyocyanin that stains the hair. The fur frequently has a clumped, spiked appearance. The skin usually exhibits alopecia, erythema, edema, hemorrhage, and ulceration in the affected areas without evidence of suppuration.

Microscopic examination of the site demonstrates ulceration, necrosis, abscessation, and bacterial colonies. The infection has been observed to spread to the cervical and pulmonary lymph nodes.

The diagnosis is confirmed on the basis of the clinical appearance and the recovery of the organism on artificial media. The colonies usually show a bluish-metallic sheen and beta-hemolysis on blood agar.

Treatment consists of careful removal of the hair from the infected site. After cleansing with a surgical scrub, gentomycin sulfate ointment may be applied topically twice daily until the infection resolves. Animals with generalized infections respond poorly to systemic antibiotics and usually die. Prevention should be aimed at removing the etiology of the continued wetness of the fur. Leaking water valves or water bottles should be replaced. Water bowls or pans should be replaced by water bottles with siper tubes. Malocclussion of the teeth should be corrected to prevent "drooling" or ptyalism. Wet bedding should be changed more frequently, or the animal may be switched to a suspended caging system.

Treponema. *Treponema cuniculi*, a slender spirochete, is the etiologic agent of a venereal disease of rabbits. It can also be transmitted by extragenital contact.[94]

Various serological surveys have indicated that more animals have been exposed to the spirochete than actually develop clinical signs. Once a rabbit becomes infected the bacteria localize and proliferate in the skin and mucosa near the mucocutaneous junctions. The acute inflammatory reaction is followed by a chronic reaction. Focal skin ulcerations may accompany the chronic stage.

The genitalia are the primary site for lesions to develop, followed later by the chin, lips, face, nostrils, eyelids, ears, legs, and feet. The spread of the organism from the genitalia to the other sites occurs by autoinfection. Local lymph nodes also become infected.

Early, the lesions are reddened and edematous. Minute vesicles form on the genitalia, which soon exude serum and form a brownish crust. Focal ulcers and hemorrhage may occur under the crusted areas. The pain associated with the genital lesions probably insures oral-genital contact as the rabbits lick the affected areas.

The hair at the site of the facial lesions may epilate but return quickly during the healing process. Chronic lesions tend to be dry, scaly, and slightly raised. After a period of several weeks the lesions usually resolve, and the rabbits appear normal except for the scaly lesions.

Microscopically, the lesions exhibit acanthosis, hyperkeratosis and exaggerated rete peg formation. The ulcerated areas contain large numbers of neutrophiles. The spirochetes can be demonstrated in the lesion with the Warthin-Starry silver stain.

Skin biopsies, dark field microscopic (400×) examination of lymph-containing scrapings from the lesions suspended in phosphate buffered saline, and serology are proven methods of diagnosis. *Treponema cuniculi* can not be grown in artificial media, embryonated eggs, or cell culture. The Venereal Disease Research Laboratory (VDRL) slide test, the rapid plasma reagin (RPR) card test, and the fluorescent treponemal antigen (FTA) test may be used for diagnostic purposes. A commercially available RPR card test has been reported to be positive with titers greater than 1:8.[96] Genital lesions preceed the development of a positive RPR test by an average of 5 to 6 weeks.

Venereal spirochetosis of rabbits can be eliminated by systemic treatment with three subcutaneous injections of benzathine penicillin G-procaine penicillin G (42,000 IU/kg) at 7-day intervals.[96] Skin lesions heal within 2 weeks of the first treatment and the RPR titers decline markedly or become negative by 6 weeks after the first treatment.

Fusobacterium. Necrobacillosis, or Schmorl's disease, is a sporadic bacterial disease of the rabbit characterized by necrosis, ulceration, and abscessation of the skin, especially in the face, head, and neck area.[94] It is caused by *Fusobacterium necrophorum*, a gram-negative, nonsporeforming, anaerobic bacterium. The organism is pleomorphic, usually occurring in long filaments or coccoid forms.

Fusobacterium necrophorum is thought to be present in the digestive tract of rabbits. Infections occur when rabbits are kept in unsanitary conditions. An open wound is a potential site for secondary colonization by *Fusobacterium* and other bacterial species. Because rabbits are naturally coprophagic, the lesions are frequently observed first around the lips and the oral cavity.

The initial acute inflammatory reaction in the subcutaneous tissue of the skin is followed by necrosis and ulceration. Excoriation of the infected sites may lead to extensive involvement of the face. Hemotogenous spread to internal organs may follow the cutaneous infection.

Fusobacterium nucleatum has been isolated from a rabbit with a recurring abscess below the left eye involving the maxilla and mandible.[97] Surgical debridement and intermittent antibiotic therapy were unsuccessful in resolving the infection of the bone.

Fusobacterium spp. are strict anaerobes, and precautions must be taken to prevent exposure to oxygen. Swabs, tissue, or purulent material must be cultured as soon as possible to insure viability. On blood agar the colonies appear as small, whitish-yellow, smooth colonies with a narrow zone of alpha- or beta-hemolysis. The initial cultures may be very pleomorphic, exhibiting both short rods or long filaments. The filaments characteristically show irregular staining with the Gram's stain.

Treatment with intramuscular procaine penicillin G (60,000 IU/kg b.i.d.) or oral tetracycline (50 mg/kg q.i.d.) should be effective. Surgical debridement of the necrotic debris and topical treatment with providine-iodine are indicated to enhance the recovery process.

Viral Diseases

The European or domestic rabbit (*Oryctolagus cuniculus*) is susceptible to several viruses that result in clinical skin disease. These viral dermatopathogens are represented by the poxviruses (myxoma virus, Shope fibroma virus, hare fibroma virus, squirrel fibroma virus, and rabbit pox) and a papovavirus (Shope papilloma virus). Only experimental infections have been recorded for hare fibroma virus and squirrel fibroma virus.[98] Although infrequently diagnosed, clinical disease due to the other viruses has been reported.

Myxoma Virus. Myxomatosis is a condition occasionally observed in domestic rabbits in southern California where the virus is enzootic in the California brush rabbit (*Sylvilagus bachmani*).[98] In the reservoir host the infection appears as a fibroma. Upon transmission to domestic rabbits by mosquitoes it presents as classical myxomatosis. Several strains of the virus exists, and the California isolate is one of the most virulent strains.

Infection of *Oryctolagus* usually results in severe disease and mortality approaching 99 percent. In the peracute form, eyelid edema and cerebral depression immediately prior to death (within 7 days of onset) may be the only signs observed. The acute form of the disease is characterized by generalized edema around the anus, genitalia, mouth, and nares after 6 to 7 days incubation. Just prior to seizure and death on day 9 to 10, the edema, hemorrhage, and inflammation are more pronounced. Rabbits that survive beyond day 10 may develop purulent blepharoconjunctivitis and edema at the base of the ears. Other strains of the virus may produce a number of variable-sized skin tumors.

At necropsy the most prominent lesion is edema, especially around the face, nares, mouth, and anus. Skin hemorrhages may also be present. Internally, hemorrhages may be observed in the subepicardium, subendocardium, and the serosal surfaces of the stomach and intestine.

The microscopic lesions may range from a proliferation of undifferentiated stellate mesenchymal cells in a homogenous matrix of mucinous material to degenerative changes. Intracytoplasmic inclusions may be observed in various cell types, especially the prickel cell layer.

The diagnosis is based upon the distinctive clinical signs. The virus can be grown in embryonated eggs and chicken embryo fibroblast. Once the virus has been cultured, fluorescent antibody procedures and plaque-neutralization tests can be performed.

No effective treatments exists for myxoma virus infection. Control of the insect vectors and screening of enclosures are of paramount importance in endemic areas.

Rabbit Pox. Rabbit pox, a virus closely related to the vaccinia virus, has been infrequently reported in the domestic rabbit. Several epidemics have been reported in colonies of research animals over the last 50 years. In each case the origin of the virus and the mode of interepidemic survival of the virus have not been determined.[98]

The initial clinical signs consist of profuse nasal discharge and fever. These signs occur 2 to 3 days after the virus has localized in the nasal mucosa. Lymphadenitis usually persists throughout the course of the disease after day 5 and an erythematous rash appears over the entire body. The rash may further develop into papules or nodules up to a centimeter in diameter. The rabbits develop an extensive edema of the face and perineal area. Conjunctivitis, blepharitis, keratitis, and corneal ulceration are observed.

Death usually occurs within 7 to 10 days after infection. The peracute form of the disease may be "pockless" or without skin lesions. Death is preceeded by fever, anorexia, and occasional blepharitis. Subcutaneous edema around the body orifices is commonly seen. The skin lesions may range from a few localized papules to confluent lesions with necrosis and hemorrhage. In the "pockless" form a few pocks may be seen in the lungs and adrenals. Otherwise, pleuritis, focal liver necrosis, and splenomegaly are the only lesions.

The predominant microscopic lesion is the papule or nodule, which occurs in the skin and many other organ systems. It consists of a central zone of necrosis surrounded by a zone of mononuclear cell infiltrate. Edema and hemorrhage may be seen in areas adjacent to the nodules. Cytoplasmic inclusions are seldom seen in rabbit pox lesions.

A diagnosis of rabbit pox can be established based upon the clinical signs.

The virus can be isolated on a variety of different cell lines. The fluorescent antibody test and the hemogglutination inhibition test have been utilized to monitor the antibody responses.

In the face of an epidemic in a large colony, vaccinating with vaccinia virus could be used to protect susceptible animals.

There is no effective treatment for rabbit pox. However, the antiviral drugs rifampicin and the isatin-B derivative of thiosemicarbazone have proven to afford some protection against poxviruses.

Shope Fibroma Virus and Shope Papilloma Virus. Both of these viruses are oncogenic and are discussed under neoplasia.

Mycotic Diseases

Dermatophytoses. When ringworm is encountered by a clinician it usually involves pet rabbits or rabbitries with poor husbandry practices. Most reports indicate that young rabbits are more susceptible than adults. A carriage rate of .05 percent has been reported for *Trichophyton* from the coats of normal rabbits.[63]

Trichophyton mentagrophytes is the dermatophyte most commonly recovered from ringworm lesions. On rare occasions *Microsporum gypseum*, *Microsporum canis*, *Microsporum audouini*, and *Trichophyton schoenleini* have been reported.[95]

The pruritic ringworm lesions first appear on the head and spread to the paws and other body areas due to the rabbit scratching the affected sites. These sites are characterized by a patchy alopecia and crusty appearance. Abscessation of the hair follicles may occur secondary to invading bacteria.

The diagnosis and treatment of ringworm in the rabbit are similar to those methods previously described for the guinea pig.

Deep Mycosis. Rabbits are very resistant to deep or systemic mycotic disease. Only a single case of cutaneous involvement with *Aspergillus* has been reported.[95] The rabbits involved were all from the same litter and were 4 weeks of age. Multiple 1 to 2 mm raised papules were present in the skin. Histologically, the papules were cystic follicles distended with necrotic debris and hyphae. *Aspergillus* spp. was isolated on Sabouraud's agar.

The animals were raised on moldy grass hay bedding material. Although *Aspergillus* was not isolated from the hay, a change in the type of nesting materials prevented a recurrence of the disease.

Ectoparasites

The rabbit is a potential host for a wider variety of ectoparasites than any of the other common nondomestic species. The diversity of ectoparasites presented by the rabbit requires the practitioner to be thorough in his examination due to the possibility of multiple infections occurring in the rabbit.

Psoroptes. Otoacariasis due to *Psoroptes cuniculi* is the most common ectoparasite encountered in the rabbit.[99] All rabbits should be considered infected until proven otherwise.

A rabbit affected by psoroptic mites may shake its head or scratch at its head and ears with its rear feet due to the intense pruritis. Alopecia and excoriations with secondary bacterial infection may be present around the head and neck.

The mites are nonburrowing parasites that chew the epidermal layers of the ear canal. The exudate and inflammation provide the nutrition and substrate upon which the mites survive and reproduce. In the early stages a dry, whitish--gray to tan crusty exudate forms inside the vertical ear canal at the bottom of the concha. Later, a dry, crusty material with a layered appearance accumulates in the ear. This detritus and exudate consist of desquamated epithelial cells, inflammatory cells, serum, mite feces, and mites. At the epithelial surface the skin is moist and inflamed. A secondary bacterial infection may complicate the otitis externa, contributing to the foul odor and pain associated with the ear mites.

The mites are primarily an inhabitant of the epithelial surface of the pinna and concha of the ear. Occasionally, these mites may be found in extraauricular sites, such as the face, head, neck, limbs, abdomen, and back. When observed in sites outside of the ear, the rabbits will have an area of alopecia surrounding a lesion covered by crusted exudate. Upon lifting the crust, the mites are readily visible.

A diagnosis of otoacariasis is made by visually observing the whitish-yellow mites in the ear, with or without an otoscope. Eggs, larvae, protonymphs, and adults may be present when specimens in mineral oil are examined with a microscope. The oval-shaped mites have well-developed legs with bell-shaped suckers or caruncles. Long pointed chelicerae project from the cephalic end of the mite.

One complete life cycle occurs in slightly less than 3 weeks. Topical treatment of the ears with mineral oil or a commercially available otic preparations are usually sufficient to eradicate the mite over a 3-to-4-week treatment period. The exudate may be softened for ease of removal by filling the ear canal with mineral oil for several minutes to hours before removal is attempted. Severe infestations may require irrigation with a disinfectant solution in warm water to effectively remove the debris to insure a complete killing of the parasites.

Antibiotics and antiinflammatory agents may be indicated. Systemic antibiotics may be required when a chronic suppurative inflammatory response is present. The ears of the rabbit are delicate, sensitive structures, and rabbits are especially sensitive to inflammation involving the ears. An allergic component of the inflammatory process is suggested by the presence in the serum of specific precipitins against mite antigens.

Ivermectins (22,23-dihydroavermectin B_1) instilled in the ear (0.5 ml of a 1 percent solution) or injected subcutaneously (100 to 500 μg/kg) have recently been reported to be effective against *Psoroptes cuniculi*.[100] In animals treated by injection only dead mites were present after 5 days.

Psoroptes are transmitted between rabbits by direct contact. Infested animals should be isolated until they are mite-free. The cage and environment should be sanitized to prevent the possibility of fomites serving as a transmission source.

Sarcoptid Mange Mites (*Sarcoptes* and *Notoedres*). Infestations by *Sarcoptes scabiei* and *Notoedres cati* are infrequently encountered in domestic rabbits. The presence of the mites is usually indicated by the presence of a tan-colored crust around the nose, lips, eyes, forehead, face, external genitalia, and the lateral surfaces of the ear. These mites have not been reported from the inner aspects of the pinna. Although single infestations are the rule, dual infections of *Sarcoptes* and *Psoroptes* have been observed.[99]

Sarcoptid mites are burrowing mites, and all stages of the life cycle may be observed on the rabbit. Larvae, nymphs, and adult males tend to emerge from existing tunnels to move freely over the skin surface to invade hair follicles, but females are active burrowers and are usually located below the skin surface.

The mites ingest epithelial cells and lymph as they burrow through the skin. Their presence in the skin incites scratching, excoriations, and alopecia of the affected sites. This continuing cycle leads to secondary bacterial infection. If allowed to spread severe infestations may develop, leading to debilitation, emaciation, and death within a matter of weeks.

The presence of sarcoptid mites are confirmed by microscopic examination of deep skin scrapings. Both mites are small and round with short legs. *Sarcoptes* are slightly larger than *Notoedres*. They can be speciated by the presence of a terminal anus in *Sarcoptes* versus a dorsally located anus for *Notoedres*. Both mites possess bell-shaped suckers on some or all legs.

Under optimum conditions adults require approximately 17 days to develop from ova into sexually mature adults. At this time they mate and the female begins to lay eggs within 4 to 5 days.

Transmission occurs by direct contact and by formites. However, the mites are very susceptable to dessication and can remain alive for only a few hours off their host.

Sponge baths with lime sulfur (1:40 dilution) weekly for 6 weeks should be effective in resolving the infestation.[70] Two to three treatments with ivermectins (400 μg/kg) at 10 day intervals is also an effective treatment. Therapy is much more successful when the condition is diagnosed early in the course of the disease.

The cage environment should be sanitized to prevent possible fomite transmission. Both species may cause temporary zoonotic infestations within the skin of humans.

Cheyletiella. *Cheyletiella parasitovorax* is a nonburrowing fur mite that lives in immediate association with the keratin layer of the epidermis.[99] The mites feed upon lymph from the host skin. The mites are confined primarily to the skin of the abdomen, back, and scapular region. Most rabbits harbor *Cheyletiella* without overt signs of disease. With heavy infestations, lesions are located primarily on the scapular area and ventral abdomen. The affected areas may be partially alopecic with the skin surface covered by a fine grayish-white oily scale. In albino or light colored rabbits the skin may be inflamed and painful to the touch. Pruritis is not a constant feature of the disease.

A diagnosis may be obtained by brushing the debris from the skin and hair with a clean surgical brush. Heavy infestations may be confirmed with a skin scraping. In both instances the mites are mounted in mineral oil for microscopic examination. *C. parasitovorax* are small saddle-shaped whitish-yellow mites characterized by piercing chelicerae and large curved palpal hooks.

All stages of the life cycle can be found on the host. After a 4-day incubation period, sexually mature adults are present within 14 days. Females can live for approximately 10 days in a cool environment without feeding. Immature stages cannot survive for more than 48 hours away from the host.

Effective treatment has been reported with a 0.5 percent malathion sponge bath and cat flea powders or spray.[70] Localized lesions have been treated with topical benzyl benzoate.[101] The cage environment must be sanitized to prevent transmission via fomites.

Rabbits may serve as a reservoir for infecting humans and other pets within the home.

Listrophus. *Listrophus gibbus* is a small fur mite of rabbits that do not seem to produce overt disease.[99] Most of the time when listrophid mites are present they go unnoticed. Although *L. gibbus* may be found primarily on the back, inguineal area, and abdomen, it may be seen in other sites.

Combing or brushing the hair of infested rabbits is an excellent way of obtaining specimens for identification. All stages of the parasite are found on the body. *Listrophus* is a small ovoid mite with short legs and a dorsal projection extending over its mouth parts. Males have a tubular clasping organ projecting from the posterior end of the males.

The same treatments and control measures described above for *Cheyletiella* should be effective against *Listrophus*.

Fleas. *Ctenocephalides felis* is the most common species of flea recovered from the rabbit. The rabbit may be treated with products and regimens considered safe for cats.[70] Aqueous based spray preparations are less likely to cause drying of the skin and scales compared to alcohol-based compounds.

Flea control measures for other pets and the household must be instituted to prevent reinfestation of the rabbit.

Myiasis. Members of the genus *Cuterebra* occasionally parasitize domestic rabbits reared out-of-doors or in nonscreened quarters.[99] The cuterebrid flies are obligatory myiosis-producing flies that must pupate on mammals.

Several species of *Cuterebra* have been reported for domestic rabbits in the United States. Among these are *C. cuniculi*, *C. honripilum*, and *C. buccata*. Each species of larvae migrate to their preferred subcutaneous body sites. *C. horripilum* prefers the ventral cervical region whereas *C. buccata* larvae localize in the interscapular, axillary, inguinal, or rump area.

In the northern United States the larvae appear in the summer and early fall. In the southern states the larvae may be present throughout the year.

The site of the initial entry of the larvae is unknown. After localizing in a subcutaneous site, the warbles enlarge and produce a hole or fistula that communicates with the skin surface. The fistula is usually surrounded by moistened matted fur. The rabbit will react as if in pain when the lesion is touched. Heavy infestations may produce debilitation and death. Secondary bacterial infections and regional lymphadenopathy may be present.

Close examination of the excysted larvae may reveal movement and black pigmented spiracular plates. Once a larvae is ready to pupate it drops to the ground where it eventually develops into a warble fly. The exodus of the larvae leaves a large hole. If uncomplicated the lesion heals leaving a scar and alopecia within 10 days.

The incidence of infestation tends to decrease as the host ages. Both immediate and delayed type skin reactions to whole-larval antigens have been demonstrated in naturally infested *Oryctologus*. This immunologic reaction to larval antigens may explain the resistance to infestation as the rabbits age.[102]

Therapy consists of surgical removal of the larvae by enlarging the fistula slightly with a sterile scapel blade. Due to the immune reaction mounted by the host, crushing of the larva should be avoided. The cavity should be cleansed with surgical soap. Lesions with secondary bacterial infections should be cultured for determination of specific antibiotic sensitivity. Speciation of the larval forms recovered from rabbits is successful less than 50 percent of the time. Prevention and control should be aimed at preventing contact with the warble fly. Screening of outdoor enclosures should be effective.

Neoplasia

Spontaneous Nonviral Neoplasms. Several studies of the naturally-occurring, nonviral-induced neoplasms of the rabbit have revealed that some families of rabbits have a genetic predisposition to neoplasia, and the incidence increases significantly with age.[103] Since the mean life span for a healthy pet rabbit is 7 to 8 years, the older rabbits should be monitored closely for evidence of neoplasia.

Aside from carcinomas of the uterus, vagina, and breast, spontaneous tumors have been rarely reported for the rabbit. Very few neoplasms involving the skin have been reported. The various types of cutaneous neoplasms observed in *Oryctolagus* are recorded in Table 10-5.[103–110]

Spontaneously occurring neoplasms should be surgically removed and evaluated by a pathologist as soon as possible. The majority of the nonviral tumors of the skin have been accompanied by metastases. As the popularity of pet rabbits increases, it is likely that the private practitioner will play an important role in our understanding of spontaneous neoplasia in the rabbit.

Viral-Induced Neoplasms. The domestic rabbit may be infected by several viruses that induce neoplastic skin diseases. For the most part, these oncogenic viruses are restricted to wild rabbits (*Sylvilagus* spp.), and their occurrence in domestic rabbits should be considered a rare event.

Shope Papilloma Virus. The Shope papilloma virus is the etiologic agent

Table 10-5. Spontaneously-Occurring Nonviral Neoplasms of the Skin of the Rabbit

Type of Neoplasm	Location	Age (Months)	Sex	Metastasis Present	Reference
Carcinoma	Right side of neck	*	*	Lymphatics near tumor	Polson[104]
Squamous cell carcinoma	Base of right ear	18	Female	Retropharyngeal lymph nodes, skin, breast, lung and spleen	Green & Brown[105]
Sebaceous gland carcinoma	Dorsum of right foot	48	Male	Axillary lymph nodes and lungs	Port & Sider[106]
Sarcoma	Scrotum	66	Male	Inguinal lymph nodes, lungs, liver, kidney, spleen, bone and inguinal fat	Brown & Pearce[107]
Spindle cell sarcoma	Subcutaneous tissues of the back	*	*	None	Kato[108]
Lymphosarcoma	Dorsal thorax between shoulders	18	Female	None	Hinton[109]
Papilloma	*	*	*	N/A	Doberstein & Tamoschke[110]

*-Not described in the reference cited.
N/A-Not applicable

of Shope papilloma in the California brush rabbit (*Sylvilagus bachmani*) and cottontail rabbits (*Sylvilagus floridanus*) in the states bordering the Mississippi River, Texas, California, and Oklahoma.[103] The virus has not been recovered from the eastern cottontail rabbit.

Infection of domestic rabbits has been reported in California. Multiple horn-like growths from a single site were observed about the eyelids and ears. The lesions were typical of papillomas, and the localization of lesions to the nearly hairless sites were compatable with insect vectors such as mosquitoes. Wild rabbits were observed on the farms where the disease occurred. The papillomas were easily scratched off by the rabbits or accidently removed during restraint. Manual removal of the papillomas usually resulted in healing without complication or recurrence. The recovered rabbits were resistant to reinfection when challenged with infectious material. However, experimental infections of domestic rabbits indicated that approximately three-fourths of the inoculation sites underwent malignant transformation to squamous cell carcinoma by 8 to 9 months postinnoculation.

The diagnosis of Shope papillomatosis is readily confirmed by the characteristic clinical appearance of the skin tumors and may be confirmed by histopathologic evaluation. The Shope papilloma should not be confused with the solitary circumscribed papillomas that are frequently observed about the ears and head of adult rabbits. Other than surgical removal there is no treatment for Shope papillomatosis. A program of screening the animal enclosures and vector control should be instituted in endemic areas. Rabbits could also be immunized by two intraperitoneal inoculations of glycerinated rabbit papilloma suspensions.

Shope Fibroma Virus. Shope fibroma virus is a naturally occurring oncogenic poxvirus of wild rabbits (*Sylvilagus* spp.) of North and South America.[103] Domestic rabbits housed in outdoor cages in an endemic area have become infected via mosquito vectors. Clinically, the adult animals appeared normal but several of the suckling rabbits were lethargic and in poor condition. All of the affected rabbits had single or multiple flat, subcutaneous skin nodules involving the vulva, perineum, ventral abdomen, foot, nose, pinna, and eyelid.

Grossly, the masses varied from small discrete subcutaneous nodules to diffuse subcutaneous indurations. On cut surface the masses were pale and glistening. In the suckling-to-weanling age rabbits the number of tumors and the degree of invasion was much more extensive. The overlying skin was eroded, and metastases were seen throughout the abdominal viscera.

Histologically, some tumors appeared myxomatous while others exhibited plump fibroblasts with large oval nuclei and abundant pink-staining cytoplasm. On rare occasion eosinophilic intracytoplasmic inclusion bodies were observed in tumor cells. An inflammatory infiltrate composed largely of lymphocytes, plasma cells, macrophages, and neutrophiles was present at the base of the fibroma.

Adult *Oryctolagus* often develop fibromas within 8 to 12 days after experimental exposure but the tumors undergo necrotic involution and slough away before day 30 postinoculation. Newborn rabbits are considerably more susceptible than older animals and develop more extensive lesions. This effect has been related to the inability of newborn rabbits to react immunologically to the virus until 12 to 13 days of age, whereas adult rabbits are able to mount an immune response within 1 to 2 days after exposure.

Diagnosis of fibroma virus can be accomplished with biopsy, virus isolation, and serology. The virus can be propagated in embryonated eggs and a variety of cell lines. Serologic confirmation may be established by evaluating paired serum samples 3 to 4 weeks apart during the course of the disease. Using the domestic rabbit intradermal assay, the titers were maximized by day 51 post-infection and undetectable by days 112 to 152.

No treatment has been developed for rabbit fibromatosis. The interferon inducer polyinosinic acid-polycytdylic acid has experimentally inhibited tumor development in domestic rabbits. Mosquito eradication and enclosure screening would be indicated to prevent infection in endemic areas.

Miscellaneous

Hair Loosening during Gestation. Several days prior to parturition, does undergo a generalized loosening of the fur all over the body.[111] The females pull out mouthfuls of hair to line the nest to enhance the maintenance of body temperature in newborn rabbits. This generalized loosening of hair is especially prominent during the last 5 days prepartum, and is mediated by the decreasing levels of progesterone.

Raised Skin Patches during Hair Growth. As rabbits become older the hair growth waves become less frequent and more patchy in their distribution.[112] The irregular patches of hair growth appear as raised, thickened islands of skin. When the fur is removed, the areas appear more reddish than the surrounding skin, and experience a rapid regrowth of hair. When injured these thickened areas bleed more readily. All of these changes are due to increasing follicular size and changes in the cutaneous vascular system during the active growth phase.

There are three main vascular networks in the skin of the rabbit, the superficial subepidermal plexus, the dermal plexus in the middermal layer, and the hypodermal plexus at the dermal-hypodermal junction. During active growth these vascular structures increase in size to provide adequate nutrients for hair growth. When the hair follicles enter telogen, the follicles and vasculature decrease in size and the skin returns to normal. These cyclic changes result in the mean full thickness of the skin ranging from 1.00 mm during telogen phase to 2.00 mm during periods of active hair growth.

The European Ferret (*Mustela putorius furo*)

Bacterial Diseases

Staphylococcus and Streptococcus. During the breeding season aggressive males bite the neck of the female as a prelude to coitus. These bite wounds may become infected. Both *S. aureus* and *Streptococcus* spp. may be isolated from the abscesses and fistulas.[113,114] Both bacteria have also been reported to be a cause of mastitis in ferrets.

Diagnosis may be made by Gram's stains of smears of the exudate and routine culturing on blood agar at 37°C.

Treatment of the abscesses or draining tracts should include surgical drainage and flushing with saline or a topical disinfectant. The results of the sensitivity testing will indicate which antibiotics should be selected for parenteral administration. Procaine penicillin G and chloramphenicol palmitate are acceptable broad spectrum antibiotics until the results of the sensitivity testing are available.

Escherichia coli. In the ferret *Escherichia coli* has been reported to be the etiologic agent of gangrenous mastitis in lactating jills.[115] Several animals were found moribund and died before treatment was instituted. Other animals developed enlarged, distended mammary glands. The swelling progressed rapidly to the adjacent mammary glands and surrounding subcutis. Antibiotic therapy alone did not alter the clinical course of the disease. A combination of surgical resection, penrose drains, and antibiotic therapy were required for survival.

Histologically, the areas of coagulative and liquefactive necrosis involved the mammary tissue as well as the adjacent adipose tissue and abdominal muscle. Thrombosis and necrosis of vessels in the adjacent areas was common. These lesions were typical of the effects of endotoxin or mammary tissue.

Diagnosis was confirmed with isolation on MacConkey agar at 37°C. All isolates were sensitive to gentamicin and cephalothin. Both gentamicin and ampicillin in combination were utilized to counter the *E. coli* infections.

The kits should be removed from the jill while she is under treatment. They may be nursed by another lactating ferret, or switched to natural or artificial replacement diets. The foster parents should be monitored for mastitis because the oral cavity of the kit was routinely colonized by the same *E. coli* species responsible for the mastitis.

Viral Diseases

The ferret is extremely susceptible to canine distemper virus. Without proper immunization, the mortality rate is almost 100 percent.

After 7 to 10 days of incubation, the ferret exhibits fever, anorexia, and mucopurulent ocular and nasal discharge.[114] By day 10 to 12 a rash appears under the chin and inguinal area. The foot pads and nasal pads may swell and exhibit hyperkeratosis. Death occurs after 12 to 16 days past exposure to ferret-adapted strains and 21 to 25 days with canine-adopted strains. Ferrets that survive the catarrhal phase may die during a CNS phase characterized by hyperexcitability, salivation, tremors, convulsions, and coma.

The diagnosis is based on the characteristic clinical signs and histopathology. Since there is no effective treatment, affected animals should be euthanitized to minimize the discomfort and distress of the animal.

Prevention can be achieved with immunization against distemper with a modified live virus vaccine attenuated in chicken embryo orgin tissue culture. Beginning at 6 to 8 weeks of age, the kits may be immunized every 2 to 3 weeks until 14 weeks of age. Boosters should be given annually.

Mycotic Disease

Microsporum. Ringworm has been infrequently reported in the ferret. *Microsporum canis* has been reported to produce the typical circumscribed lesions with crust and alopecia on all parts of the body. It occurred only in kits and young ferrets.[114]

Therapy consisted of shaving the hair from the affected areas and bathing with a keratolytic shampoo. Oral pediatric griseofulvin (2.5 mg/100 g) daily for 21 to 30 days should be an effective therapeutic agent.[113] However, resolution of the dermatophytosis has been reported to occur without antimycotic therapy.

Ectoparasites

Sarcoptes. Ferrets infested with *Sarcoptes scabiei* may exhibit two forms of disease: (1) generalized alopecia and intense pruritus or (2) localized lesions of the feet and toes. If allowed to go untreated, the ferret may lose the digits or the entire foot.[114]

Diagnosis is based upon the results of microscopic examination of skin scrapings from the affected sites. Heavily keratinized specimens may need to be cleared in 10 percent KOH first.

Treatment of the feet consists of triming the nails and removing the scabs after softening them in warm water. Lime sulfur (1:40 dilution) sponge baths or 0.5 percent carbaryl shampoos weekly for 3 to 5 weeks are reported to be curative. Organophosphate dips at a concentration and regimen prescribed for cats are also appropriate to use on ferrets.

The disease is spread by direct contact and fomites. The cage environment should be cleaned and disinfected to prevent reinfestation or transmission of the disease.

Otodectes. *Otodectes cynotis*, an ear mite common to the cat is also very common in the ferret,[114] yet ferrets show few clinical signs. The ears normally contain copious amounts of a dark brown cerumen, with or without ear mites. A diagnosis may be achieved by direct examination of the ears with an otoscope.

Standard commercial otic preparations effective against ear mites are satisfactory for the ferret. The animal should be treated for a minimum of 3 weeks to insure eradication of the mites.

Fleas. Ferrets can become infected with *Ctenocephalides* spp.[114] With heavy infestations the animals typically exhibit alopecia of the dorsal thorax and cervical area. "Flea dirt" may be evident when fleas are difficult to visualize. Compounds approved for cats are acceptable therapeutic agents to use on the ferret. Flea control measures should be instituted to prevent reinfestation.

Endocrine Disease

Female ferrets become sexually mature during the spring following their birth. They are seasonally polyestrus with the breeding season extending from March through August. If not allowed to breed, females may stay in estrus for 6 months or longer. The high level of endogenous estrogens associated with prolonged estrus can induce bone marrow depression.[114]

The clinical signs include pale mucous membranes, bilaterally symmetrical alopecia, subcutaneous hemorrhages, anorexia, and depression. Affected animals typically have low packed cell volumes (less than 20 percent), low thrombocyte counts (less than 50,000 platelets/μl) and low white blood cell counts (less than 2,000 cells/μl). The pancytopenia predisposes the ferrets to hemorrhages and secondary bacterial infections involving the lungs, uterus, and vagina. Animals exhibiting the above clinical signs usually die.

Treatment is usually unrewarding in severely affected females. Ovariohysterectomy and intravenous blood transfusions (10 ml per treatment), dexamethasone (0.25 mg/kg), the anabolic steroid stanazolol (0.5 mg b.i.d.), oral vitamins and supportive care have been reported to result in recovery.

The condition may be prevented by spaying all females not intended for breeding purposes by 6 to 8 months of age. Even animals in the first 2 to 3 weeks of estrus may be safely ovariohysterectomized without undue fear of excessive hemorrhage. However, the PCV and platelet count should be evaluated prior to surgery. For females that the owners plan to breed at a later date, human chorionic gonadotropin (1,000 USP units/week) may be given for 1 to 3 treatments to cycle the females out of estrus. The vulva usually begins to involute within 2 to 3 weeks.

Neoplasia

Neoplasia has rarely been documented in the ferret. However, reports of spontaneous neoplasms in the ferret have been dominated by descriptions of neoplasms of the skin. Other than mastocytomas and mast cell accumulations the remainder of the masses were all epithelial in origin. No mesenchymal tumors have been reported to arise in the subcutis of the ferret. The various types of cutaneous masses observed in the ferret are summarized in Table 10-6.[116–123]

The mast cell accumulations appeared as hairless, circumscribed, unpigmented, paper-surfaced lesions on the skin behind the ear and on the scapular area. These lesions were slightly elevated above the surrounding skin. Such lesions may be easily overlooked during a physical examination.

The treatment for cutaneous masses is early surgical excision and histologic classification of the tumor. Although metastases were infrequently reported, early removal usually results in lower morbidity.

Miscellaneous

Dirty Appearance of Albino Ferrets. The pellage of the ferret is thick but coarse. The skin is heavily invested with sebaceous glands that produce copious amounts of secretions, which, in addition to giving the ferret its characteristic odor, also give the coat its greasy feeling. The amount of secretions is greater in the male than in the female and can be reduced by castration.

Most clients bathe their ferrets at least once per week. If the sebaceous secretions are allowed to accumulate on albino ferrets the fur appears yellow and dirty. Castration and more frequent bathing can alter the appearance of these animals.

Pelt Cycling. The pelt of the ferret undergoes seasonal change.[114] During

Table 10-6. Spontaneous Neoplastic Masses of the Skin of the Ferret

Type of Mass	Location	Age (Years)	Sex	Metastasis Present	Reference
Adenocarcinoma	Abdomen, cranial to the prepuce	4.5	M	Yes Retroperitoneal mass	Miller, Denman, & Lewis[116]
Squamous cell carcinoma	Cranium, Digit of hind foot, tarsus, and pad of front foot	5	F	*	Englebart & Strosser[117]
Basi-squamo-sebaceous carcinoma	Lateral right rear, back of neck, ventrum of base of tail	6.0+	M	*	Rewell[119]
	Lateral aspect mid-thigh	2.0+	M	No	Symmers & Thomson[120]
	Right costral margin, left lateral abdomen	2.0+	F	No	Symmers & Thomson[121]
	Ventral midline of mandible	2.5+	F	No	Chesterman & Pomerance[122]
Mastocytoma	Caudal left hind limb	3	M	*	Poonacha & Hutton[123]
Mast cell accumulations	Behind ear and on scapula	2.0+	F	N/A	Symmers & Thomson[121]

*-Not described in the reference cited.
N/A-Not applicable.

the warmer months the pelts are thinner than the coats seem during the winter months. These seasonal changes are probably directly related to the hormonal changes induced by the changing photoperiod.

Breeding Season Alopecia. A bilaterally symmetrical alopecia of the tail, perineum and inguinal area commonly occurs in the ferret during the period of sexual activity, especially the females (March through August).[114] The season of peak sexual activity for the male is December to July. The cause of the alopecia is unknown, but undoubtedly is linked to the seasonal changes in hormone levels.

Biotin Deficiency. Raw eggs may be fed to ferrets as a dietary supplement, but diets containing over 10 percent raw eggs may result in a bilateral symmetrical alopecia.[114] Avidin, an enzyme present in the egg white, causes a biotin deficiency. The deficiency may be avoided by feeding commercially available ferret chow or cat chow.

The Mouse (*Mus musculus*) and Rat (*Rattus norvegicus*)

Since these two species are the most frequently utilized in biomedical research, we probably know more about the diseases of these animals than any other nondomestic species. However, these animals are infrequently presented to the clinician for treatment.

Bacterial Diseases

Primary bacterial diseases of the skin are rarely encountered in the pet rat or mouse.[124,125] *Staphylococcus aureus* and *Streptococcus* spp. are regularly isolated from skin wounds, and probably represent colonization by normal skin flora or oral flora.

The diagnosis and treatment of superficial wounds in the rat and mouse is the same as previously described for the gerbil.

Viral Diseases

There are no viral diseases of the skin that are likely to be encountered by the private practitioner. Ectromelia, or mouse pox, is occasionally reported in mouse research colonies, but has never been reported in pet mice in the United States.[126]

Mycotic Diseases

Ringworm is frequently isolated from the fur of mice, yet clinical disease is rare.[124] The presence of *Trichophyton mentogrophytes* in the fur of lesion-free mice in pet shops has been reported to be 60 percent. Among research mice the rate has been reported to range from 0 to 90 percent. Only 1 to 2 percent of the animals had obvious areas of alopecia and crust suggestive of dermatomycosis. *Microsporum gypseum* is experimentally pathogenic for the skin of mice but is rarely recovered from the hair coat.

Dermatomycosis is much more common in the mouse than the rat.[125] The presence of *Trichophyton mentagrophytes* in the coat of normal animals may also occur.

The diagnosis and treatment for ringworm is similar to that previously described for the guinea pig.

Ectoparasites

The mouse may play host to both lice (*Polyplax serrata*) and mite infestations. Among the mites, *Myobia musculi, Radfordia affinis, Myocoptes musculinus,* and *Trichoecius rombousti* may be recovered from animals exhibiting alopecia, pruritus, and excoriations, especially about the head, neck, and dorsal thorax.[127]

Rats may also be infested with lice (*Polyplax spinulosa*) as well as skin mites (*Radfordia ensifera*) and ear mites (*Notoedres muris*).[128] The clinical signs are similar to those observed for mice. Fleas (*Ctenocephalides* spp.) may also be recovered from pet rodents maintained in a household frequented by dogs and cats.

The diagnosis and treatment of these ectoparasites is similar to that previously reported for guinea pigs. Two subcutaneous injections of invermectins (200 μg/kg) 7 to 10 days apart have also been reported to be safe and effective against *Myocoptes* and *Myobia* infestations of laboratory mice.[129]

Neoplasia

The incidence of spontaneous tumors of the skin in mice is relatively low.[130] Squamous cell carcinomas of the cutis are the most frequently observed neoplasm. Nonmammary dermal fibromas, fibrosarcomas, and mesenchymal tumors are even less frequently reported.

Spontaneous tumors of the skin are also uncommon in rats.[131] Almost all types of tumors have been observed, but squamous cell carcinomas and papillomas are the most common epithelial tumors. In rats, subcutaneous mesenchymal tumors are more common than epithelial tumors, the most common type being fibromas, lipomas, fibrosarcomas, and undifferentiated sarcomas. The masses usually occur about the face, tail, and paws.

The most frequently-occurring mass involving the skin of mice or rats is the mammary gland tumor. The incidence in some rat colonies has been reported to be 16 percent in the males and 50 to 90 percent in the aged females.[131] The vast majority of these tumors are fibroadenomas and may be easily removed when they are small. Mammary tumors in the mouse are usually caused by an oncogenic virus, the mouse mammary tumor virus. Removal of these malignant tumors are quickly followed by a regrowth of the mass. The lungs are a frequent site of metastasis in the mouse.

The diagnosis and treatment of the cutaneous neoplasms is similar to that previously reported for the gerbil.

Behavioral

Aggression. Male mice are extremely aggressive and will fight when caged together.[125] The lesions usually occur around the tail and sacrum. The dominant male among the mice is usually lesion-free and may be solely responsible for the problem. Aggression among caged rats is rarely observed.

The procedures for reducing aggression among mice and the treatment of bite wounds are similar to those described for hamsters.

Barbering, Whisker Chewing, or Hair Chewing. Barbering is frequently observed in mice, especially among inbred mouse strains.[12] The hair loss usually occurs on the muzzle, vibrissiae, face, eyes, and head, but the entire body may be involved. The dominant animal in the cage is usually responsible for the barbering. He is usually fully furred. Removal of the dominant animal may resolve the alopecia.

Miscellaneous

Mechanical Facial Alopecia. Mice frequently abrade the skin surface as they feed through slotted feeders or wire bars.[125] The constant abrasion results in a symmetrical alopecia about the nose and muzzle, giving these areas the appearance of having the face shaved. Lesions are rarely present.

Yellowing of the Fur of Aged Albino Rats. The fur of the aged rat (18 months and older) frequently turns yellow and becomes more coarse. The etiology of this change is unknown.

REPTILES

The reptiles are a diverse group of animals with varied habitat requirements. Attempts to recreate the proper artificial environment for captive animals often fall short of desired goals and contribute to the high incidence of disease and injuries experienced by reptiles. The deficiencies may be the result of poor sanitation, malnutrition, inappropriate photoperiod, and improper environmental temperatures or humidity. Each of these deficiencies may lead to systemic illnesses, including diseases of the skin.

Bacterial Diseases

The literature detailing the normal flora of the skin of reptiles is rather meager. Although gram-positive bacteria are infrequently isolated from the skin, *Staphylococcus aureus* is commonly seen in histologic sections of the skin. Most other reports have indicated that gram-negative organisms from the family Enterobacteriaceae are the predominate organisms recovered from the skin.[132] It is unknown whether this situation represents fecal contaminations or a true resident flora.

Localized Bacterial Abscesses

Subcutaneous abscesses may result from penetrating external wounds or the hematogenous spread of bacteria.[132] They may contain a central core of caseous debris and inflammatory cells surrounded by a fibrous capsule, or contain cellular material and resemble a granuloma.

A predominatly gram-negative flora can be isolated from the abscesses. *Aeromonas, Citrobacter, Enterobacter, E. coli, Peptostreptococcus, Pasteurella, Proteus, Pseudomonas, Pseudomonas, Serratia,* and *Staphylococcus* have all been recovered from abscesses. Both pure and mixed cultures may be recovered.

The diagnosis of bacterial abscesses is dependent upon culturing aspirants or specimens of the abscess. Mycobacterial isolates should be sealed in a tube or bottle of egg media and incubated at 24°, 32°, 37°, and 45°C. The other bacterial species may be isolated on blood agar at room temperature or 37°C, but *Peptostreptococcus* requires an anaerobic environment for isolation.

Antibiotic therapy is directed by the results of the culture and sensitivity testing. Gentamicin for three treatments or chloramphenicol succinate are acceptable broad-spectrum antibiotics to utilize until the results are received (See Table 10-7). Oral or parenteral fluids should be given at the rate of 44 ml/kg to prevent nephrotoxicity each time gentamicin is administered.

Bacterial Dermatitis

Most cases of dermatitis in reptiles occur secondary to skin trauma, or secondary to suboptional environmental temperature, humidity, and poor water quality.[132] Mild cases may be represented by discolored scales (necrosis of the outer layers of keratin), whereas severe cases may be accompanied by a mixed exudate of tissue fluid, blood cells, and epithelial cells.

Septicemic cutaneous ulcerative disease (SCUD) is a clinical condition of turtles characterized by anorexia, lethargy, paralysis, and cutaneous ulceration.[132,133] *Citrobacter freundi* has been reported to be the etiologic agent. Septicemiae may permit the spread to the internal organs. The condition can be prevented by improved hygiene and prompt attention to skin wounds.

Treatment consists of debridement of the necrotic debris and cleaning the affected area with povidone-iodine. Gentamicin and chloramphenicol at the dosage given above should be satisfactory.

Mycotic Diseases

Mycotic diseases in reptiles are represented by members of all classes of fungi.[134] Although reports of mycotic disease in reptiles appear to occur less often than in mammals, the skin, digestive tract, and the respiratory tract are most frequently affected. The systemic or deep mycoses have not been reported in reptiles.

Phycomycosis

Phycomycosis is caused by members of the class Phycomycetes. The fungi possess a propensity for invading the adjacent vasculature, resulting in thrombosis and necrosis of the surrounding tissue.[134]

Organisms resembling *Mucor* have been isolated from turtles with necrosis of the shell, from an Eastern indigo snake (*Drymarchon corais couperi*) with granulomatous dermatitis and from skin lesions in a bearded lizard (*Amphibolurus barbatus*). *Rhizopus arrhizus* was recovered from skins lesions in a garter snake (*Thannophis sirtalis*). *Rhizopus*, in addition to *Aspergillus* and

Penicillium, has been isolated from the skin and scales of normal alligators (*Alligator mississippiensis*).

Aspergillosis

Aspergillus is one of the most commonly reported mycotic agents recovered from reptiles.[134] It has been observed in a musk turtle (*Sternotherus odoratus*) with chronic ulcerative lesions of the forefeet. Histologically, a typical granulomatous process with histocytes, fibroblasts, and giant cells was present. *Aspergillus*, plus *Mucor* and *Rhizopus*, have been cultured from primary bacterial lesions of an American crocodile (*Crocodylus acutus*) due to *Erysipelothrix insidiosa*.

Geotrichosis

Geotrichum is ubiquitous in the environment but rarely causes clinical disease. *G. candidum* has been isolated from caseous subcutaneous nodules of a common water snake (*Nerodia sipedon*) and from pustules on the skin of a garter snake.[134] A whole-body involvement with necrotic skin lesions has been reported in several newly-captured carpet pythons. The lesions were located primarily along the ventral and lateral body surfaces.

Fusarium

Fusarium, a common soil inhabitant, has been isolated from skin lesions from a green lizard (*Lacerta viridis*), and from the loosened scales of a tortoise subjected to radiation (*Testudo radiata*.) *F. oxysporum* has been recovered from skin lesions on a common chameleon (*Chamaelo dilepis*).[134]

Chromomycosis

These fungi include the pigmented or dematiacious forms varying in color from light brown to black. The principal genera are *Phialophora*, *Hormodendrum*, *Cladosporium*, and *Fonscaea*.

Nonspeciated cases of chromomycosis have been identified as a cause of severe ulcerative dermatitis on the ventral skin of a reticulated python (*Python reticulatus*), and a cause of localized dermatitis in a boa constrictor (*Constrictor constrictor*). *Cladosporium* have been recovered from subcutaneous granulomas in an anaconda (*Eunictes murinus*).[134]

Dermatophytosis

Dermatophytosis is uncommon in reptiles. *Microsporum cookei* has been isolated from the epidermal scales of a normal monitor (*Varanus*). *Trichophyton* has been recovered from granulomas of the foot pads of the alligator.

The diagnosis of mycotic diseases may be accomplished by culturing specimens on Sabouraud's media or other media appropriate for the isolation of fungi. Biopsies of the skin should be cleansed with organic iodine solution and 70 percent alcohol prior to the surgery. The biopsy should be macerated and cultured at 20° to 24°C. Following special staining for fungi, biopsy specimens may also be examined with Gridley's, Gomori's methenamine-silver and periodic acid-Shiff stains. The results of the culture should be interpreted in light of the results of the biopsies to rule out commensual or nonpathogenic species.

Truly effective treatments for mycotic diseases are unavailable. Localized granulomas may be surgically removed. Severe cases may respond to twice daily soakings in dilute organic iodine, followed by the topical application of tinactin.

The control of mycotic diseases should be directed toward prevention by providing the proper environment that meets the needs of each captive species. The environment should be sanitized as needed to prevent the accumulation of feces. The temperature, humidity, and water quality should meet the needs of each species.

Viral Diseases

The cataloging of the viral flora of reptiles is in its infancy. Very few viruses have been characterized, and only three agents have been reported to involve the skin.

Herpesvirus

Gray-patch disease is a clinical entity of young green sea turtles (*Chelonia mydas*) 56 to 90 days of age.[135] The disease is characterized by either circumscribed papular lesions, or spreading gray skin patches with superficial necrosis. Gram-negative bacteria and fungi secondarily infect the lesions. Mortality of 5 to 20 percent are not uncommon.

Herpes-like virus particles have been observed during electron microscopic examination of materials from the lesion sites. The virus has also been observed to replicate at 25°C in vitro when inoculated into an epitheloid cell line derived from the skin of *C. mydas*.[136]

No effective treatment exists. Lowering the water temperature to 25°C has been reported to prolong the onset and to reduce the severity of the disease.[135]

Papilloma-Associated Virus

Benign papillomas collected from the skin of the green lizard (*Lacerta viridis*) have been examined by electron microscopy.[136] Herpesvirus, papovavirus, and reovirus viral particles were observed. Although the viruses were not isolated in culture, the association of papillomas in mammals with papovaviruses argues that a similar relationship possibly exists in reptiles.

Caimain Pox-Like Virus

A skin condition characterized by papular lesions and gray-white patches has been reported in captive spectacled caimans (*Caiman sclerops*.)[137] The lesions were scattered over the skin surface, and contributed to the death of one animal. Eosinophilic intracytoplasmic inclusions were present in the epithelial cells, and a poxvirus was observed by electron microscopy.

No effective treatment has been reported. Two of the affected animals recovered spontaneously within 30 days.

Ectoparasites

Leeches occur on various reptiles such as turtles and alligators, which live in aquatic environments. Although damage by leeches is rare, large numbers may result in anemia and death.[138] When infestations are discovered the leeches should be removed due to their potential to transmit bacteria (*Aeromonas*), viruses (herpevirus, "gray-patch disease"), and protozoa (*Trypanosoma, Haemogregarina*).

Ticks are present on approximately 60 percent of the larger lizards and snakes in the wild.[138] Extensive infestations have been reported to cause anemia, resulting in death. Local damage to the skin may be present at the site of attachment. It is important to control ticks because they may be intermediate hosts of bacteria, viruses, filaria, and protozoa.

Mites are commonly found on snakes, but rarely on lizards.[138] They reduce the vitality of snakes, and heavy infestations may induce death due to blood loss and the toxic effect of the mite's saliva. The infestation is evident by the rough appearance of the skin and incomplete shedding. *Ophinyssus natricis* is the most common species affecting snakes. Under optimum conditions mites complete one life cycle in about 3 weeks.

Leeches and ticks may be removed manually and the wounds treated topically with povidone-iodine solution. Mites and ticks may be eradicated by suspending a 2-inch square of dichlorvos-impregnated plastic pest strip above the animal's cage for 2 days. The strip should be out of the reach of the reptile.[133] Open containers of water should be removed during the application of dichlorvos to prevent a possible toxicity. The application should be repeated within 10 to 14 days.

An alternative treatment for debilitated animals is soaking in tepid water for 3 hours.[133] Weak animals must be handled or observed carefully to prevent the inhalation of water.

Pentosomiasis

The pentostomids are obligate endoparasites of reptiles that the adults prefer to localize in the lungs. Sometimes the parasites localize in the dermis where rents in the skin may occur.[139] Migratory larvae or nymphs may cause an inflammatory reaction, abscessation, and mineralization. *Kiricephalus* commonly localize in the dermis of some snakes.

Other than surgical removal, no effective treatment exists for the parasites located in the skin. Antibiotics and supportive therapy are indicated if systemic illness is present.

The environment should be sanitized frequently to prevent the accumulation of eggs passed via feces or sputum. Eggs may also hatch in the intestinal tract of anorectic or weakened animals, leading to superinfection. Gloves should be worn when cleaning the environment due to the zoonotic potential for man to act as an intermediate host.

Neoplasia

Cutaneous neoplasia of the skin is more commonly reported in snakes than lizards or turtles.[140,141] This situation probably reflects the fact that snakes and lizards are more commonly kept as pets or for exhibition. It may also reflect the fact that animals kept in captive aquatic environments die at a younger age, or are less likely to encounter carcinogens than terestrial animals.

Green sea turtles have been observed to have fibropapillomas about the flippers, head, neck, and tail. Trematode larva and leeches are frequently associated with these lesions and have been suggested as an etiologic agent or promoter of the development of these masses. Papillomas have been confirmed on the tail of *Sternotherus odoratus*. A single report of a squamous cell carcinoma of the foot exists for turtles.

Papillomas of the head, tail, and body have been reported on various species of lizards. Squamous cell carcinomas have been observed on the foot of the Gila monster, and the foot and skin of other lizard species. The soft tissue tumors of the subcutis, the fibromas and myxoma have been infrequently reported.

The crocodilians have infrequently revealed papillomas as the only type of cutaneous neoplasm observed. The snakes have displayed the largest variety of tumor types. The singular occurrence of papillomas, fibropapillomas, fibromas, fibrosarcomas, lipomas, xanthomas, and undifferentiated sarcomas have been described.

The most common form of treatment in reptiles is surgical excision. A

Table 10-7. Antibiotic Dosages for Reptiles[a,b]

Drug	Species	Dosage/Unit of Body Weight	Route of Administration
Ampicillin trihydrate	All	3–6 mg/kg daily	IM, SC
Amikacin[c]	Snakes	3 mg/kg every 72 hours—also give fluids	SC
	Crocodilians	2.5 mg/kg every 72 hours—also give fluids	IM
Chloramphenicol succinate	All	40 mg/kg daily	IM, SC
Gentamicin	Snakes	2.5 mg/kg every 72 hours—also give fluids	SC
	Turtles	10 mg/kg every 48 hours—also give fluids	IM
Penicillin		20,000–80,000 IU/kg	IP, IM
Benzithine penicillin with procaine penicillin	All	10,000 IU/kg every 24–72 hours	IM
Sulfadimethoxine	All	30 mg/kg the first day, then 15 mg/kg for the next 3 days	IM, IV
Tetracycline	All	25–50 mg/kg daily	IM, SC, PO
Oxytetracycline	All	6–10 mg/kg daily	IM, IV, PO, SC
Trimethoprim/sulfa	All	30 mg/kg daily	SC
Tylosin	All	25 mg/kg	IM

[a] Jacobson ER, Kollias GV, Peters LJ: Dosages for antibiotics and parasiticides used in exotic animals. Compend Contin Educ Pract Vet 5:315, 1983.

[b] Holt PE: Drugs and dosages. p. 553. Cooper JE, Jackson OF (eds): In Diseases of the Reptilia. Vol. 2. Academic, New York, 1981.

[c] Jacobson ER, personal communication, 1986.

pathologist should evaluate the tissue to identify the tissue type and effectiveness of the excision. Supportive therapy in the form of antibiotics, (Table 10-7) fluids, and forced feeding may be indicated.

Miscellaneous

Trauma

Traumatic injuries are common in captive reptiles. Overzealous restraint or poor restraining technique using grabsticks or hooks may injure the skin, skeleton, or internal organs.[142] Cuts and abrasions may occur in poorly designed cages.[143] Snakes and lizards may damage their rostrum by rubbing or striking the surfaces of the cage. These injuries may require only topical treatment with disinfectants, or more extensive diagnostic evaluation and surgery. Nonabsorbable sutures within the skin should be left in place for 4 or more weeks to insure proper healing. Hide boxes may also prevent the snakes from damaging the rostral area.

Bite Wounds

Bite wounds from live rodents or cagemates may occur.[143] Only stunned or dead animals should be fed to reptiles to insure that they are not injured during feeding. Snakes that are not hungry may suffer severe bites from rodents. Hide boxes will provide a place for cagemates to seek shelter and reduce the risk of injury if the animals can not be separated.

The wounds should be cleaned topically with povidone-iodine. If granulomas or abscesses develop they should be treated as previously described for bacterial infections.

Shell Fracture

Fractures of the carapace or plastron are common to pet turtles and free-ranging chelonians. Under sedation, the wounds should be debrided and cleansed with povidone-iodine solution.[142] The fracture fragments should be returned to their proper sites. If the fragments are absent, a patch consisting of fiberglass with several layers of epoxy resin may be utilized to close the defects. Care should be taken to prevent the resin from contacting the exposed ends of the bone or entering the coelomic cavity. Antibiotic therapy should be instituted to combat bacterial infections.

Complete healing may require 1 to 2 years. The patches in adults may remain for the lifetime of the animal, but they may interfere with shell growth which occurs at the interface between the bony plates and scutes on immature turtles. The patch may be removed at these interface areas with a hand-held motorized brin. This can be performed as early as 6 months after the initial repair.

Burns

Snakes and lizards may be burned by incadescent light bulbs or electric heating pads placed in the primary enclosure to maintain the environmental temperature.[142] These devices should be placed so that they are inaccessible for direct contact with the animals.

The lesions may be treated by soaking in a solution of 16 cc of 2 percent chlorhexidine added to 4 liters of water, twice per day until healing occurs.[144] Mafenide acetate is an excellent ointment for topical treatment of wounds after each bath. Since pseudomonas infections are a common sequella to burns, systemic antibiotics are indicated.

Dysecdysis (Impaired Shedding of the Old Skin)

Reptiles normally renew their skin by shedding the outer keratinized skin or plates.[143] The skin of snakes and some lizards is lost as a continuous sheet or tube. Most lizards and the crocodilians lose large sheets of skin in a piecemeal fashion. Turtles and tortoises shed one or more keratin shields at a time.

Normal shedding in snakes is marked by anorexia and a light blue coloration of the eyes several days beforehand. Within 2 to 3 days the eyes clear and the snake rubs its maxillae and rostrum on rough surfaces to loosen the old skin. After loosening the skin from around the rostral area, the snake crawls out of his old skin.

Dysecdysis occurs secondary to systemic illness, endocrine dysfunction, injuries, improper humidity, ectoparasitism, and lack of suitable substrate to initiate the loosening of the skin. Treatment consists of soaking the affected animals in warm water for 1 to 2 hours, followed by gentle removal of the retained skin with a damp cloth. The water should be shallow to prevent the inhalation of water. Constricting bands of the skin being shed around the feet of iguanas or the distal tail of snakes must be removed quickly to prevent necrosis.

REFERENCES

1. Peckham JC, Cole JR, Chapman WB, et al: Staphylococcal dermatitis in Mongolian gerbils (*Meriones unguiculatus*). Lab Anim Sci 24:43, 1974
2. Reynold SL, Gainer JH: Dermatitis of Mongolian gerbils (*Meriones unguiculatus*) caused by *Demodex* sp. Abstract No. 150, Scientific sessions of the 19th Annual Meeting of the American Association for Laboratory Animal Science, Las Vegas, Nevada, October 21, 1968
3. Schwarzbratt SS, Wagner JE, Frisk CS: Demodicosis in the Mongolian gerbil (*Meriones unguiculatus*): A case report. Lab Anim Sci 24:666, 1974
4. Flynn RJ: Parasites of Laboratory Animals. Ames, Iowa The Iowa State University Press, 1973, p. 446
5. Benit KF, Kramer AW: Spontaneous tumors in the Mongolian gerbil. Lab Anim Care 15:281, 1965
6. Cramlet SH, Toft JD, Olsen NW: Malignant melonoma in a black gerbil (*Meriones unguiculatus*). Lab Anim Sci 24:545, 1974
7. Vincent AL, Porter DD, Ash LR: Spontaneous lesions and parasites of the Mongolian gerbil, (*Meriones unguiculatus*). Lab Anim Sci 25:711, 1975
8. Vincent AL, Ash LR: Further observations on spontaneous neoplasms in the Mongolian gerbil, (*Meriones unguiculatus*). Lab Anim Sci 28:297, 1978
9. Meckley PE, Zwicker GM: Naturally occurring neoplasms in the Mongolian gerbil, (*Meriones unguiculatus*). Lab Anim Sci 13:203, 1979

10. Kittrell EMW, Gregg BR, Thiessen DL: Brood patch function for the ventral scent gland of the female Mongolian gerbil, (*Meriones unguiculatus*). Develop Physchobio 15:197, 1982
11. Glen EM, Gray J: Effect of various hormones on the growth and histology, of the gerbil (*Meriones unguiculatus*) abdominal sebaceous gland pad. Endocrinology 76:1115, 1965
12. Harkness JE, Wagner JE: The Biology and Medicine of Rabbits and Rodents, 2nd Ed. Lea & Febiger, Philadelphia, 1983
13. Marston JH, Chong MC: The breeding, management and reproductive physiology of the Mongolian gerbil, (*Meriones unguiculatus*). Lab Anim Care 15:34, 1965
14. Schwentker V: Care and Maintenance of the Mongolian Gerbil. Tumblebrook Farm, Brent Lake, NY, 1967, p. 24
15. Williams CSF: Practical Guide to Laboratory Animals CV Mosby, St. Louis, 1976, p. 35
16. Bresnaham JF, Smith GD, Lentsch RH, et al: Nasal dermatitis in the Mongolian gerbil. Lab Anim Sci 33:258, 1983
17. Thiessen DD, Pendergrass M: Harderian gland involvement in facial lesions in the Mongolian gerbil. J Am Vet Med Assoc 181:1375, 1982
18. Kittrell EMW, Thiessen DD: Does removal of the Harderian gland affect the physiology of the Mongolian gerbil, (*Meriones unguiculatus*). Physiol Phychol 3:299, 1981
19. Frisk CS, Wagner JE, Ovens DR: Streptococcal mastitis in golden hamsters. Lab Anim Sci 26:97, 1976
20. Brennan PC, Fritz TE, Flynn RJ: Pasteurella pneumotropica: culture and biochemical characteristics, and its association with diseases in laboratory animals. Lab Anim Care 15:307, 1965
21. Mckenna JM, South FE, Musachia XJ: *Pasteurella* infection in irradiated hamsters. Lab Anim Care 20:443, 1970
22. Nutting WB: *Demodex aurati* sp. rov. and *D. criceti*, ectoparasites of the Golden hamster (*Mesocricetus auratus*). Parasitology 51:515, 1961
23. Nutting WB, Rauch H: Distribution of *Demodex aurati* in the host (*Mesocricetus auratus*) skin complex. J Parasitol 49:323, 1963
24. Owen D, Young C: The occurrence of *Demodex aurati* and *Demodex criceti* in the Syrian hamster, (*Mesocricetus auratus*) in the United Kingdom. Vet Rec 92:282, 1973
25. Estes PC, Richter CB, Franklin JA: Demodectic mange in the Golden hamster. Lab Anim Sci 21:825, 1971
26. Schmidt RE, Eason RL, Hubbard GB, et al: Pathology of the Aging Syrian Hamster. CRC Press, Boca Raton, FL, 1983, p. 183
27. Hanson CJ: Skin lesions in guinea pigs, mice and hamsters. Vet Rec 100:77, 1977
28. Bauck LB, Ovi JP, Lawrence KH: Hyperadrenocorticism in three teddy bear hamsters. Can Vet J 25:247, 1984
29. Cardesa A, Handler AH, Kelman AD: Tumors of the pituitary gland. p. 255. In Tursov VS (ed): Pathology of Tumors in Laboratory Animals, Vol 3. International Agency for Research on Cancer, Lyon, 1982
30. Cardesa A, Handler AH, Kelman AD: Tumors of the adrenal gland. p. 281. In Tursov VS (ed): Pathology of Tumors in Laboratory Animals, Vol 3. International Agency for Research on Cancer, Lyon, 1982
31. Fortner JG, Allen AC: Hitherto unreported malignant melanomas in the Syrian hamster: An experimental counterpart of the human malignant melanomas. Cancer Res 18:98, 1958

32. Green HSN: A spontaneous melanoma in the hamster with propensity for amelanotic alteration and sarcomatous transformation during transplantation. Cancer Res 18:422, 1958
33. Bomirski A, Dominiczak T, Nowinska L: Spontaneous transplantable melanoma in the golden hamster (*Mesocricetus auratus*). Acta Un Int Cancer 18:178, 1962
34. Mangkoewidjoyo S, Kim JCS: Malignant melanoma metastatic to the lung in a pet hamster. Lab Anim 11:125, 1977
35. Van Hoosier GL, Trentin JJ: The naturally occurring tumors of the Syrian hamster Prog exp Tumor Res 23:1, 1979
36. Kirkman H: A preliminary report concerning tumors observed in Syrian hamsters. Stanford Med Bull 20:163, 1962
37. Kirkman H, Algard FT: Spontaneous and nonviral induced neoplasms. p. 227. In Hoffman RA, Robinson PF, Magalhaes (eds): The Golden Hamster. Iowa State Press, Ames, Iowa, 1968
38. Yabe Y, Kataoka N, Kogama H: Spontaneous tumors in hamsters: Incidence, morphology, transplantation, and virus studies. Gann 63:329, 1972
39. Toth B: Studies on the incidence, morphology transplantation and cell-free filtration of malignant lymhomas in the Syrian golden hamster. Cancer Res 27:1430, 1967
40. Ambrose KR, Coggin JH Jr: An epizootic in hamsters of lymphomas of undetermined origin and mode of transmission. J Natl Cancer Inst 54:877, 1975
41. Brindley DC, Banfield WG: A contagious tumor of the hamster. J Natl Cancer Inst 26:949, 1961
42. Garcia H, Bahroni C, Rappaport H: Transplantable tumors of the Syrian hamster, (*Mesocricetus auratus*). J Natl Cancer Inst 27:1323, 1961
43. Lee KY, Toth B, Shubik P: Carcinogenic response of the Syrian hamster treated at birth with 7,12-dimethybenz(a)anthracene. Proc Soc Exp Biol Med 114:579, 1963
44. Van Hoosier BL, Spjut HJ, Trentin JJ: Spontaneous tumors of the Syrian hamster: Observation in a closed breeding colony and a review of the literature. In Defining the Laboratory Animal. National Academy of Sciences, Washington, DC, 1971, pp. 450–473
45. Kelin M: A spontaneous metastasizing fibrosarcoma in the golden hamster (*Mesocricetus auratus*) with some observations on tumor recurrence and metastasis after transplantation. J Natl Cancer Inst 26:1381, 1961
46. Marques DM, Valenstern ES: Individual differences in aggressiveness of female hamsters: Response to intact and castrated males and to females. Anim Behav 25:131, 1977
47. Vandenbergh JG: The effects of gonadal hormones on the aggressive behavior of adult golden hamsters (*Mesocricetus auratus*). Anim Behav 19:589, 1971
48. Tessler J: Vesicular lesions produced in guinea pigs by a *Staphylococcus aureus* strain. Can J Comp Med 37:323, 1973
49. Markham NP, Markam JG: Staphylococci in man and animals. J Comp Path 76:49, 1966
50. Warnick CL, Hong CC: Acute necrotizing mastitis in strain 2/N guinea pigs. Abstract Number 1, Twenty-sixth Annual Session of the American Association for Laboratory Animal Science, Boston, November 16, 1975
51. Ishihara C: An exfoliative skin disease in guinea pigs due to *Staphylococcus aureus*. Lab Anim Sci 30:552, 1980
52. Smith MW: Staphylococcal cheilitis in the guinea pig. J Small Anim Pract 18:47, 1977

53. Taylor JL, Wagner JE, Owens DR, Stuhlman RA: Chronic pododermatitis in guinea pigs, a case report. Lab Anim Sci 21:944, 1971
54. Gupta BN, Conner GH, Meyer DB: Osteoarthritis in guinea pigs. Lab Anim Sci 22:362, 1972
55. Gupta BN, Carter GR, Longham RF, Conner GH: Bacteriologic examination of guinea pig mammary gland: Preliminary report. J Diary Res 55:867, 1972
56. Gupta BN, Langham RF, Conner GH: Mastitis in guinea pigs. Amer J Vet Res 31:1703, 1970
57. Kinkler RJ, Jr, Wagner JE, Doyle RE, Owens DR: Bacterial mastitis in guinea pigs. Lab Anim Sci 26:214, 1976
58. Gandaway JR: Bacterial, mycoplasial, and rickettsial diseases. p. 121. In Wagner JE, Manning PJ (eds): The Biology of the Guinea Pig. Academic Press, New York, 1976
59. Fraunfetter FC, Schmidt RE, Beattie RJ, Garner FM: Lancefield type C Streptococcal infections in strain 2 guinea pigs. Lab Anim Sci 5:1, 1976
60. Diaz J, Soave OA: Cephaloridine treatment of cervical lymphadenitis in guinea pigs. Lab Anim Sci 8:60, 1973
61. Henderson JD: Cervical lymphadenitis in the guinea pig. Vet Med/Sm Anim Clin 71:462, 1976
62. Hampton EG, Bruce M, Jackson FL: Virus-like particles in a fibrovascular growth in guinea pigs. J Gen Virol 2:205, 1968
63. Lopez-Martiney R, Mier T, Quirante M: Dermatophytes isolated from laboratory animals. Mycopathologia 88:111, 1984
64. Fuentes CA, Aboulofia RT: Mentagrophytes from apparently health guinea pigs. Arch Dermatol 71:478, 1955
65. Sprouse RF: Mycosis. p. 153. In Wagner JE, Manning PJ: The Biology of the Guinea Pig. Academic Press, New York, 1976
66. Vogel RA, Timpe MA: Spontaneous *Microsporum audouini* infection in a guinea pig. J Invest Dermatol 28:311, 1957
67. Kuttin ES, Beemer AM, Amani H: *Trichophyton mentagrophytes* infection in rabbits successfully treated with a polyvinyl iodine solution. Lab Anim Sci 26:960, 1976
68. Post K, Saunders JR: Topical treatment of experimental ringworm in guinea pigs with griseofulvin in dimethylsulfoxide. Can Vet J 20:45, 1979
69. Ronald NC, Wagner JE: The arthropod parasites of the genus Cavia. p. 201. In Wagner JE, Manning PJ (eds): The Biology of the Guinea Pig. Academic Press, New York, 1976
70. Russell RJ, Johnson DK, Stunkard JA: A Guide to Diagnosis, Treatment and Husbandry of Pet Rabbits and Rodents. Veterinary Medicine Publishing Co., Lenexa, Kansas, 1981
71. Henderson JD: Treatment of cutaneous acariasis in the guinea pig. J Am Vet Med Assoc 163:591, 1973
72. Wagner JE, Al-Rabiai S, Rings RW: Chirodiscoides caviae infestation in guinea pigs. Lab Anim Sci 22:750, 1972
73. Kummel BA, Estes SA, Arbian LG: Trixacarus caviae infestation of guinea pigs. J Am Vet Med Assoc 177:903, 1980
74. McDonald SE, Lavioipierre MMJ: Trixacarus caviae infestation in two guinea pigs. Lab Anim Sci 30:67, 1980
75. Zojac A, Williams JF, Williams CSF: Mange caused by Trixacarus caviae in guinea pigs. J Am Vet Med Assoc 177:900, 1980

76. Manning PJ: Neoplastic diseases. p. 211. In Wagner JE, Manning PJ: The Biology of the Guinea Pig. Academic Press, New York, 1976
77. Ediger RD, Dill GS, Kovatch RM: Trichofolliculoma of the guinea pig. J Natl Cancer Inst 46:517
78. Zwart P, Mander Hage MH, Mullink JWAA, Cooper JE: Cutaneous tumors in the guinea pig. Lab Anim Sci 15:375, 1981
79. Kitcen DN, Carlton WW, Bickford AA: A report of fourteen spontaneous tumors of the guinea pig. Lab Anim Sci 25:92, 1975
80. Heston WE, Deringer MK: Induction of pulmonary tumors in guinea pigs by intravenous injection of nethylcholanthrene and dibenzanthracene. J Nat Cancer Inst 13:705, 1952
81. Stenback F: Guinea pigs and carcinogens. Acta Path Microbial Scand, Section A. 78:192, 1970
82. Dickson EC: Sarcoma occurring in the guinea pig. Proc Soc Exp Biol Med 13:26, 1915
83. Murray JA: A transplantable sarcoma of the guinea pig. J Path Bacteriol 20:260, 1916
84. Haagensen CD, Krehbiel LF: Liposarcoma produced by 1:2 benzpyrene. Amer J Cancer 27:474, 1936
85. Warren S, Gates O: Spontaneous and induced tumors of the guinea pig. Cancer Res 1:65, 1941
86. Rogers JB, Blumenthal HT: Studies on guinea pig tumors. I. Report on fourteen spontaneous guinea pig tumors, with a review of the literature. Cancer Res 20:191, 1960
87. Blumenthal HT, Rogers JB: Spontaneous and induced tumors in the guinea pig. p. 183. In Ribelin WE, McCoy JR (eds): The Pathology of Laboratory Animals. Charles C. Thomas, Springfield, Illinois, 1965
88. Wagner JE: Miscellaneous disease conditions of guinea pigs. p. 229. In Wagner JE, Manning PJ (eds): The Biology of the Guinea Pig. Academic Press, New York, 1976
89. Festing MFW: The guinea-pig or cavy. p. 237. In UFAW (ed): The UFAW Handbook on the Care and Management of Laboratory Animals. 5th Ed. Churchill Livingstone, Edinburgh, 1976
90. Breazile JE, Brown EM: Anatomy. p. 53. In Wagner JE, Manning PJ (eds): The Biology of the Guinea Pig. Academic Press, New York, 1976
91. Harper LV: Behavior. p. 35. In Wagner JE, Manning PJ (eds): The Biology of the Guinea Pig. Academic Press, New York, 1976
92. Sachser N, Prove E: Short-term effects of residence on the teststerone responses to fighting in alpha male guinea pigs. Aggres Behav 10:285, 1984
93. Lee KJ, Johnson WD, Long CM: Preputial dermatitis in male guinea pigs (*Cavia porcellus*). Lab Anim Sci 28:99, 1978
94. Flatt RE: Bacterial Disease. p. 194. In Weisbroth SH, Flatt RE, Kraus AL (eds): The Biology of the Laboratory Rabbit. Academic Press, New York, 1975
95. Flatt RE, Weisbroth SH, Kraus AL: Metabolic traumatic, mycotic, and miscellaneous diseases of rabbits. p. 435. In Weisbroth SH, Flatt RE, Kraus AL (eds): The Biology of the Laboratory Rabbit. Academic Press, New York, 1974
96. Cunliffe-Beamer TL, Fox RR: Veneral spirochetosis of rabbits: Eradication. Lab Anim Sci 31:379, 1981
97. Ward GS, Crumrine MH, Mattlock JR: Inflammatory exostosis and abscessation associated with *Fusobacterium nucleatum* in a rabbit. Lab Anim Sci 31:280, 1981

98. Mare CJ: Viral diseases. p. 237. In Weisbroth SH, Flatt RE, Kraus AL (eds): The Biology of the Laboratory Rabbit. Academic Press, New York, 1974
99. Kraus AL: Arthropod diseases. p. 287. In Weisbroth SH, Flatt RE, Kraus AL (eds): The Biology of the Laboratory Rabbit. Academic Press, New York, 1974
100. Wilkins CA, Conray JA, Ito P, et al: Treatment of psoroptic mange with ivermectins. Am J Vet Res 41:2112, 1980
101. Barr AR: A case of "mange" of the domestic rabbit due to *Cheyletiella parasitivorax* (Megnin). J Parasitol 41:323, 1955
102. Weisbroth SH, Wang R, Scher S: Immune and pathologic consequences of spontaneous *Cuterebra* myiasis in domestic rabbits (*Oryctolagus cuniculus*). Lab Anim Sci 23:241, 1973
103. Weisbroth SH: Neoplastic diseases. p. 331. In Weisbroth SH, Flatt RE, Kraus AL (eds): The Biology of the Laboratory Rabbit. Academic Press, New York, 1974
104. Polson CJ: Tumours of the rabbit. J Path Bact 30:603, 1927
105. Greene HSN, Brown WH: A transplantable squamous cell carcinoma in the rabbit. Cancer Res 3:53, 1943
106. Port CD, Sidor MA: A sebaceous gland carcinoma in a rabbit. Lab Anim Sci 28:215, 1978
107. Brown WH, Pearce L: Studies based on a malignant tumor of the rabbit. I. The spontaneous tumor and associated abnormalities. J Exp Med 37:601, 1923
108. Kato T: On a transplantable sarcoma of the rabbit. p. 933. Far East Ass Trop Med Trans Congr, 6th, 1925
109. Hinton M: Cutaneous lymphosarcoma in a rabbit. Vet Rec 103:140, 1978
110. Doberstein J, Tamoschke C: Die spontantumoren beim kanichen. p. 477. In Cohrs P, Jaffe R, Meessen H (eds): Pathologic der Laboratoritorium-stiere. Springer-Verlag, Berlin, 1958
111. Savin PB, Deneberg VH, Ross S, et al: Maternal behavior in the rabbit: Hair loosening during gestation. Am J Physiol 198:1099, 1960
112. Marcella KL, Wright EM, Foresman PA, Franzelle MG: What's your diagnosis: raised skin patches. Lab Anim 15(4):13, 1986
113. Wallach JD, Boever WJ: Mustelidae. p. 495. Diseases of Exotic Animals. WB Saunders Company, Philadelphia, 1983
114. Bernard SL, Gorham JR, Ryland LM: Biology and diseases of ferrets. p. 386. In Fox JG, Cohen BJ, Loew FM (eds): Laboratory Animal Medicine. Academic Press, New York, 1984
115. Liberson AJ, Newcomer CE, Ackerman JI, et al: Mastitis caused by hemolytic *Escherichia coli* in the ferret. J Am Vet Med Assoc 183:1179, 1983
116. Miller TA, Denman DL, Lewis GC: Recurrent adenocarcinoma in a ferret. J Am Vet Med Assoc 181:839, 1985
117. Engelbart K, Strosser H: Squamous carcinoma in the ferret. Blue Book for the Veterinary Profession, Volume 11:28, 1966
118. Olsen GH, Turk MAM, Foil CS: Disseminated cutaneous squamous cell carcinoma in a ferret. J Am Vet Med Assoc 186:702, 1985
119. Rewell RE: Multiple squamo-sebaceous carcinomas of the skin in a polecat, *Putorius putorius*. J Path Bact 61:146, 1949
120. Symmers WStC, Thomson APD: A spontaneous carcinoma of the skin of the feet (Mustela furo L) J Path Bact 62:229, 1950
121. Symmers WStC, Thomson APD: Multiple carcinomata and focal mast-cell ac-

cumulation in the skin of a ferret (Mustelo furo L) with a note on other tumors in ferrets. J Path Bact 65:481, 1953
122. Chesterman FC, Pomerance A: spontaneous neoplasms in ferrets and polecats. J Path Bact 89:529, 1965
123. Poonacha KBD, Hutton UL: Cutaneous mastocytoma in a ferret. J Am Vet Med Assoc 185:442, 1984
124. Weisbroth SH: Bacterial and mycotic diseases. p. 55. In Baker HJ, Lindsey JR, Weisbroth SH (eds): The Laboratory Rat. Vol 1. Academic Press, New York, 1979
125. Williford CB, Wagner JE: Bacterial and mycotic diseases of the integumentary system. p. 209. In Foster HL, Small JD, Fox JG (eds): The Mouse in Biomedical Research. Vol 2. Academic Press, New York, 1982
126. Fenner F: Mousepox p. 209. In Foster HL, Small JD, Fox JG (eds): The Mouse in Biomedical Research. Vol 2. Academic Press, New York, 1982
127. Weisbroth SH: Arthropods. p. 385. In Foster HL, Small JD, Fox JG (eds): The Mouse in Biomedical Research. Vol 2. Academic Press, New York, 1982
128. Kohn DF, Barthold SW: Biology and diseases of rats. p. 91. In Fox JG, Cohen BJ, Loew FM (eds): Laboratory Animal Medicine. Academic Press, Orlando, 1984
129. Wing SR, Courtney CH, Young MD: Effect of ivermectin on murine mites. J Am Vet Med Assoc 187:1191, 1985
130. Holland JM, Fry RJM: Neoplasms of the integumentary system and Harderian gland. p. 513. In Foster HL, Small JD, Fox JG (eds): The Mouse in Biomedical Research. Vol 4. Academic Press, New York, 1982
131. Altman NH, Goodman DG: Neoplastic diseases. p. 334. In Baker HH, Lindsey JR, Weisbroth SH (eds): The Laboratory Rat. Vol 1. Academic Press, New York, 1979
132. Cooper JE: Bacteria. p. 165. In Cooper JE, Jackson OF (eds): Diseases of the Reptilia. Vol 1. Academic Press, New York, 1981
133. Frye FL: Husbandry, Medicine and Surgery in Captive Reptiles. Veterinary Medicine Publishing, Bonner Springs, Kansas, 1973
134. Migaki G, Jacobson ER, Casey HW: Fungal diseases in reptiles. p. 183. In Hoff GL, Frye FL, Jacobson ER (eds): Diseases of Amphibians and Reptiles. Plenum Press, New York, 1984
135. Hoff GL, Hoff DM: Herpesviruses of Reptiles. p. 159. In Hoff GL, Frye FL, Jacobson ER (eds): Diseases of Amphibians and Reptiles. Plenum Press, New York, 1984
136. Clark HF, Lunger PD: Viruses. p. 135. In Cooper JE, Jackson OF (eds): Diseases of the Reptilia. Vol 1. Academic Press, New York, 1981
137. Jacobson ER, Popp JA, Shields RP, Gaskin JM: Pock-like skin lesions in captive caimans. J Am Vet Med Assoc 175:937, 1979
138. Frank W: Ectoparasites. p. 359. In Cooper JE, Jackson OF (eds): Diseases of the Reptiles. Vol 1. Academic Press, New York, 1981.
139. Cosgrove GE, Deakins DE, Self JT, Pentosomiasis. p. 205. In Hoff GL, Frye FL, Jacobson ER (eds): Diseases of Amphibians and Reptiles. Plenum Press, New York, 1984
140. Machotka SVL: Neoplasia in Reptiles. p. 519. In Hoff GL, Frye FL, Jacobson ER (eds): Diseases of Amphibians and Reptiles. Plenum Press, New York, 1984
141. Jacobson ER: Neoplastic Diseases. p. 429. In Cooper JE, Jackson OF (eds): Diseases of the Reptilia. Vol 2. Plenum Press, 1981

142. Cooper JE: Physical Influences. p. 607. In Hoff GL, Frye FL, Jacobson ER (eds): Diseases of Amphibians and Reptiles. Plenum Press, New York, 1984
143. Frye FL: Traumatic and Physical diseases. p. 387. In Cooper JE, Jackson OF (eds): Diseases of the Reptilia. Vol 2. Academic Press, New York, 1981
144. Jacobson ER: Pseudomonas. p. 37. In Hoff GL, Frye FL, Jacobson ER (eds): Diseases of Amphibians and Reptiles. Plenum Press, New York, 1984

11 Skin and Feather Diseases of Pet Birds

Sharron L. Martin

Pet birds are presented commonly to veterinarians for problems involving the feathers and skin. Inexperienced owners of these birds are more likely to recognize abnormalities of the feathering than they are serious internal disorders.

ANATOMY AND PHYSIOLOGY

Feathers are unique and interesting structures that are similar in derivation to reptile scales. Eight to 10 percent of the body weight of a budgerigar will be comprised of the feathers, which may number up to 3,000 in an individual bird. There are three main types of feathers: the outer contour feather that gives the shape and color to the body; plumules, the down feathers that lay close to the body; and filoplumes, hair-like feathers that terminate with a tuft of barbs. The eyelashes of a budgerigar, for instance, are filoplumes. The main functions of feathers are to provide the ability to fly and for thermal regulation. The feathers on the body surface grow in tracts (pterylae) that are named by anatomic location. Normally, there are skin areas on birds that do not contain feather follicles.

As in mammals, the skin of birds is comprised of three layers, the thin epidermis, thicker dermis, and subcutaneous tissue which, particularly in some species, may accumulate fat. The skin of birds in most areas is thin, dry, relatively inelastic, and fairly loosely attached to the deep tissues. There is a network of dermal muscles which originate and insert on feather follicles and provide a means for raising or ruffling the feathers. The epidermis and dermis give rise to such structures as the bill, claws, and scaled portion of the legs, wattles, and comb. In some species such as the budgerigar there is a soft, fleshy area at the base of the upper beak through which the nostrils open, referred to as the cere. The main skin gland of birds is not associated with feather follicles, but is a bilobed structure located at the dorsal base of the tail (uropygium) and is referred to as the uropygial gland. This gland is not present in some birds, such as pigeons and some parrots. Also known as the oil or preen gland, it secretes fatty acids, fat, and wax.[1] These materials are spread on feathers by the bird during preening and may facilitate waterproofing of the feathers.

Molting is a normal physiologic process by which birds replace feathers and is analagous to shedding in mammals. Different species of birds have different molting patterns, and many migratory birds will molt twice a year. Generally, birds do not molt during active reproductive cycles or during migration periods, as all these activities produce nutritional stress on the bird. In general, psittacine birds such as budgerigars have a less well-defined molting cycle[2] than passerine species (such as canaries). Molting is influenced by many factors including the photo period,[3] reproduction,[4] temperature, humidity, social interaction, nutrition, and sex.

As the old feathers are lost during the molt, either by dropping from the feather follicle or being picked out by the bird in its grooming activity, new feathers emerge encased in a keratin sheath and are referred to as pin feathers. During periods of heavy molt, birds will indulge in much more grooming and preening activity, which may be misinterpreted by concerned owners as abnormal behavior. Heavy molt produces nutritional stress upon the bird, as both protein and calcium are required for the formation of new feathers. Birds may be more susceptible to fractures of long bones during this period.

PARASITES OF THE SKIN AND FEATHERS

Scaly Faced Mites

The most common parasitic infestation of the skin seen in pet birds is that caused by the scaly faced mite (*Knemidokoptes pilae*). This parasite is particularly common in budgerigars,[5] but will also be observed in canaries and other caged bird species. Knemidokoptes mites apparently spend their entire life cycle on the bird and are probably spread by direct contact between birds.

Early signs of this infestation is the appearance of a powdery, white line at the junction of the cere and upper beak. As the infestation spreads, the normal shiny horn of the beak will be covered with a tannish, powdery scale and crust perforated by tiny holes. Lesions will form on the cere, beak, and commisures of the beak and gradually spread into the feathered skin. The infestation will commonly spread to the scaled portions of the legs (Fig. 11-1) and, in heavily infested birds, the vent area will become involved also. The cancellous appearance of the crust is due to the multiple burrows produced by the female mite. As the infestation becomes more severe, distortion and ab-

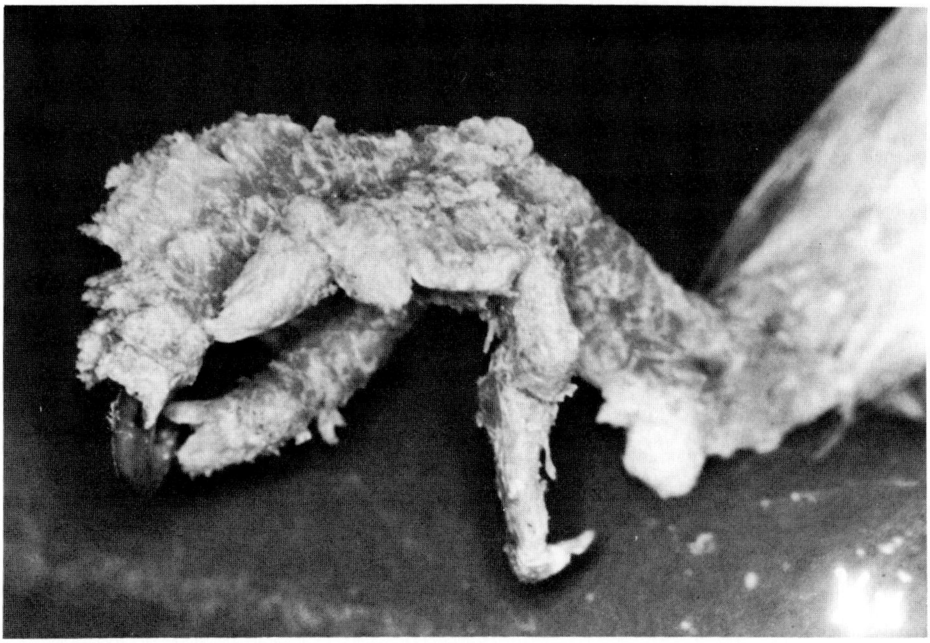

Fig. 11-1. Lower leg and foot of a budgerigar with severe *Knemidokoptes* mite infestation. There is crusting, epidermal hyperplasia, and loss of some toenails.

normal growth of the bill will occur (Fig. 11-2)[6] and eventually may cause difficulty for the bird in grasping its food.

In canaries, the scaled portion of the feet are involved in the infestation with *Knemidokoptes* mites. Typically, in severe infestations, triangular projections of keratinized tissue will form on the legs and feet (Fig. 11-3). This condition is referred to by canary breeders as "tassel foot."

Affected birds are usually not pruritic, but when the feet are severely affected they may show evidence of lameness. Loss of nails may occur in severe infestations. If affected birds are banded there may be enough swelling of the leg to result in pressure necrosis of the superficial skin beneath the band.

The diagnosis of *Knemidokoptes* infestation is usually by the observation of typical clinical signs. Confirmation of the diagnosis may be made by examining skin scrapings or crusts carefully removed from the lesions. Ten percent potassium hydroxide (KOH) may be used as a keratolytic to clear the sample, enabling easier observation of the mites and/or eggs. The *Knemidokoptes pilae* mite is typically round with short legs. The ova are relatively large and oval in shape.

In the past, *Knemidokoptes pilae* infestations in parakeets were frequently misdiagnosed as fungal infections by inexperienced veterinarians and owners. Overgrowth of the upper bill may occur secondary to liver disease; however, in these cases the surface of the bill retains its shiny normal appearance. Aging

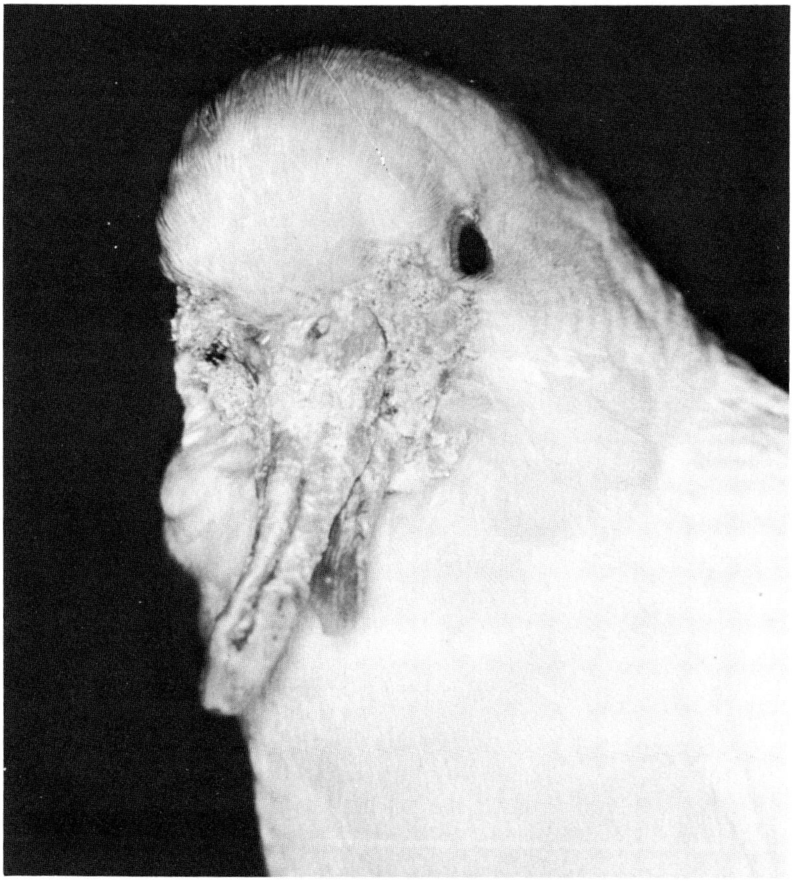

Fig. 11-2. An adult budgerigar with severe deformity of the beak as a result of *Knemidokoptes* mite infestation. The incrustations are spreading to the feathered skin adjacent to the cere and beak.

canaries and other perching birds commonly develop proliferation of the scales on the legs and feet which could be confused with scaly leg mite infestation.

Many different drugs have been used in the treatment of Knemidokoptes mite infestation in birds. One preparation that is safe and effective in the treatment of these mites in pet birds is a cream containing crotamiton (Eurex). The cream is applied twice weekly to affected areas for 4 to 6 weeks. Another topical preparation which has been recommended for treatment of this condition contains p-chloro-sym-M-xylenol and terpineol (Dettol).[7] This preparation can be obtained by owners from pet stores and should be diluted to 10 percent (50 drops of Dettol to 1 oz water). This preparation is applied to the lesions daily for 1 to 2 weeks. Nebulization with a solution of malathion, Dimethylsulfolane (DMSO), and tylosin in water has been reported to be successful in the treatment of mite infestations that do not respond to conventional therapy.[8]

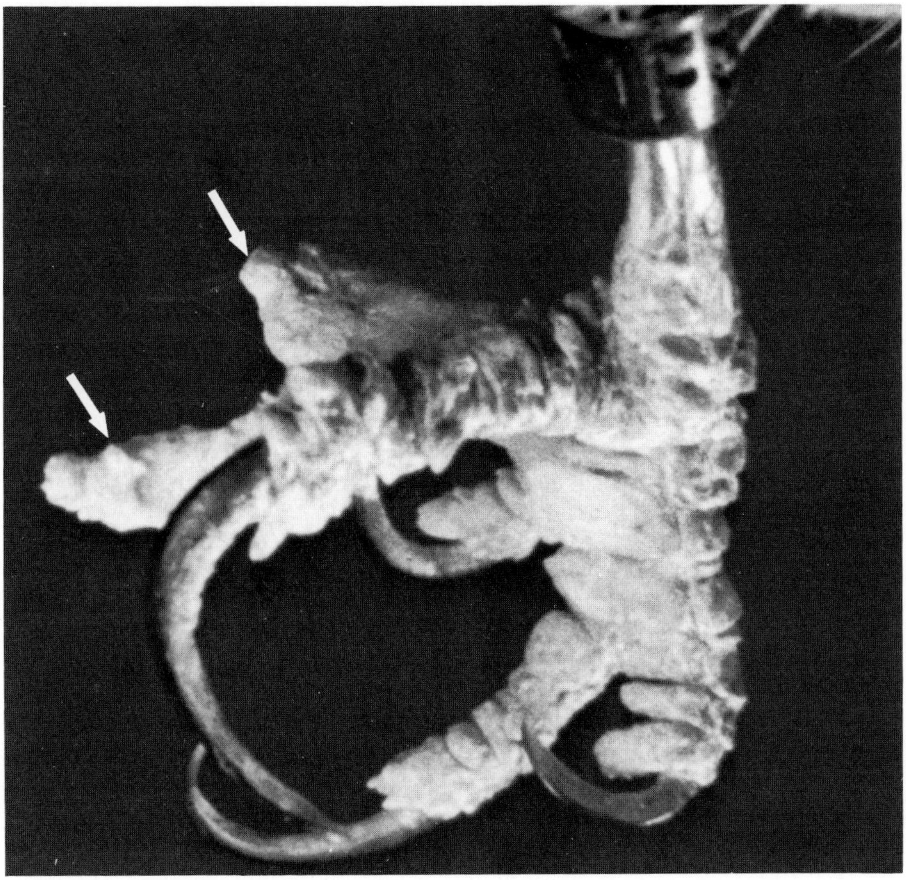

Fig. 11-3. Lower leg and foot of a canary infested with *Knemidokoptes pilae* mites. Arrows point to triangular projections of hyperplastic epidermis and crusts.

A parenteral drug which is not approved for use in birds but appears to be effective in noncontrolled studies for the treatment of Knemidokoptes mites in caged birds is ivermectin.[9] Presently this drug is available only in an injectable form labeled for use in cattle or an oral paste form for use in horses. The drug must be diluted to be able to accurately measure dosages and is unstable in aqueous diluents. This drug may be toxic in some avain species and should be used with caution.

Feather Mites

Aviaries and, occasionally, individual pet birds may become infested with either the red mite (*Dermanyssus gallinae*) or the Northern roost mite (*Ornithonyssus sylviarum*).[10] The red mite spends a good portion of its life cycle away from the avian host and is usually present on the birds only at night when it feeds. Both the adult and nymph are parasitic for birds. The northern mite, on the other hand, may spend its entire life cycle on the host. The mites are usually 0.5 mm long and may be observed without magnification.

Infestation with red mites or northern mites occurs most commonly in passerine birds such as canaries and finches and is encountered infrequently in psittacine birds. Clinical signs will vary depending on the species of mite involved in the infestation. Since red mites feed primarily at night, infested birds tend to be restless and uncomfortable during the period when the mites are crawling and feeding on them. The northern mite may stay on the bird and infested birds may show discomfort and increased preening at any time. Debilitation and anemia occur in severe infestations, particularly in fledglings. Infested birds do not usually pull out or chew on their feathers excessively.

There are several approaches to the diagnosis of red mite or northern mite infestation. In the case of red mites, clinical examination during the daytime will reveal no mites on the birds. The classic method of diagnosis is placing a white cloth over the cage at night and examining the cloth early the next morning for small moving red dots which are the engorged mites. If the birds are presented to the veterinarian in their own cages, as is most desirable, a thorough examination should be undertaken of the cage including an examination of the ends of the perches, behind and around food dishes, under the cage paper, and any other potential hiding places. Northern mites may be found on the infested birds with careful examination, ideally using some form of magnification such as a head loupe.

Treatment of pathogenic feather mites should be directed towards control in the environment and on the bird. Cages and all of the equipment in the cage should be cleaned thoroughly. In the case of red mites, it is helpful to remove the bird or birds into a different area and use an insecticide fogger in the infested room. A 4 to 5 percent malathion dust can be used in the cage and on birds if mites are found on them. A 5 percent carbaryl powder may be used also to dust infested birds.[9]

Miscellaneous Parasites

Other parasites of the skin and feathers, such as lice, fleas, and other mites are not encountered commonly in small pet birds such as canaries and budgerigars. Recently acquired birds, particularly larger birds such as parrots, macaws, and cockatoos should be thoroughly inspected for such parasites on initial physical examination. Usually, local treatment such as dusting with a carbaryl or malathion powder and environmental control will eliminate the infestation.

INFECTIOUS DISEASES

Pox Virus Infections

Many bird species may be infected with pox virus. It is not clearly understood whether viruses which affect different groups of birds, such as the canary pox virus, is a strain or variant of a single avian pox virus or a distinct, separate virus. Certain strains of canary pox virus appear to be effective only for canaries,[11] but other strains will infect other species of birds such as house sparrows.[12]

Canary pox is a well recognized and serious disease of the species. The distribution of canary pox is worldwide, and outbreaks have been reported from North and South America, Europe, and Japan.[13] Outbreaks of canary pox occur sporadically and may occur after introduction of latently infected birds into a previously unexposed aviary. Because of the slow spread of the disease once it is introduced into an aviary, it is suspected that intermediate hosts, such as mosquitoes or other parasites, may contribute to the spread of this disease.

Clinical signs associated with canary pox infection varies considerably in the face of such factors as virulence of the viral strain, resistance of the host, and management of the aviary. Virulent forms of the virus have been known to result in mortality rates of 100 percent in susceptible aviaries. Initial clinical signs are inflammation of the conjunctiva with pruritus of the eyes and the appearance of proliferative skin lesions on the eyelids. Affected birds often scratch at their eyes or rub them on perches and other objects in their cage. The skin lesions frequently extend to the commisures of the beak, the intermandibular space, and the skin of the head and neck. The birds may not appear to be seriously ill until the development of respiratory signs. At this time, ruffling of the feathers, inappetance, depression, and marked dyspnea which progresses in severity is observed in infected birds. Birds with these clinical signs usually die. The total course of the disease is usually from 5 to 9 days but birds with only skin lesions may survive for longer periods. Some infected birds do not develop skin lesions, but die very rapidly after onset of dyspnea.

Pathologic changes occuring in birds infected with canary pox also vary considerably with the degree of virulence of the virus. Birds that die rapidly from a highly virulent strain of pox virus may have congestion of the respiratory tract and lungs only. Other infected birds may have pneumonia, pericarditis, and lesions in the air sacs. Proliferative lesions of skin and mucous membrane will be found in the more chronically infected birds with less virulent virus. In these birds there is hyperplasia and ballooning degeneration of the epithelial cells. Many of these cells may contain the typical eosinophilic intracytoplasmic inclusion bodies in hematoxylin-eosin stained sections. A recent study has shown that the pox virus enters the inclusion body during its maturation process.[14] Virus multiplication does not take place in this type of inclusion body, but rather in basophilic staining areas in the cytoplasm which are pooled viral DNA.[15]

The diagnosis of canary pox should be considered in aviaries experiencing a disease problem characterized by gradual spread but high mortality and morbidity, particularly where the disease is characterized by respiratory signs and skin lesions around the head and neck. Confirmation of a diagnosis of canary pox can be based on necropsy findings and demonstration of intracytoplasmic inclusion bodies. Virus isolation studies, where available, will provide the most definitive diagnosis.

There is no effective treatment for this disease in canaries with systemic signs. It has been reported that Mercurochrome in an aqueous-alcohol base may be applied to cutaneous lesions with good response in those birds having only skin lesions.[13] Prevention of the disease through client education is important in controlling the spread of this disease. Aviculturists must be taught the importance of isolating new birds for at least 1 month before introducing them into the aviary. They should isolate any birds which they have taken out of the aviary to show or to loan to other breeders for the same period of time. It has been demonstrated that vaccination of canaries with highly attenuated strains of the canary pox virus is both safe and effective.[16,17] Unfortunately, there are no commercially available vaccines produced in this country for vaccination against canary pox.

Psittacine Pox Virus

Pox virus infections have been reported in several psitticines including Amazon parrots,[18,19] conures,[20] lovebirds,[21] and a budgerigar.[22] The disease in psitticine species has occurred as both a cutaneous form with discreet proliferative lesions occurring on the eyelids, beak, legs, and feet and a systemic (diphtheritic) form in which lesions are found in the mouth or pharynx and upper respiratory tract. Transmission and cross-challenge studies of the virus isolated from parrots demonstrated that skin lesions would develop in specific-pathogen-free chicks innoculated with the virus isolate from parrots.[23] It was also demonstrated that chickens that had been vaccinated with both fowl and pigeon pox vaccines and innoculated with the virus isolate from parrots develop lesions typical of avian pox. Also, if chickens were vaccinated with the psitticine virus they were still susceptible to fowl and pigeon pox virus infections.

Clinical signs may vary, but initial signs of the disease usually are swelling of the eyelids and conjunctiva. Some birds develop only skin lesions and recover from the disease. Other birds develop the diphtheritic form, in which extensive fibronecrotic lesions occur in the mucous membranes of the mouth, pharynx, trachea, and esophagus. A high mortality rate is associated with this form of the disease. Secondary bacterial and/or fungal infections probably contribute to this mortality rate. Infected birds will exhibit severe respiratory distress, anorexia, and weight loss.

Pathologic changes observed in psitticine pox virus infections are similar to those seen in other avian species. There is epidermal hyperplasia with ballooning degeneration of cells, intraepithelial vesicles, and eosinophilic intracytoplasmic inclusions. Lesions in the mouth and esophagus, which appear grossly as plaque-like lesions, are usually areas of central necrosis covered with cellular debris with the typical proliferative epithelial changes seen primarily at the periphery of some lesions. The tracheal and bronchial epithelium may be thickened in some birds. In these areas, there is usually severe necrosis of epithelium.

Diagnosis of pox virus infection may be confirmed by biopsy of cutaneous lesions and demonstration of typical eosinophilic intracytoplasmic inclusion bodies and, where available, virus isolation studies using embryonated chicken eggs.

There is no specific treatment for pox virus infections. Isolation of infected birds and good general supportive care may be of some benefit; however, the prognosis is poor if there are respiratory signs.

Papovavirus of Fledgling Budgerigars

In 1980, a disease which affected 1- to 3-week-old budgerigars involving aviaries in Georgia and Texas was reported by Davis et al.[24] Subsequently, this disease problem was reported in other parts of the United States, Canada,[25] and Germany.[26] In 1984, a report of a similar disease associated with a papova-like virus involving conures and macaws was reported by Jacobson et al.[27] In the reported outbreaks, the mortality rate ranged from 30 to 80 percent in young birds. The highest mortality rates have been in budgerigars between 1 and 20 days of age. This disease has been named budgerigar fledgling disease (BFD) and the etiologic agent was named budgerigar fledgling disease virus (BFDV); however, in view of this recent report of a similar disease occurring in conures and macaws, this name may be too limited in describing this disease.

The most consistent sign of disease in younger birds is abdominal distension and reddening of the skin. Birds less than 2 weeks of age usually do not exhibit feathering disorders. Infected birds over 15 days of age fail to grow down feathers on the back and abdomen and contour feathers on the back of the head and neck, and there was sparse feathering of the wings and tail. There is a retarded growth of primary wing and tail feathers in birds that survive the infection. Poor development of the feathers and lack of proximal barbs of the contour feathers were observed in surviving 4 to 7-week-old birds.[25]

Gross pathologic changes were most severe and widespread in birds that died shortly after hatching. Common lesions observed in these birds included hydropericardium, enlarged and congested livers with white or yellow foci of varying sizes and petechial hemorrhages, congested or pale kidneys with multiple small white foci and petechial hemorrhages, and enlarged hearts with white foci. Some birds exhibited ascites. Histologic examination of involved tissues reveal varying degrees of vacuolar degeneration and large pleomorphic intranuclear inclusion bodies.[28] Most of these inclusion bodies have a clear center containing very small, slightly basophillic granules. Lesions are found in the feather follicles in which there is ballooning degeneration of cells and large numbers of intranuclear inclusion bodies. These changes are also found in the epidermal cells of the skin. Examination of the inclusion bodies by transmission electron microscope have identified the causative virus as a papova virus. Isolation studies with the budgerigar papova virus have shown that it does not replicate on cell culture derived from chickens, but will replicate in cell cultures using budgerigar cells.[29] Experimental chicken embryo innoculation studies show that the isolated virus was pathogenic for 10-day-old chick embryos, but not at 11 and 12 days. The latter embryos produced antibodies to the virus that were detectable 2 weeks after hatching by agar gel immunodiffusion tests.[30] In recent studies, the DNA of this papova virus has been purified; however, attempts to characterize the proteins of the virus were unsuccessful, apparently due to the close association of the virus and the host cell components.[31]

The tentative clinical diagnosis of this disease is based on a history of loss of young fledgling psitticines with the clinical signs and gross necropsy findings described previously. The diagnosis is verified by identification of the virus with electromicroscopy or cell cultures using budgerigar cells.

There is no known treatment for this disease, nor is there a vaccine available for prevention of the infection in susceptible aviaries. In controlling the disease in breeding aviaries, it has been necessary to depopulate the aviary and then to wait 6 months before restocking.

Psitticine Beak and Feather Disease

Psitticine beak and feather disease syndrome is characterized by progressive loss of feathers and growth of abnormally developed feathers often accompanied by abnormal growth of the beak. This problem has been recognized most commonly in cockatoos,[32] but also has been reported in lovebirds.[33] It has been suggested by Pass and Perry[33] that French molt, as seen in fledgling budgerigars, is a form of this disease. The disease occurs in both captive birds, either kept in aviaries or as pets, and in wild birds.[34] Psitticine beak and feather disease occurs in both male and female birds and appears to be more common in young adults. When it occurs in pet birds, it is a particularly frustrating situation for both the veterinarian and the owner. The course of the disease is slowly progressive over a period of months and sometimes years and is invariably fatal.

The initial clinical sign of the disease is feather loss. Both contour and down feathers are involved (Fig. 11-4) and the pattern of feather loss may vary from bird to bird. In wild cockatoos the feathers of the crest and tail were affected most commonly. New feathers that grow to replace the feathers that have been lost, perhaps during a normal molt, are abnormal. They are quite short and retain the outer feather sheath that is normally removed or shed as the feather grows. The feathers may be deformed or curled and many times there is a constriction of the shaft of the feather close to the feather follicle. These abnormal feathers are easily dislodged and blood is often observed in the proximal feather shaft. These birds are not ''feather pickers'' and are rarely observed indulging in excessive grooming.

As the disease progresses, changes in both the upper and lower beaks occur in many birds. The beak may grow abnormally and develop cracks and splits on the surface. There is often a secondary infection along the inner surface of the beak and affected birds may have difficulty cracking shelled seeds or nuts. Similar changes may occur in the claws.[33] It has been observed that some sulfur crested cockatoos, particularly those in the wild, develop darkly pigmented skin.[34]

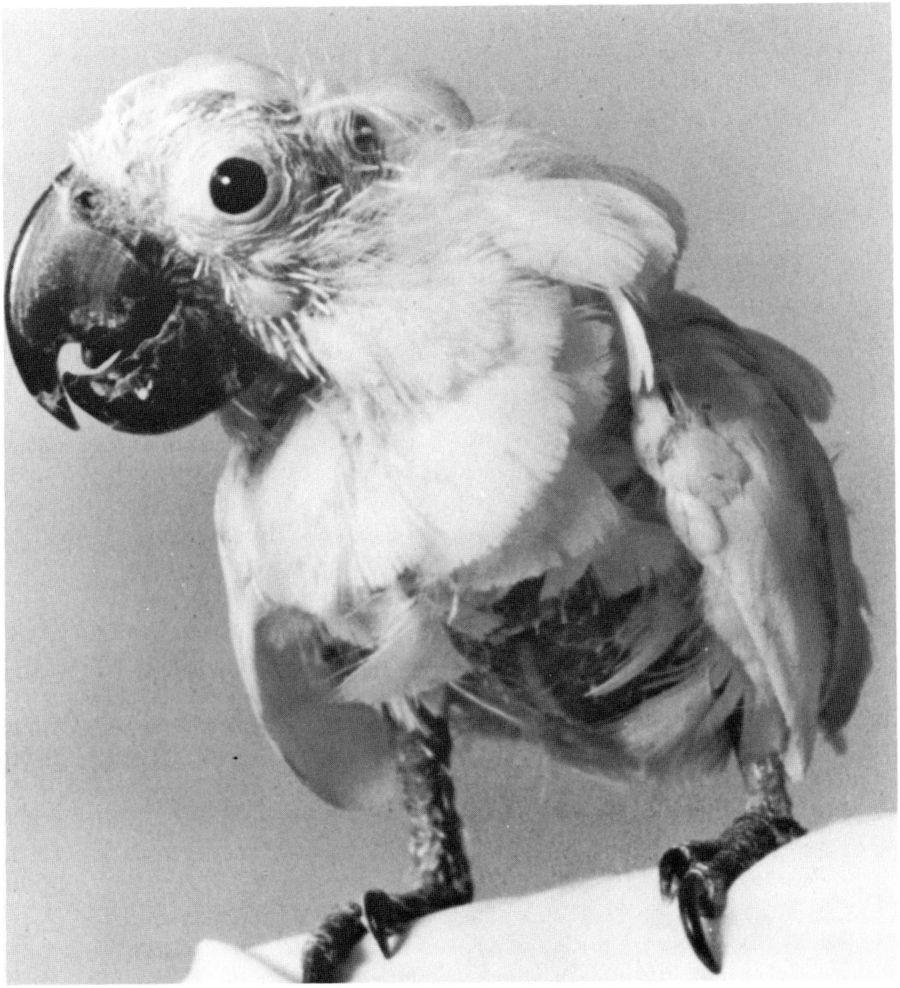

Fig. 11-4. An adult umbrella cockatoo with psittacine beak and feather syndrome. There is a loss of feathers involving the head, body, and tail. Note the cracking and peeling of the lower bill.

Pathologic changes are found in the developing feather and feather follicle. Focal neurosis of epithelial cells occurs in the epidermal collar and in the basalar and intermediate zones of the epidermis of the developing rachis (feather shaft).[35] There is disruption of the basal cell layer due to the presence of necrotic cells and cells with large nuclei. Focal hyperplasia may also occur in the basal cell layer. Intracytoplasmic inclusions of variable size have been observed in cells within the pulp of the feather shaft and epidermal layers. In many feathers, there is necrosis of the distal pulp and epithelium with hemorrhage into the distal feather shaft.

There are similar changes in the beak with necrosis of the basal epidermis. Associated with the necrosis is separation of the overlying lamina from the epidermis. The intracytoplasmic inclusion bodies that have been observed in these birds resemble a parvovirus on evaluation by transmission electron microscopy.[34]

Examination of internal organs has not revealed any consistent systemic abnormalities. Although one case report in 1981 incriminated chronic endocrine disorders (hypothyroidism and hypoadrenocorticism) in a sulfur crested cockatoo with beak and feather abnormalities,[36] subsequent studies have shown no consistent abnormalities of the endocrine system in affected birds.[33]

There is no known effective treatment for this disease and the prognosis for long-term survival is poor. Good supportive care with a high level of nutrition and a protected environment may prolong the life span of affected birds.

NONINFECTIOUS DISEASES

Feather Cysts (Hypopteronosis Cystica)

Feather cysts occur most commonly in canaries. Although the exact pathogenesis of this condition is not understood, it is suspected to be a genetic disorder. It is most common in canaries of the Norwich breed.[37] Feather cysts are seen sporadically in other species such as budgerigars and parrots. As the name implies, feather cysts develop in feather follicles, most commonly on the wings in canaries and initially involving a single feather follicle. The feather does not emerge from the feather follicle during the active growing phase, but instead curls within the follicle. This produces a cystic mass in the subcutaneous tissue. As the mass enlarges, caseous material collects within the follicle and a large, firm, palpable mass develops. Feather cysts can reach considerable size, sometimes 2 cm or more in diameter, and may ulcerate through the epithelium (Fig. 11-5). Once ulceration has occurred, the dry, caseous, yellowish-white material may be observed within the cyst. Sometimes portions of the feather may also be seen protruding from the ulcerated area. Some birds develop multiple feather cysts at one time.

Diagnosis of feather cysts is usually by observation and palpation of thse typical firm masses in a canary. A differential diagnosis would be a cutaneous tumor, which would be encountered infrequently in canaries. Treatment of a single cyst can be accomplished by the removal of exudate and the abnormal feather within the feather cyst; then, after controlling hemorrhage which may be a problem, cauterization of the lining of the follicle should be performed to destroy the feather follicle. In cases of very large, nonulcerated feather cysts, surgical removal of the entire cystic structure and suturing of the skin wound may be accomplished successfully. Many of the canaries thus treated will continue to develop new feather cysts as they go through molting periods. The prognosis is guarded to poor for a bird with multiple cysts. Although there have not been extensive studies done on the genetics of this disease, it is advisable

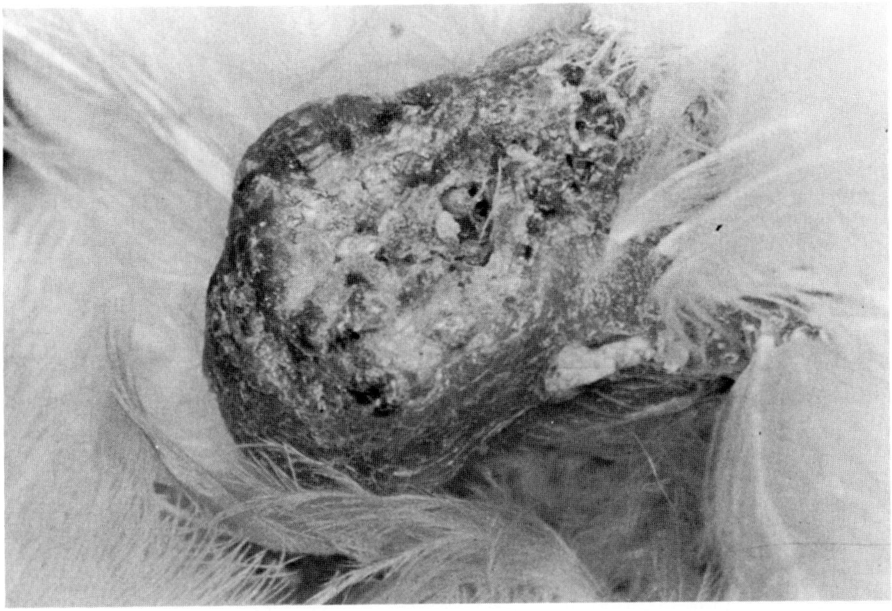

Fig. 11-5. A large feather cyst in the skin of a canary. There is ulceration of the overlying epidermis and dermis with exposure of the dry caseous keratin and debris filling the abnormal feather follicle.

for breeders to eliminate those bloodlines which produce a high percentage of affected birds from their breeding stock.

French Molt

French molt is a well recognized but poorly understood disease of the feathers that affects budgerigar fledglings primarily. French molt has been recognized in budgerigars almost from the time they were first bred in captivity and derives its name from the fact that French breeders first described the problem. This problem probably occurs in wild flocks also.

In spite of a long-standing interest in this disease among aviculturists and veterinarians treating pet birds, the pathogenesis remains unclear. Breeding studies have indicated that French molt is not a genetic disease.[38] The possibility of a nutritional deficiency causing the disease has been studied without definitive results; however, it has been shown that birds fed a high level of vitamin A produced a higher percentage of affected young than birds fed low to normal levels of vitamin A.[38] In this study, however, there was a 35 percent incidence of affected young in those birds fed the lower levels of vitamin A. Recent authors have implicated viral infections as the cause of the disease, including the papovavirus infection of fledgling budgerigars[25] and the suspected

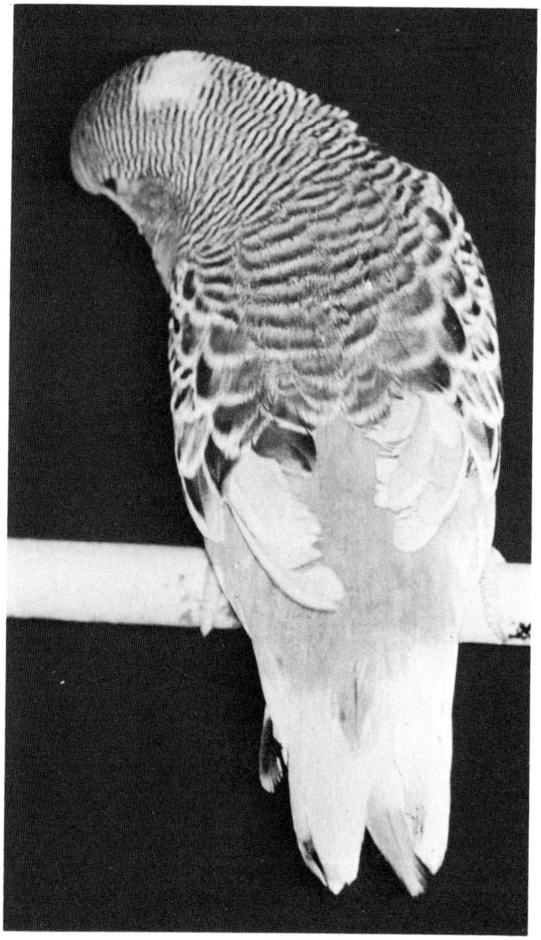

Fig. 11-6. A 4-month-old budgerigar with moderate French molt. Note the absence of flight feathers and long primary tail feathers. The contour feathers on the body appear normal.

virus involved in psitticine beak and feather disease.[33] Further studies are needed to clarify the relationship between these viruses and the disease French molt. It has been suggested that this disease may be the result of multiple factors and not attributable to a single etiology.[38]

The clinical signs of the disease are observed most commonly in young budgerigars at the time they leave the nest or shortly thereafter. Clinical signs vary considerably. Some mildly affected birds may only lose two tail feathers, while others will lose most of their flight feathers and longer primary tail feathers (Fig. 11-6). In severely affected birds, not only are the flight feathers lost but most of the contour feathers of the body may also fall out during normal activities (Fig. 11-7). Feathers most susceptible to being lost are those in the active growing stage. These feathers are often misshapen and shorter than the corresponding feathers from normal budgerigar fledglings (Fig. 11-8). It has been observed that many of the abnormal feathers that are lost will contain blood within the tip of the calamus (Fig. 11-9). This may be due to increased

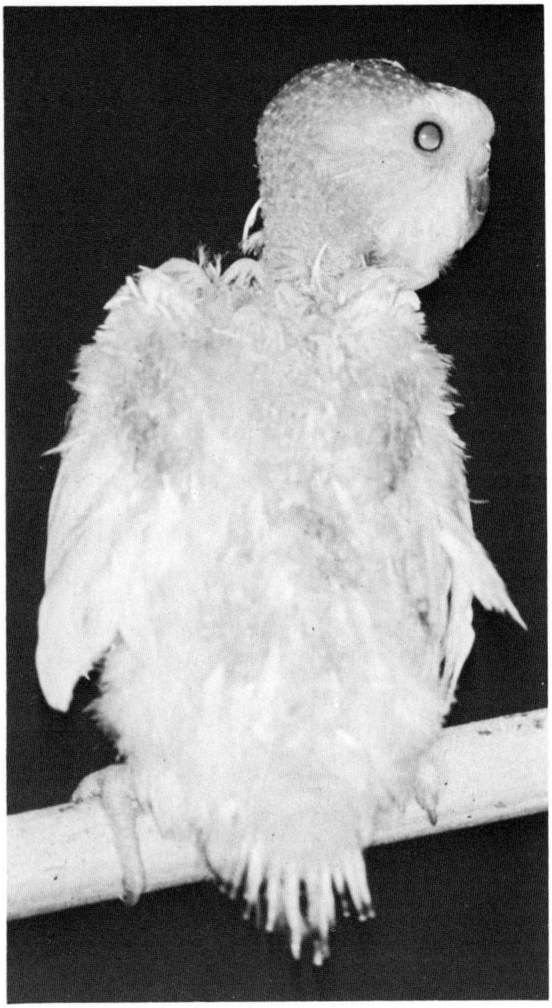

Fig. 11-7. Four-month-old budgerigar with severe French molt. There is severe involvement of all contour feathers and flight feathers.

capillary fragility and bleeding within the quill. The birds that lose many of the flight feathers are unable to sustain flight and are thus referred to by the breeders as "creepers" or "runners." In affected aviaries, the incidence of the disease tends to increase as the breeding season progresses. For commercial breeders this represents a considerable financial loss.

The diagnosis of the disease is made usually by the observation of typical clinical signs of feather loss in young fledgling budgerigars. Differential diagnoses to be considered include feather picking by adult birds. In these cases the main feather loss is usually on the back of the head. Papovavirus infection should also be considered a differential diagnosis, particularly if there is an associated death loss in young budgerigar nestlings.

There is no specific treatment for French molt in the fledgling. Mildly

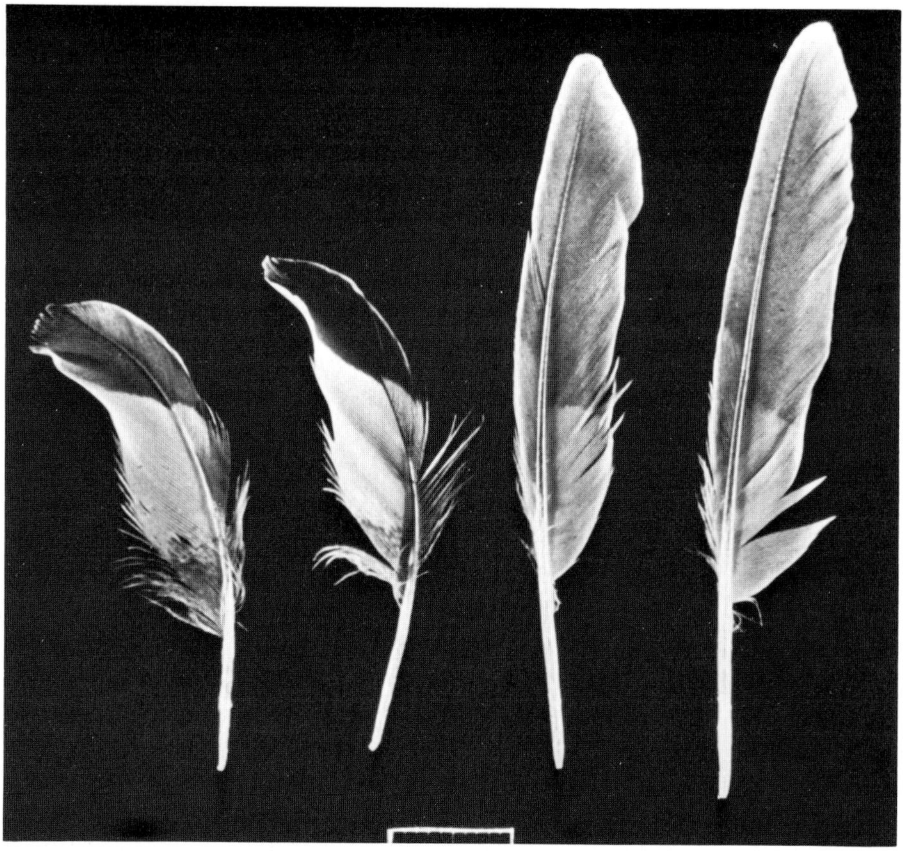

Fig. 11-8. Two primary flight feathers (left) from a bird with French molt compared to primary flight feathers in the same location on the wing of a normal budgerigar on the right. The feathers are short and mishapen.

affected birds may recover with time and good nutrition. More severely affected birds with loss of body contour feathers will not recover and should be destroyed. Because of the uncertainty about the pathogenesis of the disease, it is difficult to give extensive advise to breeders experiencing this problem. Obviously, breeding birds should be on a good nutritional program and excessive levels of vitamin A in the diet should be avoided. If it is late in the breeding season and the incidence of the disease is increasing in an aviary, it is advisable to stop further breeding for the season and to cull those pairs of birds that have produced a high incidence of affected young.

Feather Picking

Birds that chronically chew or pull their feathers are presented commonly to avian practitioners. Most of the birds that develop this problem are in the Psitticiformes order, and cockatiels and African gray parrots are particularly

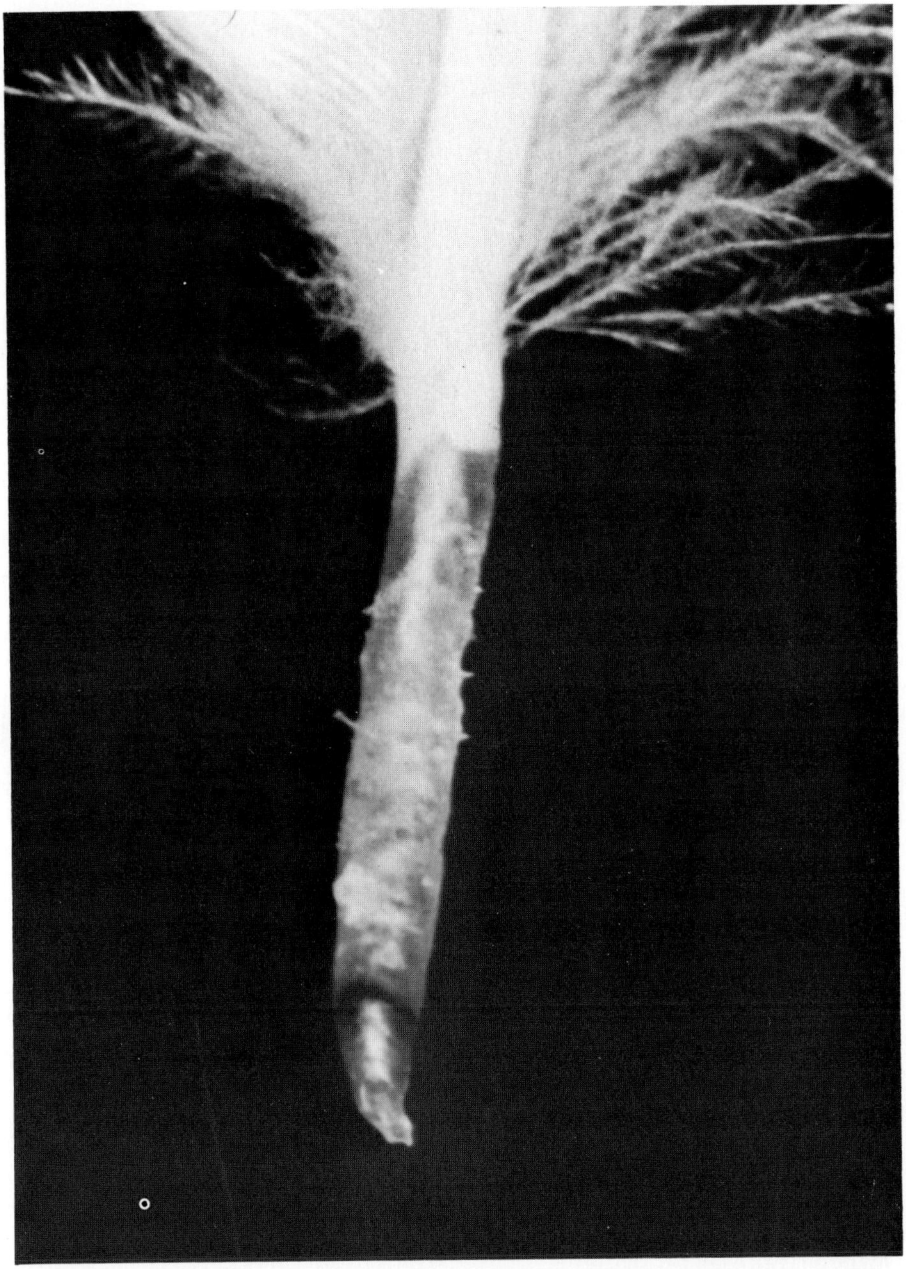

Fig. 11-9. The proximal end of the calamus of a feather from a bird with French molt. Note the darkened appearance due to dried blood within the interior of the shaft.

notorious feather pickers. This disorder is usually psychogenic in origin and represents an aberrant behavioral pattern. In the wild state, psitticines form flocks in which there is a high degree of social interaction and the formation of pair bonds within the flock. These birds undergo considerable stress when they are captured and separated from the flock and their mates, and, if they survive the intermediate stages of captivity, end up as an individual isolated pet in a home. Out of frustration and/or boredom, they may begin to excessively groom their feathers and eventually destroy the structure of the feather or actually pluck it from the skin. Cockatiels have been successfully bred in captivity for many generations, and it is theorized by Harrison[39] that this species, after being developed for high reproductive capabilities, exhibit feather picking as a sign of frustration when kept as isolated, nonbreeding pets. Some of these birds may feel threatened in the home situation by either other pets, children, or adults who try to handle them and they may become feather pullers in reaction to the high stress level. Some birds develop a strong attachment to their owner and develop a feather picking habit when separated from their human companion. In some cases an event that seems minor to the owner, such as moving the location of the cage, will elicit this behavioral abnormality in a pet bird. It has been suggested that psitticines are more likely to pick their feathers during the breeding season or when the bird is in active breeding condition.[39]

As the name suggests, the main clinical sign of this disorder is feather picking; however, there is a considerable variation in the pattern of behavior among affected birds. Some birds will pluck a few feathers from the ventral sternal area, while others will completely pluck feathers from most of the body surfaces. Others birds do not actually pull their feathers, but chew and fray them, destroying the normal vane pattern. In many birds the head feathering remains normal, as the bird cannot reach the area with its bill (Fig. 11-10). In a minority of cases the bird will actually chew on its skin, producing wounds and blood loss. The abnormal behavior of feather pulling or feather biting may either be continuous or intermittent.

The diagnosis of psychogenic feather picking is based on the signalment (i.e., psitticine type bird), a careful and detailed history in regard to the environment, time of onset, and type of behavior, and a thorough physical examination to exclude other etiologies. Differential diagnoses that should be considered in cases of feather picking include feather folliculitis,[40] parasitic infections such as mites and lice, mycotic infections of the feathers,[41] nesting behavior in some female birds, and feather plucking by other birds in the cage. Diagnostic tests that may be helpful in making a diagnosis of psychogenic feather picking and eliminating other causes include examination of growing contour feathers by performing a Gram's stain of the pulp of the quill and then performing cultures on the pulp. In one case, a pure culture of *Aeromonas* sp. was isolated from a bird showing acute onset of discomfort and feather pulling.[40] Fungal cultures can be made from feathers plucked from areas of active feather pulling. Careful examination of skin and feathers, including microscopic examination of feather quills should determine the presence of parasitic infes-

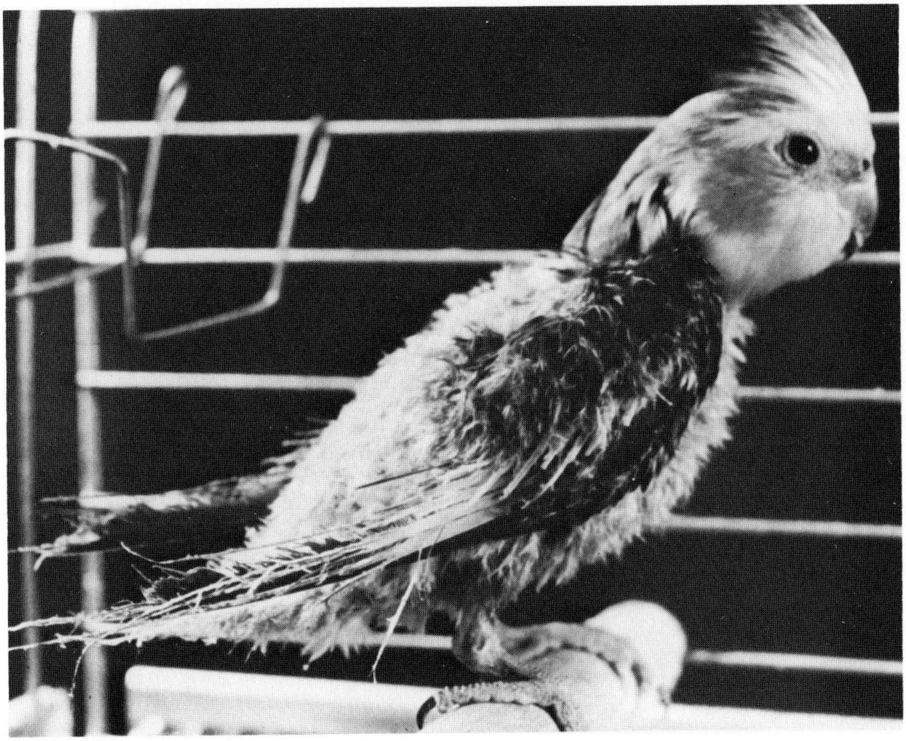

Fig. 11-10. An adult male cockatiel that developed a psychogenic feather-chewing behavior after its owner had returned to work. Note the normal appearance of the head feathering and the frayed appearance of all other feathers on the body.

tations. Nest building behavior by some birds may include plucking feathers from the ventral abdominal area and inner thighs. This difference in behavior should be recognized by careful observation or questioning of the owner. In some species of birds there may be feather pulling activity by dominant cage mates. This is particularly true of cockatoos and zebra finches. Many times feathers are plucked from the back of the head in these species.

There is no simple solution to the problem of psychogenic feather pulling. In many birds, this behavior has become quite patterned and is indeed a vice. As in all caged birds, the first step should be to ensure adequate nutrition and to supplement minerals, particularly calcium, vitamins, and protein as needed. Mechanical restraints such as Elizabethan collars or tube collars may be helpful in some birds in preventing further feather loss. It is important to use them in those birds that are actually damaging the skin. These collars do represent an additional stress factor for the bird. If collars are used, they should be adjusted carefully and the edges padded to prevent injury to the skin. One needs to analyze the environmental situation which is influencing the birds behavior and attempt to correct the environmental problems. In some cases, increased stimulation of the bird through providing toys and objects which they may chew on is helpful. Obviously, any material put in the cage should be nontoxic. Soft woods, rawhide bones, and other bones such as chicken bones may be provided to the birds.[42] Increased attention to the bird by the owner may be helpful in some cases; however, if the bird is afraid of the owner, increased attention may increase the stress situation. Owners must be careful not to reinforce the undesirable behavior by giving the bird attention only when it indulges in the feather picking/pulling activity. The use of environmental sounds such as music, radio programs, or television programs may be helpful in some cases. Spraying or misting the bird with warm water may help in inducing more normal preening behavior. Some birds may be stressed by their cage being located in an area of marked activity late into the night. These birds may benefit by being placed in a quiet, darkened area and covering the cage at night. Providing another bird for companionship may be helpful in some cases, but this approach is very unpredictable as the bird may not relate to a new bird, particularly a bird of another species. The correction of this behavioral problem requires patience and diligence on the part of both owner and veterinarian and, despite all efforts, some birds will continue to pull their feathers.

NEOPLASMS

Lipomas

Lipomas are the most common tumors of the integumentary system in pet birds and are commonly observed in budgerigars. These tumors form in the subcutis, most commonly over the ventral sternal area, but also occur in the ventral abdominal and intra-abdominal regions and over dorsal areas. These benign tumors occur in birds from 1 year of age upwards. Petrak and Gilmore[43] found the majority of tumors were in birds between 2 and 7 years of age. In their study, males predominated over females (29 males:9 females); however, the overall sex ratio of birds presented to that hospital was not discussed in the paper. Lipomas occur in other psitticine species, but appear to be rare in passerine species.

Lipomas vary in size considerably, with those occurring over the sternal area attaining the largest size (up to 4 cm in diameter). These masses present no particular problem to the bird, but as they enlarge they may interfere with the bird's ability to fly or perch normally (Fig. 11-11). The overlying skin often becomes thickened and yellowish in color. These changes in the skin are referred to as xanthomatous, a term which refers to the fact that cholesterol clefts are found in the dermal area of the skin with a surrounding foreign body reaction. Frequently, the feathers are lost from the affected skin, which becomes quite friable. In an exposed area, the bird may traumatize the area with its nails with resulting bleeding or there may be ulceration of skin due to irritation from the perch or other cage structures (Fig. 11-4). Lipomas that occur in these subcutaneous tissues near the thoracic inlet may result in dyspnea and/or dys-

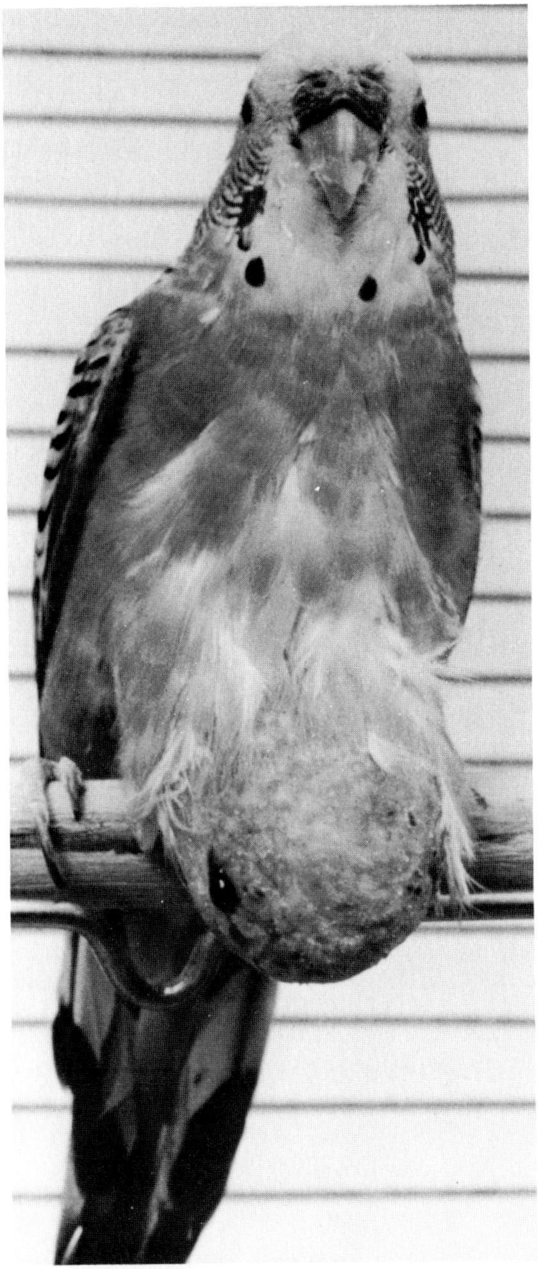

Fig. 11-11. A large dependent lipoma in an adult female budgerigar. The skin overlying the tumor is xanthomatous. Note the blood on the surface of the tumor and on the perch. The bird's nails repeatedly traumatize the friable skin, resulting in blood loss.

phagia due to mechanical obstruction. In budgerigars, lipomas appear to occur more commonly in obese birds.[44] These birds may also have fatty infiltration or degeneration of the liver, making them poor surgical candidates. As these tumors enlarge, they often undergo central necrosis and liquefaction. At this time, they may appear to grow quite rapidly and attract an unobservant owner's attention.

The diagnosis of lipoma is based initially on the finding of a typical, somewhat firm, subcutaneous mass in a budgerigar. Differential diagnoses to be considered include simple obesity. The fat in obese birds should be bilaterally symmetrical and not firm. Other tumors arising from deeper structures, such as fibrosarcomas, are quite smooth on palpation and have a wide base of attachment. Lipomas occurring at the thoracic inlet may mimic iodine deficient goiter in affected birds. Careful palpation of the ventral cervical area and lack of clinical response to iodine supplementation would help in the diagnosis of lipoma. There may be problems differentiating xanthomas occurring in the extremities from a lipoma with overlying xanthomatous skin. A biopsy should help differentiate these two tumors.

Surgical excision is the treatment of choice for subcutaneous lipomas. Although these tumors are benign and are readily removable by surgery, it must be kept in mind that these birds may not be good anesthetic and surgical risks. Because of the potential liver problem, anesthesia must be approached with great care. The surgical techniques used in removing such tumors has been well described.[45–47]

Upon examination after surgical removal, lipomas are usually globular, well encapsulated masses with a fatty appearance on cut surfaces and a yellowish color. In many instances the central part of the tumor will be necrotic and may contain hemorrhage. The necrotic center may be either casseous in texture or liquified. Histologically, these tumors are composed of large cells with foamy cytoplasm and some viable fat cells. In some tumors, there are thin, fibrous trabeculae dividing the tumor into lobules. In many tumors there is central necrosis and hemorrhage. As previously described, if the overlying skin is submitted with the tumor, it is likely to be xanthomatous.

Liposarcoma

Liposarcomas are encountered less frequently in pet birds than are lipomas.[43] These tumors may have a variable clinical course and appearance, but tend to resemble lipomas in their location and gross appearance. Hemorrhages are more likely to be present within the tumor than in lipomas.[43] The treatment of choice for these tumors is wide surgical excision. The definitive diagnosis is made on histologic examination of the tumor. Obviously, if there is extension of tumor cells to the surgical margin, the prognosis is guarded.

Xanthoma

The occurrence of xanthomas has been reported in budgerigars ranging in age from 1 to 11 years and in a 39-year-old roseate cockatoo.[43] The author has observed this tumor in budgerigars and a female cockatiel. These tumors may either appear as diffuse thickening of the skin or as distinct masses. Xanthomas occur in the dermis and subcutis and have been observed over the dorsal cervical upper back, dorsal and distal wing, uropygial,[43] and intraoral areas.[48] As previously described, skin overlying subcutaneous lipomas often undergo lipomatous xanthomatous changes. Xanthomatous skin is quite friable and prone to injury from the bird's sharp toenails, beak or other trauma (Fig. 11-11). Resulting hemorrhage may be a significant problem.

Xanthomas and xanthomatous skin are yellowish in color and are characterized by a diffuse infiltration of large foam cells into the dermis. These cells are either reticuloendothelial cells or macrophages filled with droplets of fat. A characteristic of xanthomas is the presence of cholesterol clefts appearing as elliptical spaces in the tissue surrounded by macrophages and multinucleated giant cells. Surgical excision is the treatment of choice for both tumors and xanthomatous changes in the skin. Since the tissue bleeds readily, very careful hemostasis is required to successfully remove these masses. It may be necessary to amputate the distal extremity of the wing in those cases where the xanthoma is in the metacarpal region and is infiltrated deeply around the primary feather follicles in the region.

Papillomas

Papillomas are benign tumors which can occur in caged birds. This tumor has been reported to occur in budgerigars,[43,49,50] Amazon parrots,[43] African gray parrots,[43,49,51] European chaffinches,[52] a cockatiel,[43] and a Quaker parakeet.[43] Intranuclear inclusion bodies suggestive of papilloma virus were found in lesions from one African gray parrot[51] and from papillomas found on the feet of chaffinches.[53]

Papillomas have been found on various areas of the body, including the commissure of the bill, the region of the uropygial gland, and the feet. There is usually a dried crust covering the surface of the tumor which projects above the surface of the skin. The bird may pick or rub at the lesion, producing surface ulceration and hemorrhage. If the crust is removed, the underlying tissue is often soft, moist, and irregular in contour and of variable colors. These tumors tend to be friable and vascular so that there may be a history of recurrent hemorrhage from the area.

A definitive diagnosis is made by the surgical removal or biopsy of the mass and submission of the tissue to a pathologist for histopathologic diagnosis. Histologically these tumors have hyperplastic epidermis often thrown up in multiple long, thin folds or fronds. These folds of epidermis are supported by a thin dermis and a core of loose vascular connective tissue.

The treatment of choice for papillomas is surgical excision, but if the lesions are very extensive this may not be feasible. It is not known if these lesions will spontaneously regress as is the case in many virus-induced papillomas occurring in mammals.

Adenomas and Adenocarcinomas of the Uropygial Gland

Both adenomas and adenocarcinomas of the uropygial gland occur in pet birds; they have been observed most commonly in the budgerigar[43] but have also been described in a canary[50] and parrot.[52] Tumors arising in the uropygial gland vary in clinical appearance. If the mass is producing pain or discomfort to the bird, it may pick and ulcerate the surface of the tumorous mass. Diagnosis of a uropygial gland tumor is based on a histopathologic examination of the tissue after either biopsy or surgical removal. Careful hemostasis is important when performing surgery near the uropygial gland, as the tissue may be quite vascular.[43,54] Differential diagnoses for swelling of the uropygial gland include impaction, infections or abscesses, and other tumors. A number of other tumors located in the region of the uropygial gland have been described in pet birds, especially budgerigars, including squamous cell carcinomas, liposarcomas, fibrosarcomas, papillomas, keratoacanthoma and epidermal cysts.[43] The prognosis following recovery from surgery for tumors of the uropygial gland depends on the nature of the neoplasm and whether it was possible to completely excise the mass.

Other Tumors

Besides those tumors described in more detail, a variety of other neoplasms both benign and malignant occur in pet birds, particularly in psitticine species.[43,44,49,50] Squamous cell carcinomas occur in birds. These tumors are raised above the surface of skin and are firm on palpation and frequently ulcerated. Wide surgical excision is required and these tumors may recur after surgical removal.

Fibrosarcomas may originate in the subcutaneous or deeper tissues. They are most commonly located over the extremities[43] and are usually covered by intact skin. Fibrosarcomas may enlarge very rapidly and cause difficulty in locomotion or flying. If the tumor is detected before it has invaded surrounding tissue extensively, it may be possible to remove it by wide surgical excision. Amputation of the extremity is also a surgical consideration. The prognosis is guarded to poor in cases of fibrosarcoma.

REFERENCES

1. Evans HE: Anatomy of the budgerigar. p. 111. In Petrak ML (ed): Diseases of Cage and Aviary Birds. 2nd Ed. Lea & Febiger, Philadelphia, 1982
2. Wyndham E: Moult of budgerigars *Melopsittacus undulatus*. Ibis 123:145, 1981
3. Victor DR, Gaurilov VM: Photoperiodic control of the molt cycle in the chaffinch (*Fringilla coelebs*). The Auk 97:50, 1980
4. LaFeber TJ: Feather problems in caged birds: Molting. Anim Hosp 2:122, 1966
5. Mainster ME: Scaly face in budgerigars. p. 626. In Kirk RW (ed): Current Veterinary Therapy. VIII Small Animal Practice. WB Saunders, Philadelphia, 1983

6. Wichmann RW, Vincent DJ: Cnemidocoptic mange in the budgerigar (*Melopsittacus undulatus*). J Am Vet Med Assoc 133:522, 1958
7. Keymer IF: Parasitic diseases. p. 535. In Petrak ML (ed): Diseases of Cage and Aviary Birds. 2nd Ed. Lea & Febiger, Philadelphia, 1982
8. Tierney F, Baillie J: Malathion aerosol for treatment of scaly face mites in caged birds. VM/SAC 74:69, 1979
9. Stauber E, Schussman S: Parasites of pet and aviary birds—Part 2. Mod Vet Pract 66:539, 1985
10. Dodd K: Northern mite (*Ornithonyssus sylviarum*) infestation in canaries. Vet Rec 113:259, 1983
11. Antoniotto D, Romat A: Contribucion al estudio del epithelioma contagioso del canario. Revta Med Vet Buenos Aires 26:326, 1940
12. Giddens WE, Swango LJ, Henderson JD, et al: Canary pox in sparrows and canaries and in weavers. Vet Pathol 8:260, 1971
13. Cavill JP: Viral diseases. p. 515. In Petrak ML (ed): Diseases of Cage and Aviary Birds. 2nd Ed. Lea & Febiger, Philadelphia, 1982
14. Sadasiv EC, Chang PW, Gulka G: Morphogenesis of canary poxvirus and its entrance into inclusion bodies. Am J Vet Res 46:529, 1985
15. Tajima M, Ushijima T: Electron microscopy of avian pox virus with special reference to the significance of inclusion bodies in viral replication. Jpn J Vet Sci 28:107, 1966
16. Hitchner SB: Canary pox vaccination with live embryo-attenuated virus. Avian Dis 25:874, 1981
17. Munz E, Reimann M, Sailer H: Vergleichende Untersuchungen zur parenteralen und nicht-parenteralen Immulnigierung gegen Kanarienpocken. Zbl Vet Med B 21:442, 1974
18. McDonald SE, Lowenstine LJ, Ardans AA: Avian pox in blue-fronted amazon parrots. J Am Vet Med Assoc 179:1218, 1981
19. Graham CLG: Poxvirus infection in a spectacled amazon parrot (*Amazona albiforns*). Avian Dis 22:340, 1978
20. Emanuelson S, Carney J, Saito J: Avian pox in two black-masked conures. J Am Vet Med Assoc 173:1250, 1978
21. Kraft V, Teufel P: Nachuveis eines pockvirus be zwerspapaseien (*Agapoinis personata* and *Agapornis roseicollis*). Berl Muench Tieraerztl Wochenscher 84:83, 1971
22. Sharma UK, Simon J, Hanson LE: Histologic study of tissue reaction in canaries, and chicken embryos infected with a pox agent, isolated from parakeets. Avian Dis 12:594, 1968
23. Boosinger TR, Winterfield RW, Feldman DS, Dhillon AS: Psittacine pox virus: Virus isolation and identification, transmission and cross-challenge studies in parrots and chickens. Avian Dis 26:437, 1982
24. Davis RB, Bozeman LH, Gaudny D, et al: Case report—A viral disease of fledgling budgerigars. Avian Dis 25:179, 1980
25. Bernier G, Morin M, Marsolais G: Research note—A generalized inclusion body disease in the budgerigar (*Melopsittacus undulatus*) caused by a papovavirus-like agent. Avian Dis 25:1083, 1981
26. Kaleta VEF, Herbst W, Kaup FJ, et al: Untersuchangen zur virusaetiologie einer mit hepatitis und beFiederungsstoerungen einhergehender Krankheit bei wellensittich-nestlingen (*Melopsittacus undulatus*). Zentralbl Veterinarmed[B] 31:219, 1984
27. Jacobson ER, Hines SA, Quesenberry K, et al: Epornitic of papova-like virus-associated disease in a psittacine nursery. J Am Vet Med Assoc 185:1337, 1984

28. Dykstra MJ, Bozeman LH: A light and electron microscopic examination of budgerigar fledgling disease in tissue and in cell culture. Avian Pathol 11:11, 1982
29. Bozeman LH, Davis RB, Gaudry D, et al: Characterization of a papovavirus isolated from fledgling budgerigars. Avian Dis 25:972, 1981
30. Lynch J. Swinton J, Pettit J, Key D: Pet bird medicine—Isolation and experimental chicken-embryo-inoculation studies with budgerigar papovavirus. Avian Dis 28:1135, 1984
31. Dykstra MJ, Dykstra CC, Lukert PD, Bozeman LH: Investigations of budgerigar fledgling-disease virus. Am J Vet Res 45:1883, 1984
32. Perry RA: A psittacine combined beak and feather disease syndrome. p. 81. In Hungerford TG (ed): Cage and Aviary Birds. Proceedings No. 55 of Courses for Veterinarians. The Post-Graduate Committee in Veterinary Science, Sydney, Australia, 1981
33. Pass DA, Perry RA: The pathology of psittacine beak and feather disease. Austr Vet J 61:69, 1984
34. McOrist S, Black DG, Pass DA, et al: Beak and feather dystrophy in wild sulfur-crested cockatoos (*Cacatua galerita*). J Wildl Dis 20:120, 1984
35. Ruebel VA, Hauser B, Mettler F, Isenbuegel E: Verlust der Ferdern und Kerneinschlusskoerperchen in leberzellen beim gelbwangenkakadu (*Kakatoe sulphurea*). Der Praktische Tierarzt 8:681, 1984
36. Rosskopf WJ, Woerpel RW: Chronic endocrine disorder associated with inclusion body hepatitis in a sulfur-crested cockatoo. J Am Vet Med Assoc 179:1273, 1981
37. Altman RB: Conditions involving the integumentary system. p. 368. In Petrak ML (ed): Diseases of Cage and Aviary Birds. 2nd Ed. Lea & Febiger, Philadelphia, 1982
38. Taylor GT: French molt. p. 361. In Petrak ML (ed): Diseases of Cage and Aviary Birds. 2nd Ed. Lea & Febiger, Philadelphia, 1982
39. Harrison GJ: Feather disorders. Vet Clin North Am [Small Anim Pract] 14:179, 1984
40. Rosskopf WJ, Woerpel RW, Sievers MJ, Pater C: Treatment of feather folliculitis in a lovebird. Mod Vet Pract 64:923, 1983
41. Tudor DC: Mycotic infection of feathers as the cause of feather-pulling in pigeons and psittacine birds. VM/SAC 78:249, 1983
42. Galvin C: The feather picker. Calif Vet 33:12, 1979
43. Petrak ML, Gilmore CE: Neoplasms. p. 606. In Petrak ML (ed): Diseases of Cage and Aviary Birds. 2nd Ed. Lea & Febiger, Philadelphia, 1982
44. Blackmore DK: The clinical approach to tumors in cage birds—I. The pathology and incidence of neoplasia in cage birds. J Small Anim Pract 7:217, 1966
45. Gandal CP, Saunder LZ: The surgery of subcutaneous tumors in parakeets (*Melopsittacus undulatus*). J Am Vet Med Assoc 134:212, 1959
46. Murray JW: Surgery of cage-birds. Aust Vet J 43:514, 1967
47. Arnall L: The clinical approach to tumours in cage birds—IV: Treatment of cage bird tumours. J Small Anim Pract 7:241, 1966
48. Ridgway RL: Oral xanthoma in a budgerigar *Melopsittacus undulatus*. VM/SAC 72:266, 1977
49. Beach JE: Diseases of budgerigars and other cage birds. A survey of post-mortem findings. Vet Rec 74:10, 63 and 134, 1962
50. Arnall L: Further experiences with cagebirds. Vet Rec 73:1146, 1961
51. Jacobson ER, Mladinich CR, Clubb S, et al: Papilloma-like virus infection in an African gray parrot. J Am Vet Med Assoc 183:1307, 1983

52. Blackmore, DK: The pathology and incidence of neoplasia in cage birds. J Small Anim Pract 6:217, 1965
53. Lina PHC, Noord MJ, Groot FG: Detection of virus in squamous papillomas of the wild bird species *Fringilla coelebs* (chaffinch). J Natl Cancer Inst 50:567, 1973
54. Wise RD: Surgical removal of uropygial gland tumor in budgerigars. VM/SAC 75:1601, 1980

Index

Page numbers followed by t denote tables; those followed by f denote figures.